VETERINARY SCIENCE AND MEDICINE

Edited by
Nada Ben Abdallah

ArclerPress

Veterinary Science and Medicine

Edited by Nada Ben Abdallah

Edition 2018

ArclerPress

Published by
Arcler Press LLC
708 3rd Avenue, 6th Floor
New York
NY 10017
United States of America
www.arclerpress.com

ISBN: 978-1-68094-592-8 (Hardback)

Printed in United States of America

Library of Congress Control Number: 2017933193

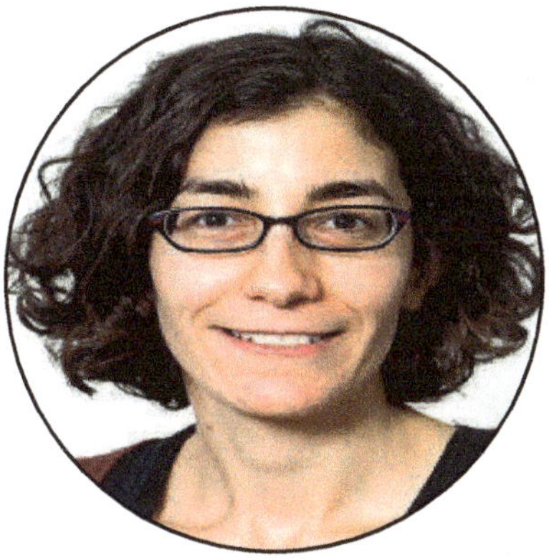

About the Editor

Nada Ben Abdallah

Nada graduated from the University of Zurich in 2010 and holds a PhD in neuroscience. Her research focuses on elucidating the processes of learning and memory as well as the affective processes and their underlying neural mechanisms. Her work so far involved normal and diseased animal models with a main interest in neurodegenerative diseases. She is currently working as a freelance researcher and science editor.

Table of Contents

2 VETERINARY MEDICINE

3 VETERINARY PHYSICIAN

6 VETERINARY ETHICS

7 VETERINARY SURGERY

8 VETERINARY VIROLOGY

List of Abbreviations

BSE	Bovine Spongiform Encephalopathy
CSIRO	Cattle in Dry Landscape North of Alice Springs, Australia
CAFOs	Concentrated Animal Feeding Operations
EPA	Environmental Protection Agency
FAO	Food and Agriculture Organization
N-S	North-South
QTLs	Quantitative trait loci
AAVA	American Academy of Veterinary Acupuncture
AAHA	American Animal Hospital Association
AAFP	American Association of Feline Practitioners
ABAA	American Board of Animal Acupuncture
AVMA	American Veterinary Medical Association
AR	Antibiotic Resistance
AMR	Antimicrobial Resistance
CGRP	Calcitonin Gene-Related Peptide
DDD	Defined Daily Doses
ESBL	Extended Spectrum Beta-Lactamase
fMRI	Functional Magnetic Resonance Imaging
IVAS	International Veterinary Acupuncture Society
MRSA	Methicillin-Resistant Staphylococcus Aureus
MDR	Multidrug Resistant
MRAB	Multidrug-Resistant a. Baumannii
PET	Positron Emission Tomography

TCVM	Traditional Chinese Veterinary Medicine
VRE	Vancomycin-Resistant Enterococcus
WHO	World Health Organization
BVNA	British Veterinary Nursing Association
DVM	Doctor Veterinariae Medicinae
CPD	Continuing Professional Development
OVs	Official Veterinarians,
PDSA	People's Dispensary for Sick Animals
PDP	Professional Development Phase
RVNs	Registered Veterinary Nurses
RCVS	Royal College of Veterinary Surgeons
RSPCA	Royal Society for the Prevention of Cruelty to Animals
VMD	Veterinary Medicines Directorate
PHS	Public Health Service
USDA	U.S. Department of Agriculture
UDAW	Universal Declaration on Animal Welfare
IACUC	Institutional Animal Care and Use Committee

Preface

Veterinary science is the application of medical, diagnostic, and therapeutic principles to companion, domestic, exotic, wildlife, and production animals. Veterinary science is vital to the study and protection of animal production practices, herd health, and monitoring the spread of widespread diseases. It requires the acquisition and application of scientific knowledge in multiple disciplines and uses technical skills towards disease prevention in both domestic and wild animals. Veterinary medicine is the branch of medicine that deals with the prevention, diagnosis, and treatment of disease, disorder, and injury in non-human animals. The scope of veterinary medicine is wide, covering all animal species, both domesticated and wild, with a wide range of conditions that can affect different species. Veterinary medicine is widely practiced, both with and without professional supervision. Professional care is most often led by a veterinary physician (also known as a vet, veterinary surgeon, or veterinarian), but also by paraveterinary workers such as veterinary nurses or technicians. This can be augmented by other paraprofessionals with specific specialisms such as animal physiotherapy or dentistry, and species relevant roles such as farriers. Veterinary science helps human health through the monitoring and control of zoonotic disease (infectious disease transmitted from non-human animals to humans), food safety, and indirectly through human applications from basic medical research. They also help to maintain food supply through livestock health monitoring and treatment, and mental health by keeping pets healthy and long living. Veterinary scientists often collaborate with epidemiologists, and other health or natural scientists depending on the type of work. Paraveterinary workers, including veterinary nurses, technicians and assistants, either assist vets in their work, or may work within their own scope of practice, depending on skills and qualifications, including in some cases, performing minor surgery. The role of paraveterinary workers is less homogeneous globally than that of a vet, and qualification levels, and the associated skill mix, vary widely. Ethically, veterinarians are usually obliged to look after animal welfare. Veterinarians assist in ensuring the quality, quantity, and security of food supplies by working to maintain the health of livestock.

Content Coverage

Chapters One and *Two* introduce animal diseases and veterinary medicine, respectively. Veterinarians work to ensure a safe food supply by maintaining the health of agricultural animals and by inspecting food processing industries.

Chapters Three and *Four* present the role of veterinary physician, and paraveterinary workers, respectively. Most veterinary physicians work in clinical settings, treating animals directly. These veterinarians may be involved in a general practice, treating animals of all types they, may be specialized in a specific group of animals such as companion animals, livestock, zoo animals, or equines. They also may specialize in a narrow medical discipline such as surgery, dermatology or internal medicine.

Chapters Five and *Six* emphasize on animal welfare and veterinary ethics, respectively. Veterinary ethics encompasses its practical application in clinical settings as well as work on its history, philosophy, theology, and sociology. It combines veterinary professional ethics and the subject of animal ethics. It can be interpreted as a critical reflection on the provision of veterinary services in support of the profession's responsibilities to animal kind and mankind.

Chapters Seven clarifies the goal of veterinary surgery, which may be quite different in pets and in farm animals. Veterinary surgery is surgery performed on animals by veterinarians, whereby the procedures fall into three broad categories: orthopedics (bones, joints, muscles), soft tissue surgery (skin, body cavities, cardiovascular system, gastrointestinal/urogenital/respiratory tracts), and neurosurgery.

Chapter Eight introduces veterinary virology, which is the study of viruses causing diseases and disorders in animals.

CHAPTER 1

Animal Diseases

Chapter Contents

INTRODUCTION

Alopecia is a condition that can affect other animals besides humans. Development of alopecia in animals is usually the sign of an underlying disease. Some animals may be genetically predisposed to hair loss, while in some it may be caused by hypersensitivity or nutritional factors.

Canine pinnal alopecia is most common in dachshunds, but other dog breeds, such as Chihuahuas, Boston terriers, Whippets and Italian greyhounds, may also be vulnerable. Certain skin conditions in animals can also cause loss of fur.

Ferret adrenal disease is extremely common and is the most common cause of alopecia in ferrets, typically affecting middle-aged specimens between three and seven years old. Bacterial pyoderma, dermatophytosis, and parasites can also cause the condition. In rabbits, dermatophytosis is a prime cause of alopecia in young, newly weaned specimens. Moreover, dermatophytosis as a cause of alopecia is common in cats, and in long-haired varieties, dermatophytic pseudomycetomas may be to blame. Alopecia areata has been studied in laboratory mice. In horses, patches of hair loss may be the result of human contact and the rubbing of the saddle across the mane.

ANTHROPONOTIC DISEASE

An anthroponotic disease, or anthroponosis, is an infectious disease in which a disease causing agent carried by humans is transferred to other animals. It may cause the same disease or a different disease in other animals. Since humans do not generally inflict bite wounds on other animals, the method of transmissions is always a "soft" contact such as skin to skin transmission. An example is chytridiomycosis, which can be spread to frogs that are handled by the bare hands of humans suffering from skin fungus.

The reverse situation, a disease transmitted from animals to humans, is known as zoonotic.

It can also be defined as a human-to-human infection with no animal vector.

Known Anthroponotic Diseases

Many human diseases can be transmitted to other primates, due to their extensive biological similarities. As a result, centers that hold, treat, or involve close proximity to primates and some other kinds of animals (for example zoos, researchers, and animal hospitals), often take steps to ensure animals are not exposed to human diseases they can catch. In some cases, animals are routinely immunized with the same vaccines given to humans.

- Leishmaniasis - both zoonotic and anthroponotic.
- Influenza, Measles, pneumonia, and various other pathogens - many primates.

Berserk Llama Syndrome

Berserk llama syndrome or Berserk male syndrome (as it is more pronounced in males) is a psychological condition suffered by human-raised llamas and alpacas that can cause them to exhibit dangerously aggressive behavior toward humans. The term has been overused, however, and is sometimes inappropriately applied to llamas with aggressive personalities that are not truly "berserk".

The condition is a result of the llama imprinting on its human handlers to such a degree that it considers them to be fellow llamas. Imprinting can be caused by bottle feeding and by isolation from other llamas. Llamas are strongly territorials, and adult male inter-llama interactions can be rough, including chest ramming and biting. Male llamas suffering from this condition become dangerous when their aggressive behavior is directed toward humans: and they usually have to be euthanised. Female llamas can also suffer from berserk llama syndrome, but their behavior is usually limited to spitting and difficult handling.

Berserk llama syndrome can be prevented in males through castration before puberty.

BESNOITIOSIS

Besnoitiosis is "a protozoan disease of the skin, subcutis, blood vessels, mucous membranes, and other tissues of animals. It is endemic in tropical and sub-tropical regions with high infection rate but low mortality, however it is rare in other regions.

The causative organisms of the cutaneous disease, and the affected animals include:

- Besnoitia besnoiti in cattle (swelling of the lymph nodes, subcutaneous swellings, diarrhea, abortion and infertility)
- Besnoitia bennetti in horses and donkeys (characterized by a widespread, serious dermatitis)
- Besnoitia jellisoni and B. wallacei in rodents
- Besnoitia tarandi in reindeer and caribou
- Besnoitia darlingi in lizards, opossums, and snakes
- Besnoitia sauriana in lizards
- Viscerotropic strains of B. besnoiti in African antelopes
- An unidentified Besnoitia species in goats in Iran, New Zealand, and Kenya

CATTLE

Cattle—colloquially cows—are the most common type of large domesticated ungulates. They are a prominent modern member of the subfamily Bovinae, are the most widespread species of the genus Bos, and are most commonly classified collectively as Bos taurus. Cattle are raised as livestock for meat (beef and veal), as dairy animals for milk and other dairy products, and as draft animals (oxen or bullocks that pull carts, plows and other implements). Other products include leather and dung for manure or fuel. In some regions, such as parts of India, cattle have significant religious meaning. From as few as 80 progenitors domesticated in southeast Turkey about 10,500 years ago, according to an estimate from 2011, there are 1.4 billion cattle in the world. In 2009, cattle became one of the first livestock animals to have a fully mapped genome. Some consider cattle the oldest form of wealth, and cattle raiding consequently one of the earliest forms of theft.

Taxonomy

Cattle were originally identified as three separate species: Bos taurus, the European or "taurine" cattle (including similar types from Africa and Asia); Bos indicus, the zebu; and the extinct Bos primigenius, the aurochs. The aurochs is ancestral to both zebu and taurine cattle. Now, these have been reclassified as one species, Bos taurus, with three subspecies: Bos taurus primigenius, Bos taurus indicus, and Bos taurus taurus.

Complicating the matter is the ability of cattle to interbreed with other closely related species. Hybrid individuals and even breeds exist, not only between taurine cattle and zebu (such as the sanga cattle, Bos taurus africanus), but also between one or both of these and some other members of the genus Bos – yaks (the dzo or yattle), banteng, and gaur. Hybrids such as the beefalo breed can even occur between taurine cattle and either species of bison, leading some authors to consider them part of the genus Bos, as well. The hybrid origin of some types may not be obvious – for example, genetic testing of the Dwarf Lulu breed, the only taurine-type cattle in Nepal, found them to be a mix of taurine cattle, zebu, and yak. However, cattle cannot successfully be hybridized with more distantly related bovines such as water buffalo or African buffalo.

The aurochs originally ranged throughout Europe, North Africa, and much of Asia. In historical times, its range became restricted to Europe, and the last known individual died in Masovia, Poland, in about 1627. Breeders have attempted to recreate cattle of similar appearance to aurochs by crossing traditional types of domesticated cattle, creating the Heck cattle breed.

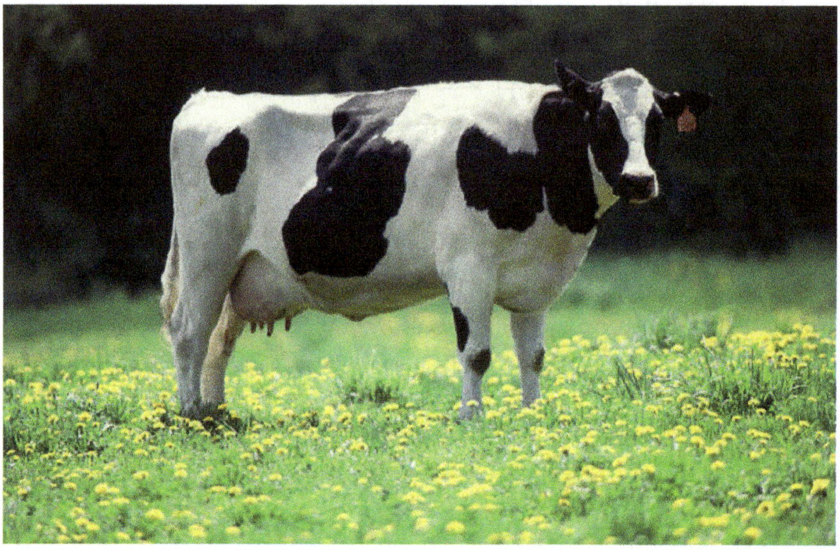

A Holstein Fresian cow, a typical member of the Bos taurus taurus sub-species

Cattle did not originate as the term for bovine animals. It was borrowed from Anglo-Norman catel, itself from medieval Latin capitale ‘principal sum of money, capital’, itself derived in turn from Latin caput ‘head’. Cattle originally meant movable personal property, especially livestock of any kind, as opposed to real property (the land, which also included wild or small free-roaming animals such as chickens — they were sold as part of the land). The word is a variant of chattel (a unit of personal property) and closely related to capital in the economic sense. The term replaced earlier Old English feoh ‘cattle, property’, which survives today as fee (cf. German: Vieh, Dutch: vee, Gothic: faihu).

The word “cow” came via Anglo-Saxon cū, from Common Indo-European gʷōus= “a bovine animal”, compare Persian gâv, Sanskrit go-, Welsh buwch. The plural cȳ became ki or kie in Middle English, and an additional plural ending was often added, giving kine, kien, but also kies, kuin and others. This is the origin of the now archaic English plural, "kine. The Scots language singular is coo or cou, and the plural is kye.

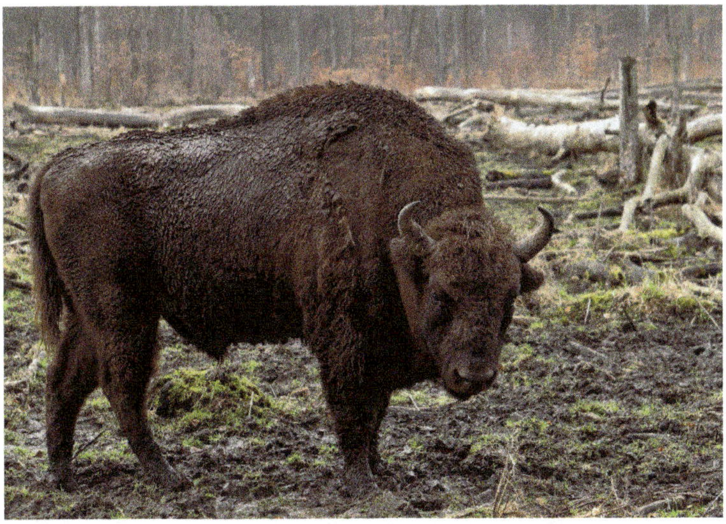

Żubroń, a wisent and cattle hybrid

Etymology

In older English sources such as the King James Version of the Bible, cattle refers to livestock, as opposed to deer which refers to wildlife. Wild cattle may refer to feral cattle or to undomesticated species of the genus Bos. Today, when used without any other qualifier, the modern meaning of "cattle" is usually restricted to domesticated bovines.

Terminology

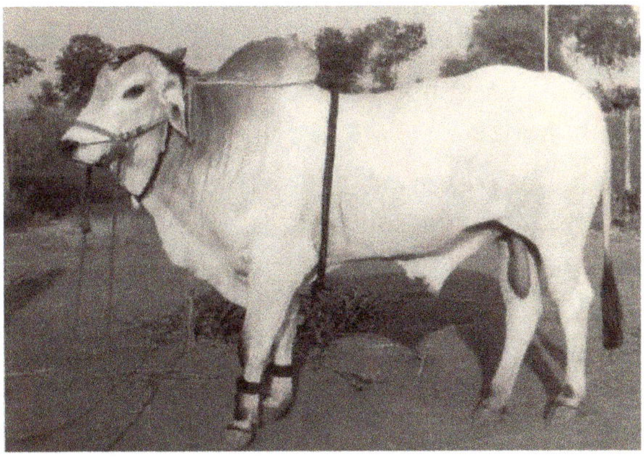

An Ongole bull

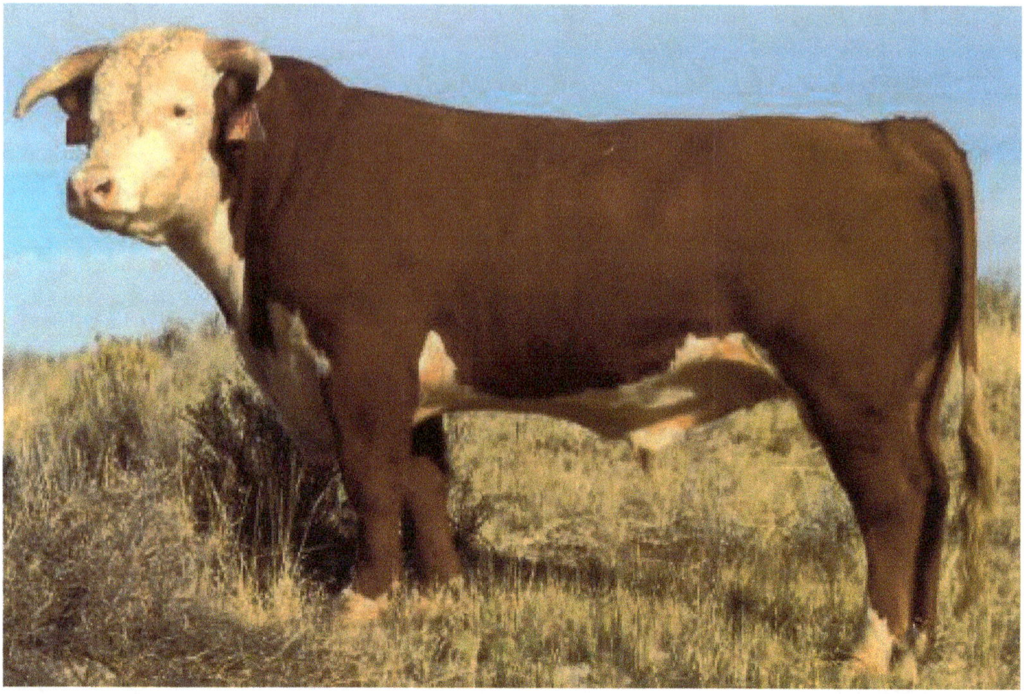

A Hereford bull

In general, the same words are used in different parts of the world, but with minor differences in the definitions. The terminology described here contrasts the differences in definition between the United Kingdom and other British-influenced parts of the world such as Canada, Australia, New Zealand, Ireland and the United States.

- An "intact" (i.e., not castrated) adult male is called a bull. A wild, young, unmarked bull is known as a "micky" in Australia. An unbranded bovine of either sex is called a "maverick" in the USA and Canada.
- An adult female that has had a calf (or two, depending on regional usage) is a cow.
- A young female before she has had a calf of her own and is under three years of age is called a heifer. A young female that has had only one calf is occasionally called a first-calf heifer.
- Young cattle of both sexes are called calves until they are weaned, then weaners until they are a year old in some areas; in other areas, particularly with male beef cattle, they may be known as feeder calves or simply feeders. After that, they are referred to as yearlings or stirks if between one and two years of age.
- A castrated male is called a steer in the United States; older steers are often called bullocks in other parts of the world, but in North America this term

refers to a young bull. Piker bullocks are micky bulls (uncastrated young male bulls) that were caught, castrated and then later lost. In Australia, the term Japanese ox is used for grain-fed steers in the weight range of 500 to 650 kg that are destined for the Japanese meat trade. In North America, draft cattle under four years old are called working steers. Improper or late castration on a bull results in it becoming a coarse steer known as a stag in Australia, Canada and New Zealand. In some countries, an incompletely castrated male is known also as a rig.

- A castrated male (occasionally a female or in some areas a bull) kept for draft purposes is called an ox (plural oxen); "ox" may also be used to refer to some carcass products from any adult cattle, such as ox-hide, ox-blood, oxtail, or ox-liver.
- A springer is a cow or heifer close to calving.
- In all cattle species, a female twin of a bull usually becomes an infertile partial intersex, and is called a freemartin.
- Neat (horned oxen, from which neatsfoot oil is derived), beef (young ox) and beefing (young animal fit for slaughtering) are obsolete terms, although poll, pollard or polled cattle are still terms in use for naturally hornless animals, or in some areas also for those that have been disbudded or dehorned.
- Cattle raised for human consumption are called beef cattle. Within the American beef cattle industry, the older term beef (plural beeves) is still used to refer to an animal of either sex. Some Australian, Canadian, New Zealand and British people use the term beast.
- Cattle bred specifically for milk production are called milking or dairy cattle; a cow kept to provide milk for one family may be called a house cow or milker. A fresh cow is a dairy term for a cow or first-calf heifer who has recently given birth, or "freshened."
- The adjective applying to cattle in general is usually bovine. The terms bull, cow and calf are also used by extension to denote the sex or age of other large animals, including whales, hippopotamuses, camels, elk and elephants.

Singular Terminology Issue

Cattle can only be used in the plural and not in the singular: it is a plurale tantum. Thus one may refer to "three cattle" or "some cattle", but not "one cattle". No universally used singular form in modern English of "cattle" exists, other than the sex- and age-specific terms such as cow, bull, steer and heifer. Historically, "ox" was not a sex-specific term for adult cattle, but generally this is now used only for draft cattle, especially adult castrated males. The term is also incorporated into the names of other species, such as the musk ox and "grunting ox" (yak), and is used in some areas to describe certain cattle products such as ox-hide and oxtail.

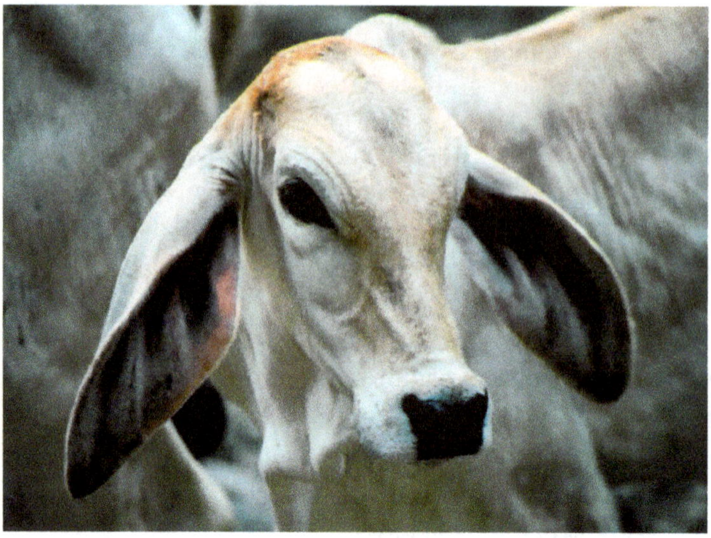

A Brahman calf

"Cow" is in general use as a singular for the collective "cattle", despite the objections by those who insist it to be a female-specific term. Although the phrase "that cow is a bull" is absurd from a lexicographic standpoint, the word "cow" is easy to use when a singular is needed and the sex is unknown or irrelevant – when "there is a cow in the road", for example. Further, any herd of fully mature cattle in or near a pasture is statistically likely to consist mostly of cows, so the term is probably accurate even in the restrictive sense. Other than the few bulls needed for breeding, the vast majority of male cattle are castrated as calves and slaughtered for meat before the age of three years. Thus, in a pastured herd, any calves or herd bulls usually are clearly distinguishable from the cows due to distinctively different sizes and clear anatomical differences. Merriam-Webster, a US dictionary, recognizes the sex-nonspecific use of "cow" as an alternate definition, whereas Collins, a UK dictionary, does not.

Colloquially, more general nonspecific terms may denote cattle when a singular form is needed. Australian, New Zealand and British farmers use the term "beast" or "cattle beast". "Bovine" is also used in Britain. The term "critter" is common in the western United States and Canada, particularly when referring to young cattle. In some areas of the American South (particularly the Appalachian region), where both dairy and beef cattle are present, an individual animal was once called a "beef critter", though that term is becoming archaic.

Other Terminology

Cattle raised for human consumption are called "beef cattle". Within the beef cattle industry in parts of the United States, the term "beef" (plural "beeves") is still used in its archaic sense to refer to an animal of either sex. Cows of certain breeds that are kept for the milk they give are called "dairy cows" or "milking cows" (formerly "milch cows"). Most young male offspring of dairy cows are sold for veal, and may be referred to as veal calves.

The term "dogies" is used to describe orphaned calves in the context of ranch work in the American West, as in "Keep them dogies moving". In some places, a cow kept to provide milk for one family is called a "house cow". Other obsolete terms for cattle include "neat" (this use survives in "neatsfoot oil", extracted from the feet and legs of cattle), and "beefing" (young animal fit for slaughter).

An onomatopoeic term for one of the most common sounds made by cattle is "moo" (also called lowing). There are a number of other sounds made by cattle, including calves bawling, and bulls bellowing. Bawling is most common for cows after weaning of a calf. The bullroarer makes a sound similar to a bull's territorial call.

Characteristics

Anatomy

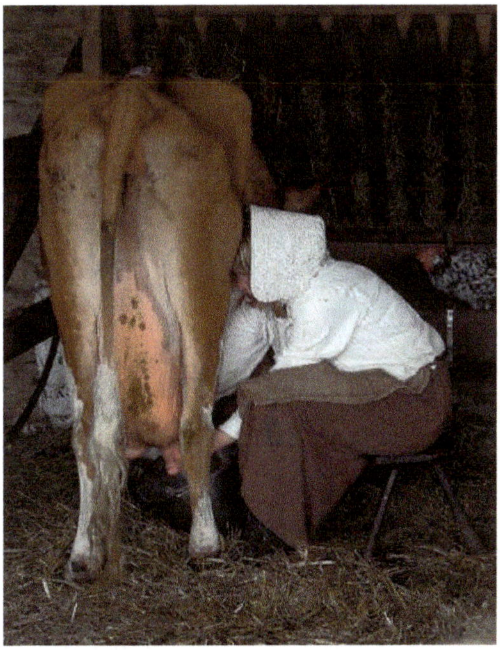

Dairy farming and the milking of cattle was once performed largely by hand, but is now usually replaced by machine

Cattle are large quadrupedal ungulate mammals with cloven hooves. Most breeds have horns, which can be as large as the Texas Longhorn or small like a scur. Careful genetic selection has allowed polled (hornless) cattle to become widespread.

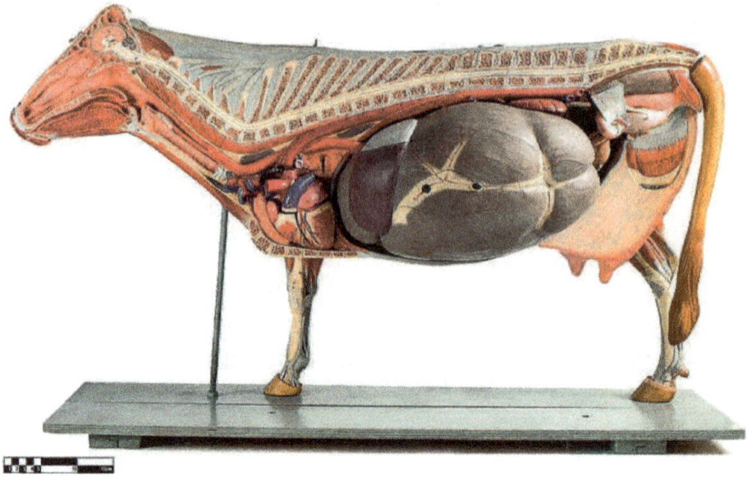

Anatomy model of a bovine (cow)

Cattle are ruminants, meaning their digestive system is highly specialized to allow the use of poorly digestible plants as food. Cattle have one stomach with four compartments, the rumen, reticulum, omasum, and abomasum, with the rumen being the largest compartment. The reticulum, the smallest compartment, is known as the "honeycomb". Cattle sometimes consume metal objects which are deposited in the reticulum and irritation from the metal objects causes hardware disease. The omasum's main function is to absorb water and nutrients from the digestible feed. The omasum is known as the "many plies". The abomasum is like the human stomach; this is why it is known as the "true stomach".

Cattle are known for regurgitating and re-chewing their food, known as cud chewing, like most ruminants. While the animal is feeding, the food is swallowed without being chewed and goes into the rumen for storage until the animal can find a quiet place to continue the digestion process. The food is regurgitated, a mouthful at a time, back up to the mouth, where the food, now called the cud, is chewed by the molars, grinding down the course vegetation to small particles. The cud is then swallowed again and further digested by specialized microorganisms in the rumen. These microbes are primarily responsible for decomposing cellulose and other carbohydrates into volatile fatty acids cattle use as their primary metabolic fuel. The microbes inside the rumen also synthesize amino acids from non-protein nitrogenous sources, such as urea and ammonia. As these microbes reproduce in the rumen, older generations die and their cells continue on through the digestive tract. These cells are then partially digested in the small intestines, allowing cattle to gain a high-quality protein source. These features allow cattle to thrive on grasses and other tough vegetation.

Gestation and Size

The gestation period for a cow is about nine months long. A newborn calf's size can vary among breeds, but a typical calf weighs between 25 to 45 kg (55 to 99 lb). Adult size and weight vary significantly among breeds and sex. The world record for the heaviest bull was 1,740 kg (3,840 lb), a Chianina named Donetto, when he was exhibited at the Arezzo show in 1955. The heaviest steer was eight-year-old 'Old Ben', a Shorthorn/ Hereford cross weighing in at 2,140 kg (4,720 lb) in 1910. Steers are generally killed before reaching 750 kg (1,650 lb). Breeding stock may be allowed a longer lifespan, occasionally living as long as 25 years. The oldest recorded cow, Big Bertha, died at the age of 48 in 1993.

Udder

A cow's udder contains two pairs of mammary glands, (commonly referred to as teats) creating four "quarters". The front ones are referred to as fore quarters and the rear ones rear quarters.

Male Genitalia

Bulls become fertile at about seven months of age. Their fertility is closely related to the size of their testicles, and one simple test of fertility is to measure the circumference of the scrotum: a young bull is likely to be fertile once this reaches 28 centimetres (11 in); that of a fully adult bull may be over 40 centimetres (16 in).

Bulls have a fibro-elastic penis. Given the small amount of erectile tissue, there is little enlargement after erection. The penis is quite rigid when non-erect, and becomes even more rigid during erection. Protrusion is not affected much by erection, but more by relaxation of the retractor penis muscle and straightening of the sigmoid flexure.

Weight

The weight of adult cattle always depends on the breed. Smaller kinds, such as Dexter and Jersey adults, range between 272 to 454 kg (600 to 1,000 lb). Large Continental breeds, such as Charolais, Marchigiana, Belgian Blue and Chianina, adults range from 635 to 1,134 kg (1,400 to 2,500 lb). British breeds, such as Hereford, Angus, and Shorthorn, mature between 454 to 907 kg (1,000 to 2,000 lb), occasionally higher, particularly with Angus and Hereford.

Bulls will be a bit larger than cows of the same breed by a few hundred kilograms. Chianina bulls can weigh up to 1,500 kg (3,300 lb); British bulls, such as Angus and Hereford, can weigh as little as 907 kg (2,000 lb) to as much as 1,361 kg (3,000 lb).

It is difficult to generalize or average out the weight of all cattle because different kinds have different averages of weights. However, according to some sources, the average weight of all cattle is 753 kg (1,660 lb). Finishing steers in the feedlot average about 640 kg (1,410 lb); cows about 725 kg (1,600 lb), and bulls about 1,090 kg (2,400 lb).

In the United States, the average weight of beef cattle has steadily increased, especially since the 1970s, requiring the building of new slaughterhouses able to handle larger carcasses. New packing plants in the 1980s stimulated a large increase in cattle weights. Before 1790 beef cattle averaged only 160 kg (350 lb) net; and thereafter weights climbed steadily.

Cognition

In laboratory studies, young cattle are able to memorize the locations of several food sources and retain this memory for at least 8 hours, although this declined after 12 hours. Fifteen-month-old heifers learn more quickly than adult cows which have had either one or two calvings, but their longer-term memory is less stable. Mature cattle perform well in spatial learning tasks and have a good long-term memory in these tests. Cattle tested in a radial arm maze are able to remember the locations of high-quality food for at least 30 days. Although they initially learn to avoid low-quality food, this memory diminishes over the same duration. Under less artificial testing conditions, young cattle showed they were able to remember the location of feed for at least 48 days. Cattle can make an association between a visual stimulus and food within 1 day – memory of this association can be retained for 1 year, despite a slight decay.

Calves are capable of discrimination learning and adult cattle compare favourably with small mammals in their learning ability in the Closed-field Test.

They are also able to discriminate between familiar individuals, and among humans. Cattle can tell the difference between familiar and unfamiliar animals of the same species (conspecifics). Studies show they behave less aggressively toward familiar individuals when they are forming a new group. Calves can also discriminate between humans based on previous experience, as shown by approaching those who handled them positively and avoiding those who handled them aversively. Although cattle can discriminate between humans by their faces alone, they also use other cues such as the color of clothes when these are available.

In audio play-back studies, calves prefer their own mother's vocalizations compared to the vocalizations of an unfamiliar mother.

In laboratory studies using images, cattle can discriminate between images of the heads of cattle and other animal species. They are also able to distinguish between familiar and unfamiliar conspecifics. Furthermore, they are able to categorize images as familiar and unfamiliar individuals.

When mixed with other individuals, cloned calves from the same donor form subgroups, indicating that kin discrimination occurs and may be a basis of grouping behaviour. It has also been shown using images of cattle that both artificially inseminated and cloned calves have similar cognitive capacities of kin and non-kin discrimination.

Cattle can recognize familiar individuals. Visual individual recognition is a more complex mental process than visual discrimination. It requires the recollection of the learned idiosyncratic identity of an individual that has been previously encountered and the formation of a mental representation. By using 2-dimensional images of the heads of one cow (face, profiles, ¾ views), all the tested heifers showed individual recognition of familiar and unfamiliar individuals from their own breed. Furthermore, almost all the heifers recognized unknown individuals from different breeds, although this was achieved with greater difficulty. Individual recognition was most difficult when the visual features of the breed being tested were quite different from the breed in the image, for example, the breed being tested had no spots whereas the image was of a spotted breed.

Cattle use visual/brain lateralisation in their visual scanning of novel and familiar stimuli. Domestic cattle prefer to view novel stimuli with the left eye, i.e. using the right brain hemisphere (similar to horses, Australian magpies, chicks, toads and fish) but use the right eye, i.e. using the left hemisphere, for viewing familiar stimuli.

Temperament and Emotions

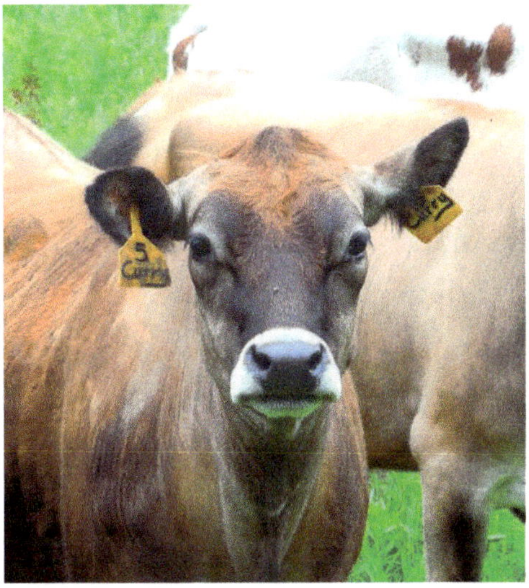

Ear postures of cows are studied as indicators of their emotional state and overall animal welfare.

In cattle, temperament can affect production traits such as carcass and meat quality or milk yield as well as affecting the animal's overall health and reproduction. Cattle temperament is defined as "the consistent behavioral and physiological difference observed between individuals in response to a stressor or environmental challenge and is used to describe the relatively stable difference in the behavioral predisposition of an animal, which can be related to psychobiological mechanisms". Generally, cattle temperament is assumed to be multidimensional. Five underlying categories of temperament traits have been proposed:

- shyness-boldness
- exploration-avoidance
- activity
- aggressiveness
- sociability

In a study on Holstein–Friesian heifers learning to press a panel to open a gate for access to a food reward, the researchers also recorded the heart rate and behavior of the heifers when moving along the race towards the food. When the heifers made clear improvements in learning, they had higher heart rates and tended to move more vigorously along the race. The researchers concluded this was an indication that cattle may react emotionally to their own learning improvement.

Negative emotional states are associated with a bias toward negative (pessimistic) responses towards ambiguous cues in judgement tasks – as encapsulated in the question of "is the glass half empty or half full?". After separation from their mothers, Holstein calves showed such a cognitive bias indicative of low mood. A similar study showed that after hot-iron disbudding (dehorning), calves had a similar negative bias indicating that post-operative pain following this routine procedure results in a negative change in emotional state.

In studies of visual discrimination, the position of the ears has been used as an indicator of emotional state. When cattle are stressed, this can be recognised by other cattle as it is communicated by alarm substances in the urine.

Cattle are very gregarious and even short-term isolation is considered to cause severe psychological stress. When Aubrac and Fresian heifers are isolated, they increase their vocalizations and experience increased heart rate and plasma cortisol concentrations. These physiological changes are greater in Aubracs. When visual contact is re-instated, vocalisations rapidly decline, regardless of the familiarity of the returning cattle, however, heart rate decreases are greater if the returning cattle are familiar to the previously-isolated individual. Mirrors have been used to reduce stress in isolated cattle.

Senses

Cattle use all of the five widely recognized sensory modalities. These can assist in some complex behavioural patterns, for example, in grazing behaviour. Cattle eat mixed diets, but when given the opportunity, show a partial preference of approximately 70% clover and 30% grass. This preference has a diurnal pattern, with a stronger preference for clover in the morning, and the proportion of grass increasing towards the evening.

Vision

Vision is the dominant sense in cattle and they obtain almost 50% of their information visually.

Cattle are a prey animal and to assist predator detection, their eyes are located on the sides of their head rather than the front. This gives them a wide field of view of 330° but limits binocular vision (and therefore stereopsis) to 30° to 50° compared to 140° in humans. This means they have a blind spot directly behind them. Cattle have good visual acuity (1/20) but compared to humans, the visual accommodation of cattle is poor.

Cattle have two kinds of color receptors in the cone cells of their retinas. This means that cattle are dichromatic, as are most other non-primate land mammals. There are two to three rods per cone in the fovea centralis but five to six near the optic papilla. Cattle can distinguish long wavelength colors (yellow, orange and red) much better than the shorter wavelengths (blue, grey and green). Calves are able to discriminate between long (red) and short (blue) or medium (green) wavelengths, but have limited ability to discriminate between the short and medium. They also approach handlers more quickly under red light. Whilst having good color sensitivity, it is not as good as humans or sheep.

A common misconception about cattle (particularly bulls) is that they are enraged by the color red (something provocative is often said to be like a red flag to a bull). This is a myth. In bullfighting, it is the movement of the red flag or cape that irritates the bull and incites it to charge.

Taste

Cattle have a well-developed sense of taste and can distinguish the four primary tastes (sweet, salty, bitter and sour). They possess around 20,000 taste buds. The strength of taste perception depends on the individual's current food requirements. They avoid bitter-tasting foods (potentially toxic) and have a marked preference for sweet (high calorific value) and salty foods (electrolyte balance). Their sensitivity to sour-tasting foods helps them to maintain optimal ruminal pH.

Plants have low levels of sodium and cattle have developed the capacity of seeking salt by taste and smell. If cattle become depleted of sodium salts, they show increased locomotion directed to searching for these. To assist in their search, the olfactory and gustatory receptors able to detect minute amounts of sodium salts increase their sensitivity as biochemical disruption develops with sodium salt depletion.

Audition

Cattle hearing ranges from 23 Hz to 35 kHz. Their frequency of best sensitivity is 8 kHz and they have a lowest threshold of −21 db (re 20 $\mu N/m^{-2}$), which means their hearing is more acute than horses (lowest threshold of 7 db). Sound localization acuity thresholds are an average of 30°. This means that cattle are less able to localise sounds compared to goats (18°), dogs (8°) and humans (0.8°). Because cattle have a broad foveal fields of view covering almost the entire horizon, they may not need very accurate locus information from their auditory systems to direct their gaze to a sound source.

Vocalisations are an important mode of communication amongst cattle and can provide information on the age, sex, dominance status and reproductive status of the caller. Calves can recognize their mothers using vocal and vocal behaviour may play a role by indicating estrus and competitive display by bulls.

Olfaction and Gustation

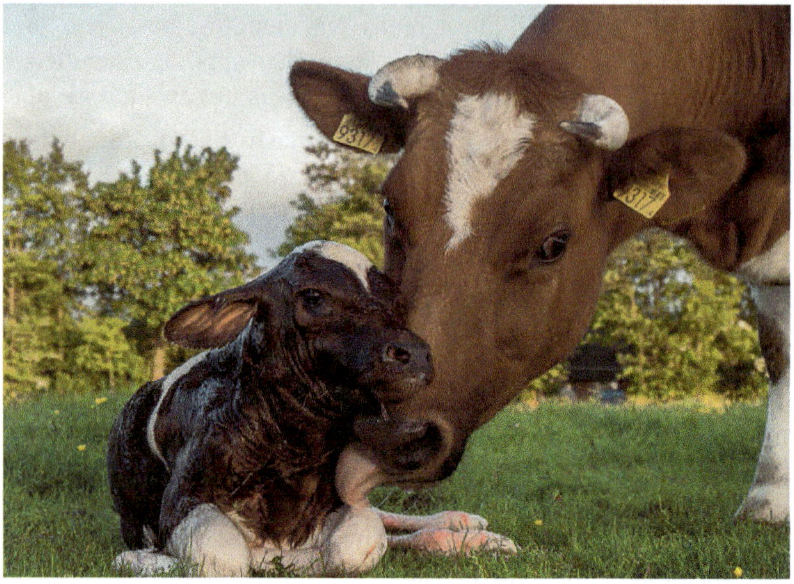

Several senses are used in social relationships between cattle

Cattle have a range of odiferous glands over their body including interdigital, infraorbital, inguinal and sebaceous glands, indicating that olfaction probably plays a large role in their social life. Both the primary olfactory system using the olfactory bulbs, and the secondary olfactory system using the vomeronasal organ are used. This latter olfactory system is used in the flehmen response. There is evidence that when cattle are stressed, this can be recognised by other cattle and this is communicated by alarm substances in the urine. The odour of dog faeces induces behavioural changes prior to cattle feeding, whereas the odours of urine from either stressed or non-stressed conspecifics and blood have no effect.

In the laboratory, cattle can be trained to recognise conspecific individuals using olfaction only.

In general, cattle use their sense of smell to "expand" on information detected by other sensory modalities. However, in the case of social and reproductive behaviours, olfaction is a key source of information.

Touch

Cattle have tactile sensations detected mainly by mechanoreceptors, thermoreceptors and nociceptors in the skin and muzzle. These are used most frequently when cattle explore their environment.

Magnetoreception

There is conflicting evidence for magnetoreception in cattle. One study reported that resting and grazing cattle tend to align their body axes in the geomagnetic North-South (N-S) direction. In a follow-up study, cattle exposed to various magnetic fields directly beneath or in the vicinity of power lines trending in various magnetic directions exhibited distinct patterns of alignment. However, in 2011, a group of Czech researchers reported their failed attempt to replicate the finding using Google Earth images.

Behavior

Under natural conditions, calves stay with their mother until weaning at 8 to 11 months. Heifer and bull calves are equally attached to their mothers in the first few months of life. Cattle are considered to be "hider" type animals, but in the artificial environment of small calving pens, close proximity between cow and calf is maintained by the mother at the first three calvings but this changes to being mediated by the calf after these. Primiparous dams show a higher incidence of abnormal maternal behavior.

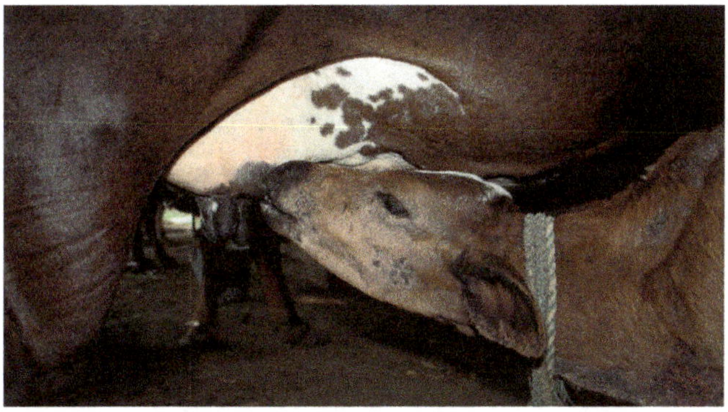

Video of a calf suckling

Beef-calves reared on the range suckle an average of 5.0 times every 24 hours with an average total time of 46 min spent suckling. There is a diurnal rhythm in suckling activity with peaks between 05:00–07:00, 10:00–13:00 and 17:00–21:00.

Studies on the natural weaning of zebu cattle (Bos indicus) have shown that the cow weans her calves over a 2-week period, but after that, she continues to show strong affiliatory behavior with her offspring and preferentially chooses them for grooming and as grazing partners for at least 4–5 years.

Reproductive Behavior

Semi-wild Highland cattle heifers first give birth at 2 or 3 years of age and the timing of birth is synchronized with increases in natural food quality. Average calving interval is 391 days, and calving mortality within the first year of life is 5%.

Dominance and Leadership

One study showed that over a 4-year period, dominance relationships within a herd of semi-wild highland cattle were very firm. There were few overt aggressive conflicts and the majority of disputes were settled by agonistic (non-aggressive, competitive) behaviors that involved no physical contact between opponents (e.g. threatening and spontaneous withdrawing). Such agonistic behavior reduces the risk of injury. Dominance status depended on age and sex, with older animals generally being dominant to young ones and males dominant to females. Young bulls gained superior dominance status over adult cows when they reached about 2 years of age.

As with many animal dominance hierarchies, dominance-associated aggressiveness does not correlate with rank position, but is closely related to rank distance between individuals.

Dominance is maintained in several ways. Cattle often engage in mock fights where they test each other's strength in a non-aggressive way. Licking is primarily performed by subordinates and received by dominant animals. Mounting is a playful behavior shown by calves of both sexes and by bulls and sometimes by cows in estrus, however, this is not a dominance related behavior as has been found in other species.

The horns of cattle are "honest signals" used in mate selection. Furthermore, horned cattle attempt to keep greater distances between themselves and have fewer physical interactions than hornless cattle. This leads to more stable social relationships.

In calves, the frequency of agonistic behavior decreases as space allowance increases, but this does not occur for changes in group size. However, in adult cattle, the number of agonistic encounters increases as the group size increases.

Grazing Behavior

When grazing, cattle vary several aspects of their bite, i.e. tongue and jaw movements, depending on characteristics of the plant they are eating. Bite area decreases with the density of the plants but increases with their height. Bite area is determined by the sweep of the tongue; in one study observing 750-kilogram (1,650 lb) steers, bite area reached a maximum of approximately 170 cm^2 (30 sq in). Bite depth increases with the height of the plants. By adjusting their behavior, cattle obtain heavier bites in swards that are tall and sparse compared with short, dense swards of equal mass/area. Cattle adjust other aspects of their grazing behavior in relation to the available food; foraging velocity decreases and intake rate increases in areas of abundant palatable forage.

Cattle avoid grazing areas contaminated by the faeces of other cattle more strongly than they avoid areas contaminated by sheep, but they do not avoid pasture contaminated by rabbit faeces.

Genetics

In the 24 April 2009, edition of the journal Science, a team of researchers led by the National Institutes of Health and the US Department of Agriculture reported having mapped the bovine genome. The scientists found cattle have about 22,000 genes, and 80% of their genes are shared with humans, and they share about 1000 genes with dogs and rodents, but are not found in humans. Using this bovine "HapMap", researchers can track the differences between the breeds that affect the quality of meat and milk yields.

Behavioral traits of cattle can be as heritable as some production traits, and often, the two can be related. The heritability of fear varies markedly in cattle from low (0.1) to high (0.53); such high variation is also found in pigs and sheep, probably due to differences in the methods used. The heritability of temperament (response to isolation during handling) has been calculated as 0.36 and 0.46 for habituation to handling. Rangeland assessments show that the heritability of aggressiveness in cattle is around 0.36.

Quantitative trait loci (QTLs) have been found for a range of production and behavioral characteristics for both dairy and beef cattle.

Domestication and Husbandry

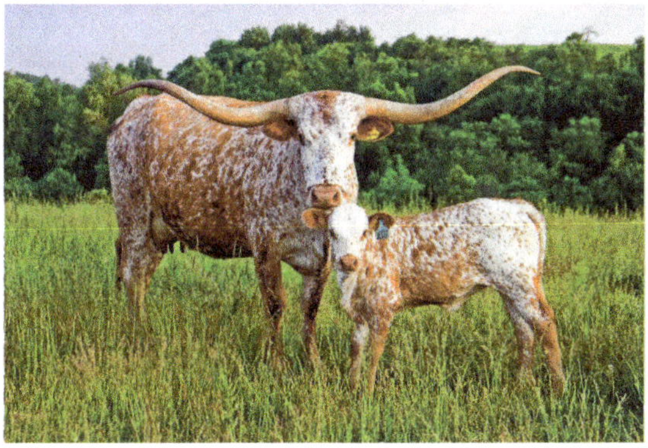

Texas Longhorns are a US breed

Cattle occupy a unique role in human history, having been domesticated since at least the early neolithic age.

Archeozoological and genetic data indicate that cattle were first domesticated from wild aurochs (Bos primigenius) approximately 10,500 years ago. There were two major areas of domestication: one in the area that is now Turkey, giving rise to the taurine line, and a second in the area that is now Pakistan, resulting in the indicine line. Modern mitochondrial DNA variation indicates the taurine line may have arisen from as few as 80 aurochs tamed in the upper reaches of Mesopotamia near the villages of Çayönü Tepesi in southeastern Turkey and Dja›de el-Mughara in northern Iraq.

Although European cattle are largely descended from the taurine lineage, gene flow from African cattle (partially of indicine origin) contributed substantial genomic components to both southern European cattle breeds and their New World descendants. A study on 134 breeds showed that modern taurine cattle originated from Africa, Asia, North and South America, Australia, and Europe. Some researchers have suggested that African taurine cattle are derived from a third independent domestication from North African aurochsen.

Usage as Money

As early as 9000 BC both grain and cattle were used as money or as barter (Davies) (the first grain remains found, considered to be evidence of pre-agricultural practice date to 17,000 BC). Some evidence also exists to suggest that other animals, such as camels and goats, may have been used as currency in some parts of the world. One of the advantages of using cattle as currency is that it allows the seller to set a fixed price. It even created the standard pricing. For example, two chickens were traded for one cow as cows were deemed to be more valuable than chickens.

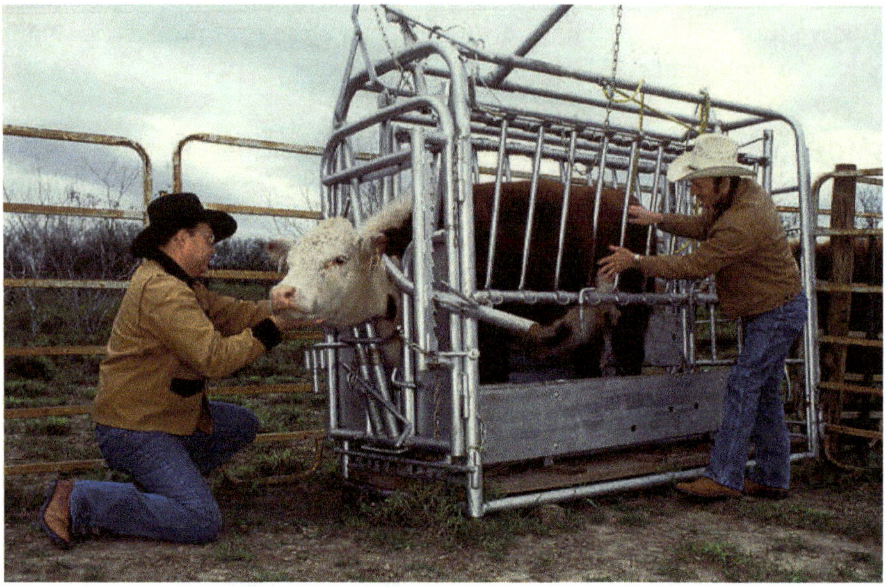

This Hereford is being inspected for ticks; cattle are often restrained or confined in cattle crushes (squeeze chutes) when given medical attention.

Modern Husbandry

Cattle are often raised by allowing herds to graze on the grasses of large tracts of rangeland. Raising cattle in this manner allows the use of land that might be unsuitable for growing crops. The most common interactions with cattle involve daily feeding, cleaning and milking. Many routine husbandry practices involve ear tagging, dehorning, loading, medical operations, vaccinations and hoof care, as well as training for agricultural shows and preparations. Also, some cultural differences occur in working with cattle; the cattle husbandry of Fulani men rests on behavioral techniques, whereas in Europe, cattle are controlled primarily by physical means, such as fences. Breeders use cattle husbandry to reduce M. bovis infection susceptibility by selective breeding and maintaining herd health to avoid concurrent disease.

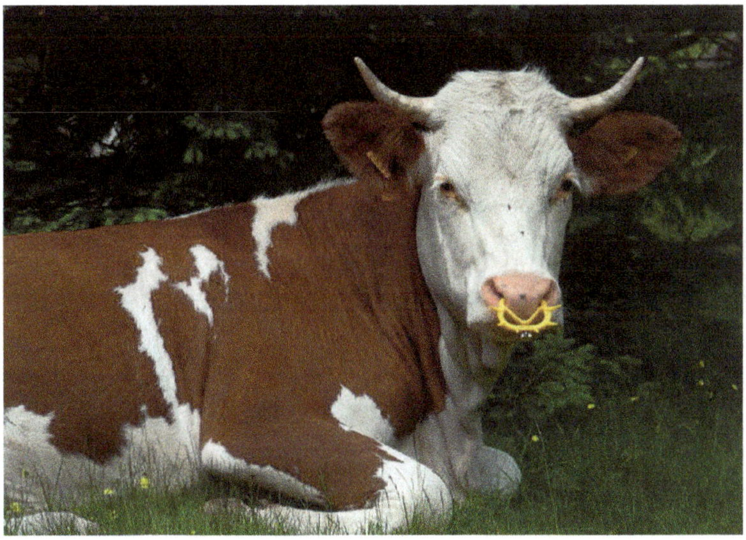

This young bovine has a nose ring to prevent it from suckling, which is usually to assist in weaning.

Cattle are farmed for beef, veal, dairy, and leather, and they are less commonly used for conservation grazing, simply to maintain grassland for wildlife – for example, in Epping Forest, England. They are often used in some of the most wild places for livestock. Depending on the breed, cattle can survive on hill grazing, heaths, marshes, moors and semidesert. Modern cattle are more commercial than older breeds and, having become more specialized, are less versatile. For this reason, many smaller farmers still favor old breeds, such as the Jersey dairy breed. In Portugal, Spain, southern France and some Latin American countries, bulls are used in the activity of bullfighting; Jallikattu in India is a bull taming sport radically different from European bullfighting, humans are unarmed and bulls are not killed. In many other countries bullfighting is illegal. Other activities such as bull riding are seen as part of a rodeo, especially in North America. Bull-leaping, a central ritual in Bronze Age Minoan culture (see Bull (mythology)), still exists in southwestern France. In modern times, cattle are also entered into agricultural competitions. These competitions can involve live cattle or cattle carcases in hoof and hook events.

In terms of food intake by humans, consumption of cattle is less efficient than of grain or vegetables with regard to land use, and hence cattle grazing consumes more area than such other agricultural production when raised on grains. Nonetheless, cattle and other forms of domesticated animals can sometimes help to use plant resources in areas not easily amenable to other forms of agriculture.

Sleep

The average sleep time of a domestic cow is about four hours a day. Cattle do have a stay apparatus, but do not sleep standing up, they lie down to sleep deeply. In spite of the urban legend, cows cannot be tipped over by people pushing on them.

Economy

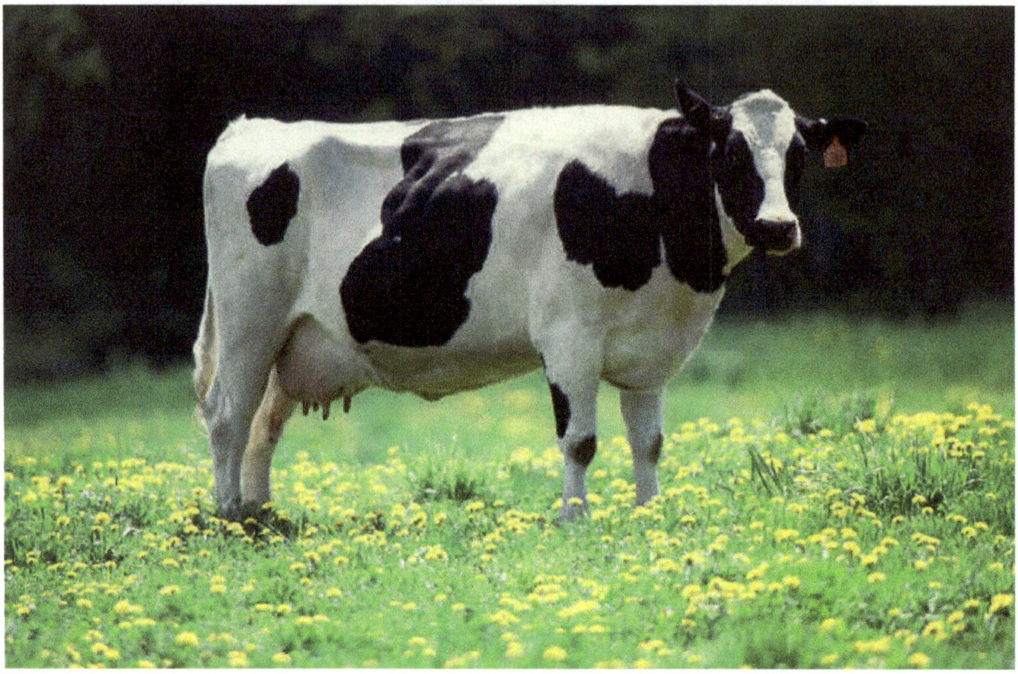

Holstein cattle are the primary dairy breed, bred for high milk production.

The meat of adult cattle is known as beef, and that of calves is veal. Other animal parts are also used as food products, including blood, liver, kidney, heart and oxtail. Cattle also produce milk, and dairy cattle are specifically bred to produce the large quantities of milk processed and sold for human consumption. Cattle today are the basis of a multibillion-dollar industry worldwide. The international trade in beef for 2000 was over $30 billion and represented only 23% of world beef production. The production of milk, which is also made into cheese, butter, yogurt, and other dairy products, is comparable in economic size to beef production, and provides an important part of the food supply for many of the world's people. Cattle hides, used for leather to make shoes, couches and clothing, are another widespread product. Cattle remain broadly used as draft animals in many developing countries, such as India. Cattle are also used in some sporting games, including rodeo and bullfighting.

Cattle Meat Production

Cattle meat production (kt)

Country ▲	2008 ♦	2009 ♦	2010 ♦	2011 ♦
Argentina	3132	3378	2630	2497
Australia	2132	2124	2630	2420
Brazil	9024	9395	9115	9030
China	5841	6060	6244	6182
Germany	1199	1190	1205	1170
Japan	520	517	515	500
USA	12163	11891	12046	11988

Source: Helgi Library, World Bank, FAOSTAT

About half the world's meat comes from cattle.

Dairy

Certain breeds of cattle, such as the Holstein-Friesian, are used to produce milk, which can be processed into dairy products such as milk, cheese or yogurt. Dairy cattle are usually kept on specialized dairy farms designed for milk production. Most cows are milked twice per day, with milk processed at a dairy, which may be onsite at the farm or the milk may be shipped to a dairy plant for eventual sale of a dairy product. For dairy cattle to continue producing milk, they must give birth to one calf per year. If the calf is male, it generally is slaughtered at a young age to produce veal. They will continue to produce milk until three weeks before birth. Over the last fifty years, dairy farming has become more intensive to increase the yield of milk produced by each cow. The Holstein-Friesian is the breed of dairy cow most common in the UK, Europe and the United States. It has been bred selectively to produce the highest yields of milk of any cow. Around 22 litres per day is average in the UK.

Hides

Most cattle are not kept solely for hides, which are usually a by-product of beef production. Hides are most commonly used for leather which can be made into a variety of product including shoes. In 2012 India was the world's largest producer of cattle hides.

Feral Cattle

Feral cattle are defined as being 'cattle that are not domesticated or cultivated'. Populations of feral cattle are known to come from and exist in: Australia, United States of America, Colombia, Argentina, Spain, France and many islands, including New Guinea, Hawaii, Galapagos, Juan Fernández Islands, Hispaniola (Dominican Republic and Haiti), Tristan da Cunha and Île Amsterdam, two islands of Kuchinoshima and Kazura Island next to

Naru Island in Japan. Chillingham cattle is sometimes regarded as a feral breed. Aleutian wild cattles can be found on Aleutian Islands. The "Kinmen cattle" which is dominantly found on Kinmen Island, Taiwan is mostly domesticated while smaller portion of the population is believed to live in the wild due to accidental releases.

Environmental Impact

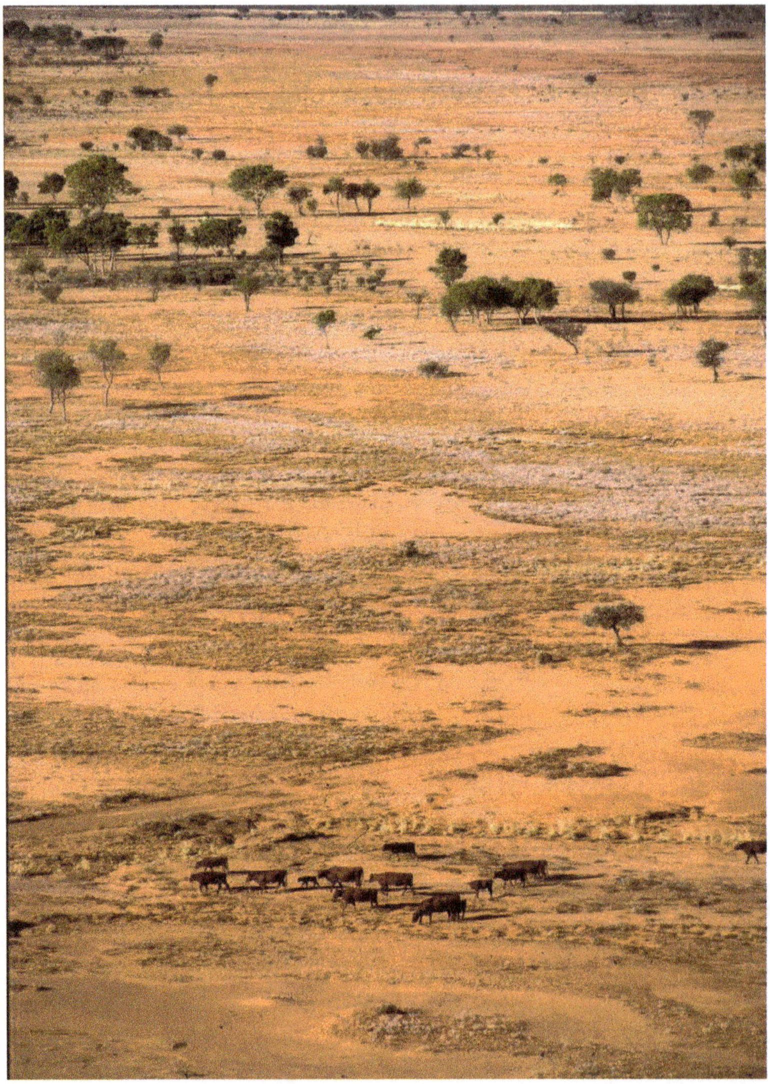

Cattle in dry landscape north of Alice Springs, Australia (CSIRO)

Cattle near the Bruneau River in Elko County, Nevada

A report from the Food and Agriculture Organization (FAO) states that the livestock sector is "responsible for 18% of greenhouse gas emissions". The report concludes, unless changes are made, the damage thought to be linked to livestock may more than double by 2050, as demand for meat increases. Another concern is manure, which if not well-managed, can lead to adverse environmental consequences. However, manure also is a valuable source of nutrients and organic matter when used as a fertilizer. Manure was used as a fertilizer on about 15.8 million acres of US cropland in 2006, with manure from cattle accounting for nearly 70% of manure applications to soybeans and about 80% or more of manure applications to corn, wheat, barley, oats and sorghum. Substitution of manure for synthetic fertilizers in crop production can be environmentally significant, as between 43 and 88 megajoules of fossil fuel energy would be used per kg of nitrogen in manufacture of synthetic nitrogenous fertilizers. A cow does on overage release between 70 and 120 kg of Methane per year. Methane is a greenhouse gas like carbon dioxide (CO_2). But the negative effect on the climate of Methane is 23 times higher than the effect of CO2.

One of the cited changes suggested to reduce greenhouse gas emissions is intensification of the livestock industry, since intensification leads to less land for a given level of production. This assertion is supported by studies of the US beef production system, suggesting practices prevailing in 2007 involved 8.6% less fossil fuel use, 16.3% less greenhouse gas emissions, 12.1% less water use, and 33.0% less land use, per unit mass of beef produced, than those used in 1977. The analysis took into account not only practices in feedlots, but also feed production (with less feed needed in more intensive production systems), forage-based cow-calf operations and back-grounding before cattle enter a feedlot (with more beef produced per head of cattle from those sources, in more intensive systems), and beef from animals derived from the dairy industry.

The number of American cattle kept in confined feedlot conditions fluctuates. From 1 January 2002 through 1 January 2012, there was no significant overall upward or downward trend in the number of US cattle on feed for slaughter, which averaged about 14.046 million head over that period. Previously, the number had increased; it was 12.453 million in 1985. Cattle on feed (for slaughter) numbered about 14.121 million on 1 January 2012, i.e. about 15.5% of the estimated inventory of 90.8 million US cattle (including calves) on that date. Of the 14.121 million, US cattle on feed (for slaughter) in operations with 1000 head or more were estimated to number 11.9 million. Cattle feedlots in this size category correspond to the regulatory definition of large concentrated animal feeding operations (CAFOs) for cattle other than mature dairy cows or veal calves. Significant numbers of dairy, as well as beef cattle, are confined in CAFOs, defined as new and existing operations which stable or confine and feed or maintain for a total of 45 days or more in any 12-month period more than the number of animals specified where "crops, vegetation, forage growth, or post-harvest residues are not sustained in the normal growing season over any portion of the lot or facility. They may be designated as small, medium and large. Such designation of cattle CAFOs is according to cattle type (mature dairy cows, veal calves or other) and cattle numbers, but medium CAFOs are so designated only if they meet certain discharge criteria, and small CAFOs are designated only on a case-by-case basis.

A CAFO that discharges pollutants is required to obtain a permit, which requires a plan to manage nutrient runoff, manure, chemicals, contaminants, and other wastewater pursuant to the US Clean Water Act. The regulations involving CAFO permitting have been extensively litigated. Commonly, CAFO wastewater and manure nutrients are applied to land at agronomic rates for use by forages or crops, and it is often assumed that various constituents of wastewater and manure, e.g. organic contaminants and pathogens, will be retained, inactivated or degraded on the land with application at such rates; however, additional evidence is needed to test reliability of such assumptions . Concerns raised by opponents of CAFOs have included risks of contaminated water due to feedlot runoff, soil erosion, human and animal exposure to toxic chemicals, development of antibiotic resistant bacteria and an increase in E. coli contamination. While research suggests some of these impacts can be mitigated by developing wastewater treatment systems and planting cover crops in larger setback zones, the Union of Concerned Scientists released a report in 2008 concluding that CAFOs are generally unsustainable and externalize costs.

An estimated 935,000 cattle operations were operating in the USA in 2010. In 2001, the US Environmental Protection Agency (EPA) tallied 5,990 cattle CAFOs then regulated, consisting of beef (2,200), dairy (3,150), heifer (620) and veal operations (20). Since that time, the EPA has established CAFOs as an enforcement priority. EPA enforcement highlights for fiscal year 2010 indicated enforcement actions against 12 cattle CAFOs for violations that included failures to obtain a permit, failures to meet the terms of a permit, and discharges of contaminated water.

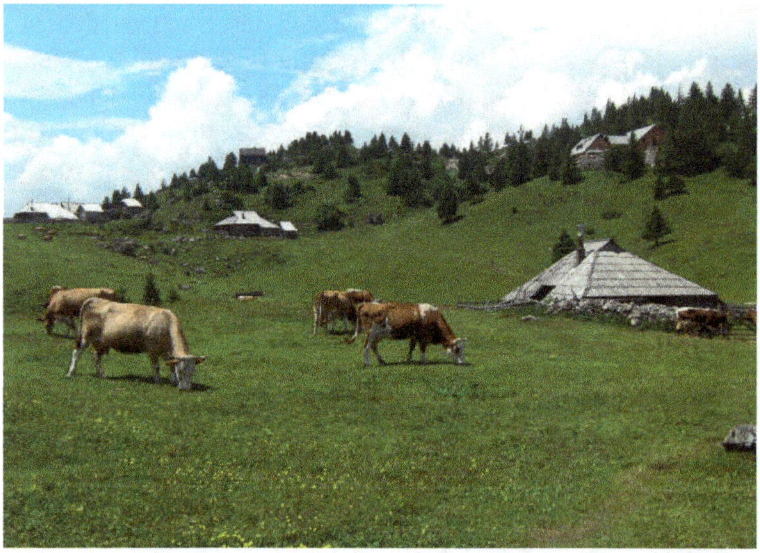

Cattle grazing in a high-elevation environment at the Big Pasture Plateau, Slovenia

Grazing by cattle at low intensities can create a favourable environment for native herbs and forbs; in many world regions, though, cattle are reducing biodiversity due to overgrazing. A survey of refuge managers on 123 National Wildlife Refuges in the US tallied 86 species of wildlife considered positively affected and 82 considered negatively affected by refuge cattle grazing or haying.Proper management of pastures, notably managed intensive rotational grazing and grazing at low intensities can lead to less use of fossil fuel energy, increased recapture of carbon dioxide, fewer ammonia emissions into the atmosphere, reduced soil erosion, better air quality, and less water pollution.

Some microbes in the cattle gut carry out anaerobic process known as methanogenesis, which produces methane. Cattle and other livestock emit about 80 to 93 Tg of methane per year, accounting for an estimated 37% of anthropogenic methane emissions, and additional methane is produced by anaerobic fermentation of manure in manure lagoons and other manure storage structures. The 100-year global warming potential of methane, including effects on ozone and stratospheric water vapor, is 25 times as great as that of carbon dioxide. Methane's effect on global warming is correlated with changes in atmospheric methane content, not with emissions. The net change in atmospheric methane content was recently about 1 Tg per year, and in some recent years there has been no increase in atmospheric methane content. Mitigation options for reducing methane emission from ruminant enteric fermentation include genetic selection, immunization, rumen defaunation, diet modification and grazing management, among others. While cattle fed forage actually produce more methane than grain-fed cattle, the increase may be offset by the increased carbon recapture of pastures, which recapture three times the CO_2 of cropland used for grain.

Health

The veterinary discipline dealing with cattle and cattle diseases (bovine veterinary) is called buiatrics. Veterinarians and professionals working on cattle health issues are pooled in the World Association for Buiatrics, founded in 1960. National associations and affiliates also exist.

Cattle diseases were in the center of attention in the 1980s and 1990s when the Bovine spongiform encephalopathy (BSE), also known as mad cow disease, was of concern. Cattle might catch and develop various other diseases, like blackleg, bluetongue, foot rot too.

In most states, as cattle health is not only a veterinarian issue, but also a public health issue, public health and food safety standards and farming regulations directly affect the daily work of farmers who keep cattle. However, said rules change frequently and are often debated. For instance, in the U.K., it was proposed in 2011 that milk from tuberculosis-infected cattle should be allowed to enter the food chain. Internal food safety regulations might affect a country's trade policy as well. For example, the United States has just reviewed its beef import rules according to the "mad cow standards"; while Mexico forbids the entry of cattle who are older than 30 months.

Cow urine is commonly used in India for internal medical purposes. It is distilled and then consumed by patients seeking treatment for a wide variety of illnesses. At present, no conclusive medical evidence shows this has any effect. However, an Indian medicine containing cow urine has already obtained U.S. patents.

Digital dermatitis is caused by the bacteria from the genus Treponema. It differs from foot rot and can appear under unsanitary conditions such as poor hygiene or inadequate hoof trimming, among other causes. It primarily affects dairy cattle and has been known to lower the quantity of milk produced, however the milk quality remains unaffected. Cattle are also susceptible to ringworm caused by the fungus, Trichophyton verrucosum, a contagious skin disease which may be transferred to humans exposed to infected cows.

Mycobacterium vaccae is a non pathogenic, possibly even beneficial bacteria, that is seen naturally in soil; that was first isolated from cow dung.

Effect of High Stocking Density

Stocking density refers to the number of animals within a specified area. When stocking density reaches high levels, the behavioural needs of the animals may not be met. This can negatively influence health, welfare and production performance.

The effect of overstocking in cows can have a negative effect on milk production and reproduction rates which are two very important traits for dairy farmers. Overcrowding of cows in barns has been found to reduced feeding, resting and rumination. Although they consume the same amount of dry matter within the span of a day, they consume the food at a much more rapid rate, and this behaviour in cows can lead to further complications. The feeding behaviour of cows during their post-milking period is very important as it has been proven that the longer animals can eat after milking, the longer they will be standing up and therefore causing less contamination to the teat ends. This is necessary to reduce the risk of mastitis as infection has been shown to increase the chances of embryonic loss. Sufficient rest is important for dairy cows because it is during this period that their resting blood flow increases up to 50%, this is directly proportionate to milk production. Each additional hour of rest can be seen to translate to 2 to 3.5 more pounds of milk per cow daily. Stocking densities of anything over 120% have been shown to decrease the amount of time cows spend lying down.

Cortisol is an important stress hormone; its plasma concentrations increase greatly when subjected to high levels of stress. Increased concentration levels of cortisol have been associated with significant increases in gonadotrophin levels and lowered progestin levels. Reduction of stress is important in the reproductive state of cows as an increase in gonadotrophin and lowered progesterone levels may impinge on the ovulatory and lutenization process and to reduce the chances of successful implantation. A high cortisol level will also stimulate the degradation of fats and proteins which may make it difficult for the animal to sustain its pregnancy if implanted successfully.

Oxen

Oxen (singular **ox**) are cattle trained as draft animals. Often they are adult, castrated males of larger breeds, although females and bulls are also used in some areas. Usually, an ox is over four years old due to the need for training and to allow it to grow to full size. Oxen are used for plowing, transport, hauling cargo, grain-grinding by trampling or by powering machines, irrigation by powering pumps, and wagon drawing. Oxen were commonly used to skid logs in forests, and sometimes still are, in low-impact, select-cut logging. Oxen are most often used in teams of two, paired, for light work such as carting, with additional pairs added when more power is required, sometimes up to a total of 20 or more.

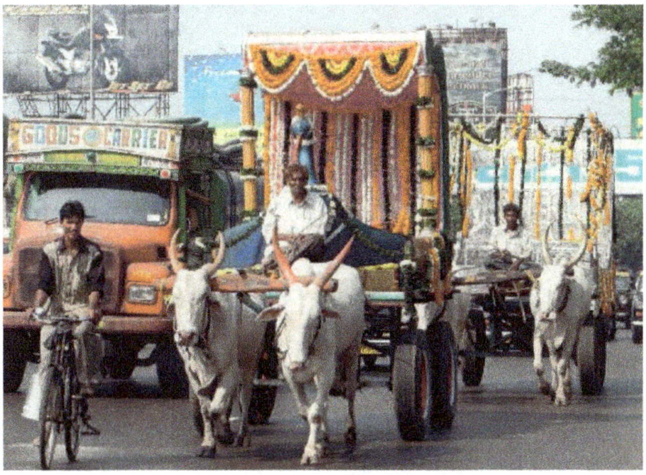

Draft Zebus in Mumbai, Maharashtra, India

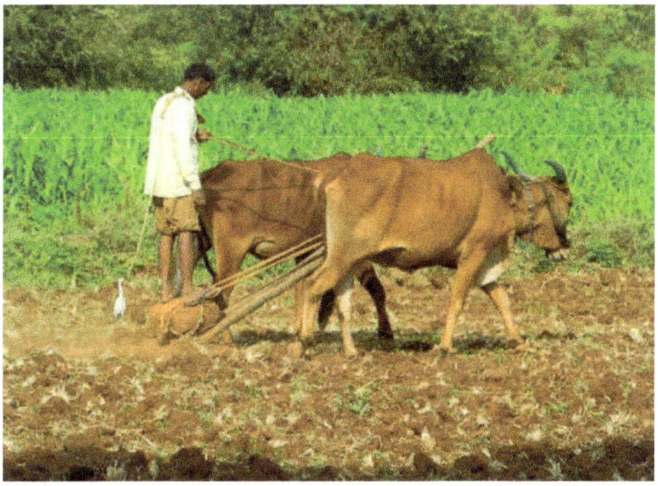

Oxen used in Plowing

An ox is a mature bovine which has learned to respond appropriately to a teamster's signals. These signals are given by verbal commands or by noise (whip cracks). Verbal commands vary according to dialect and local tradition. In one tradition in North America, the commands are:

- "Back up": go backwards
- "Gee": turn right
- "Get up": walk forward
- "Haw": turn left
- "Whoa": stop

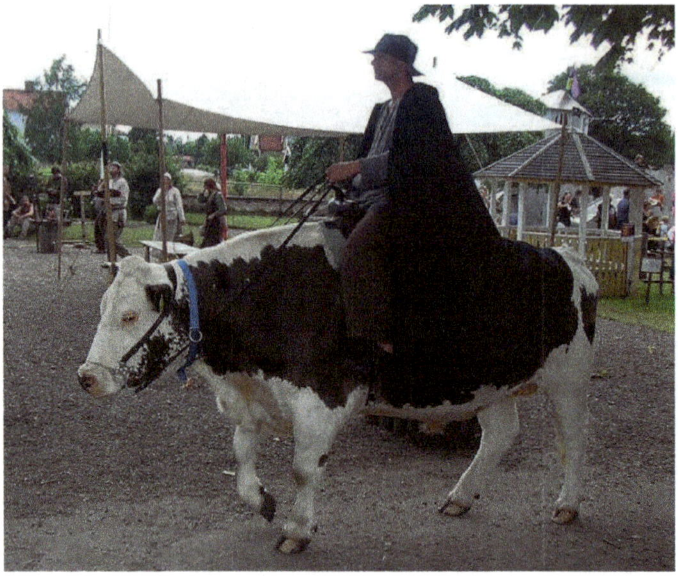

Riding an ox in Hova, Sweden

Oxen can pull harder and longer than horses. Though not as fast as horses, they are less prone to injury because they are more sure-footed.

Many oxen are used worldwide, especially in developing countries. About 11.3 million draft oxen are used in sub-Saharan Africa. In India, the number of draft cattle in 1998 was estimated at 65.7 million head. About half the world's crop production is thought to depend on land preparation (such as plowing) made possible by animal traction.

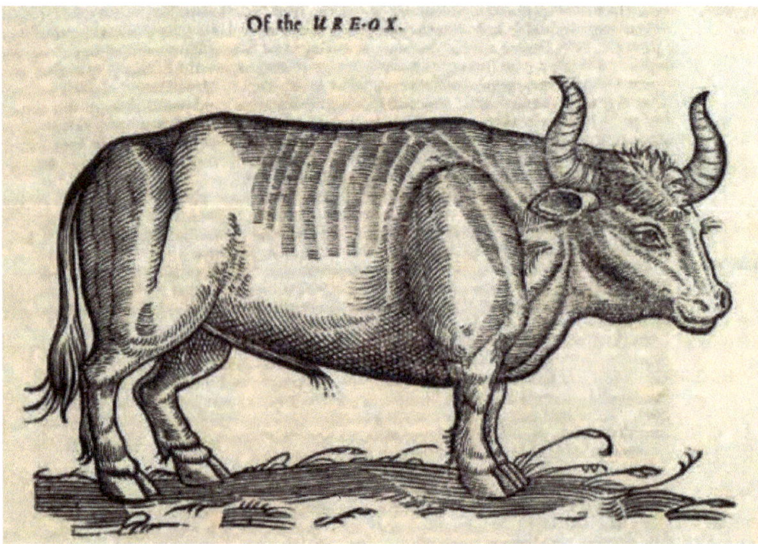

The "Ure-Ox" (Aurochs) by Edward Topsell, 1658

Religion, Traditions and Folklore

Hindu Tradition

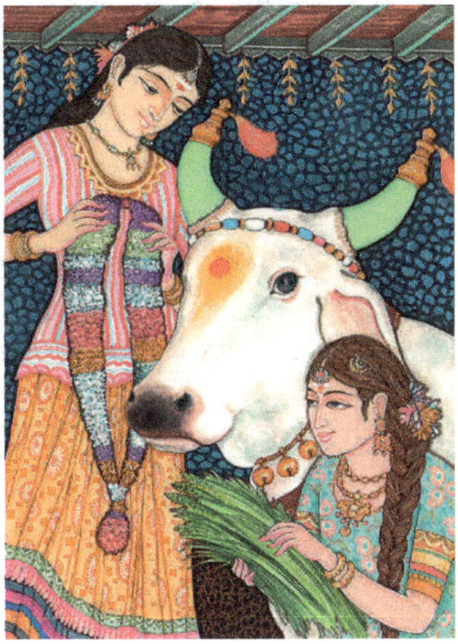

In Hinduism, the cow is a symbol of wealth, strength, abundance, selfless giving and a full Earthly life.

Cattle are venerated within the Hindu religion of India. In the Vedic period they were a symbol of plenty and were frequently slaughtered. In later times they gradually acquired their present status. According to the Mahabharata they are to be treated with the same respect 'as one's mother'. In the middle of the first millennium, the consumption of beef began to be disfavoured by lawgivers. Although there has never been any cow-goddesses or temples dedicated to them, cows appear in numerous stories from the Vedas and Puranas. The deity Krishna was brought up in a family of cowherders, and given the name Govinda (protector of the cows). Also, Shiva is traditionally said to ride on the back of a bull named Nandi.

Milk and milk products were used in Vedic rituals. In the postvedic period products of the cow – milk, curd, ghee, but also cow dung and urine (gomutra), or the combination of these five (panchagavya) – began to assume an increasingly important role in ritual purification and expiation.

Veneration of the cow has become a symbol of the identity of Hindus as a community, especially since the end of the 19th century. Slaughter of cows (including oxen, bulls and calves) is forbidden by law in several states of the Indian Union. McDonalds outlets in India do not serve any beef burgers. In Maharaja Ranjit Singh›s empire of the early 19th century, the killing of a cow was punishable by death.

Other Traditions

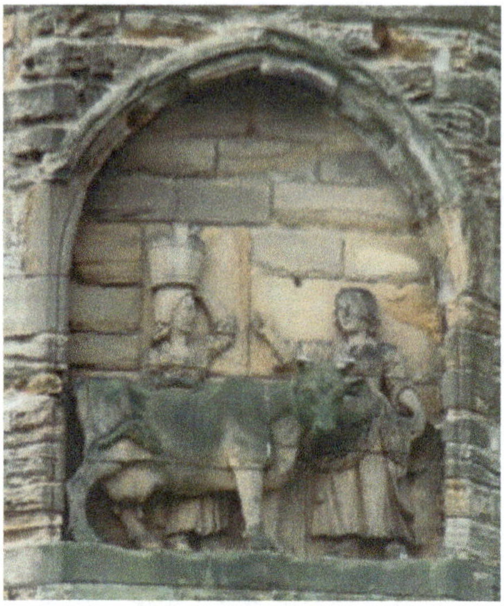

Legend of the founding of Durham Cathedral is that monks carrying the body of Saint Cuthbert were led to the location by a milk maid who had lost her dun cow, which was found resting on the spot.

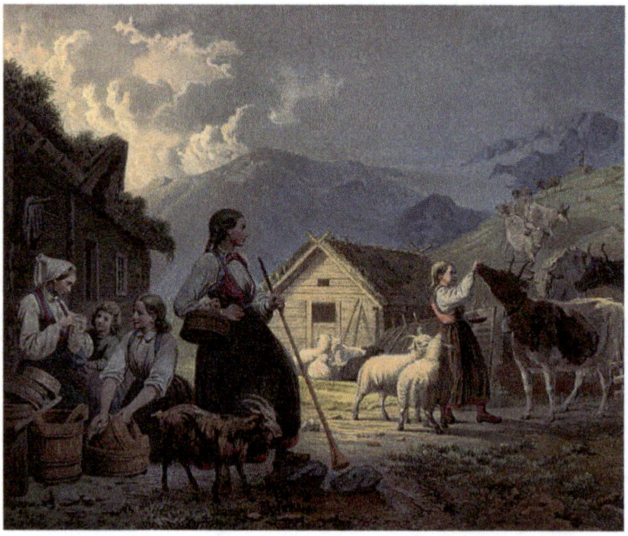

An idealized depiction of girl cow herders in 19th-century Norway by Knud Bergslien.

- The Evangelist St. Luke is depicted as an ox in Christian art.
- In Judaism, as described in Numbers 19:2, the ashes of a sacrificed unblemished red heifer that has never been yoked can be used for ritual purification of people

who came into contact with a corpse.

- The ox is one of the 12-year cycle of animals which appear in the Chinese zodiac related to the Chinese calendar.: Ox (Zodiac).
- The constellation Taurus represents a bull.
- An apocryphal story has it that a cow started the Great Chicago Fire by kicking over a kerosene lamp. Michael Ahern, the reporter who created the cow story, admitted in 1893 that he had fabricated it for more colorful copy.
- On 18 February 1930, Elm Farm Ollie became the first cow to fly in an airplane and also the first cow to be milked in an airplane.
- The first known law requiring branding in North America was enacted on 5 February 1644, by Connecticut. It said that all cattle and pigs had to have a registered brand or earmark by 1 May 1644.
- The akabeko is a traditional toy from the Aizu region of Japan that is thought to ward off illness.
- The case of Sherwood v. Walker—involving a supposedly barren heifer that was actually pregnant—-first enunciated the concept of mutual mistake as a means of destroying the meeting of the minds in contract law.
- The Fulani of West Africa are the world's largest nomadic cattle-herders.
- The Maasai tribe of East Africa traditionally believe their god Engai entitled them to divine rights to the ownership of all cattle on earth.

In Heraldry

Cattle are typically represented in heraldry by the **bull**.

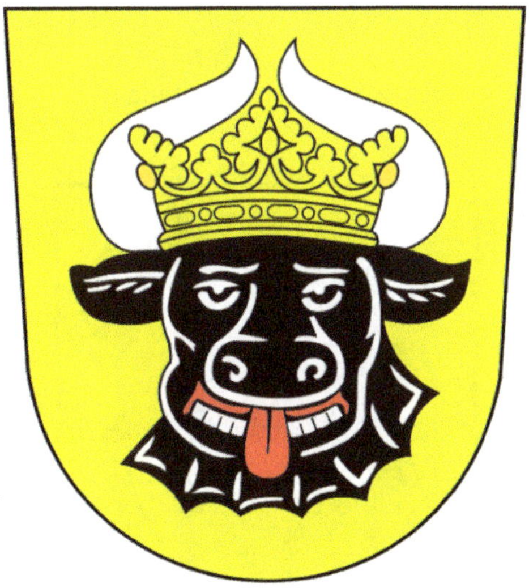

Arms of Mecklenburg region, Germany

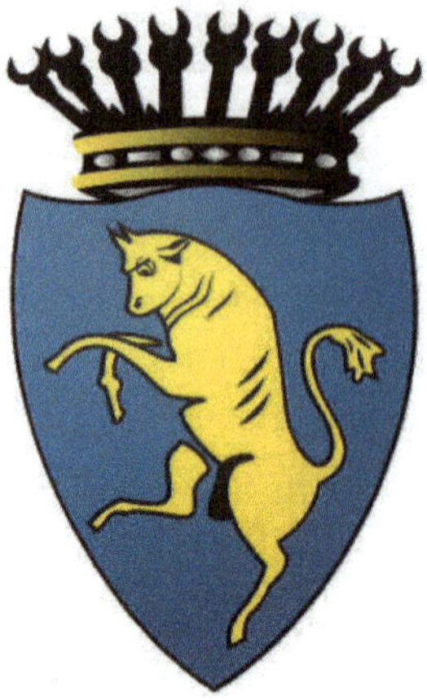

Arms of Turin, Italy

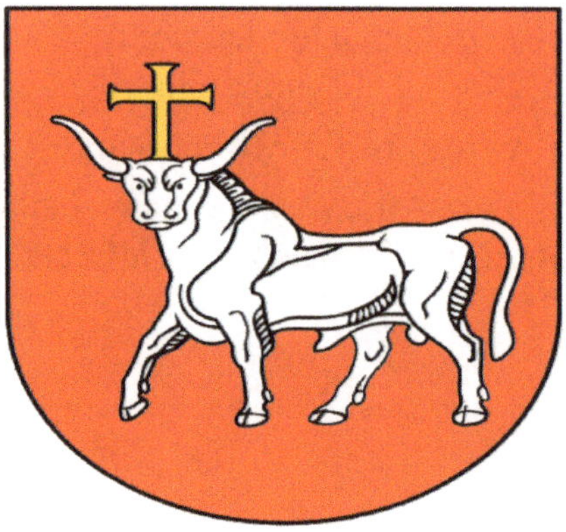

Arms of Kaunas, Lithuania

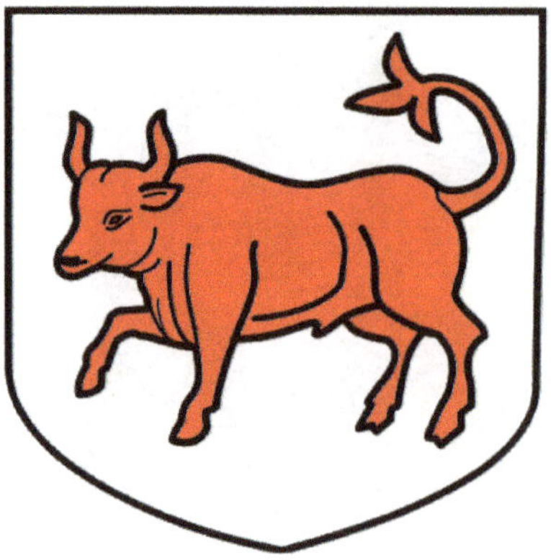

Arms of Turek, Poland

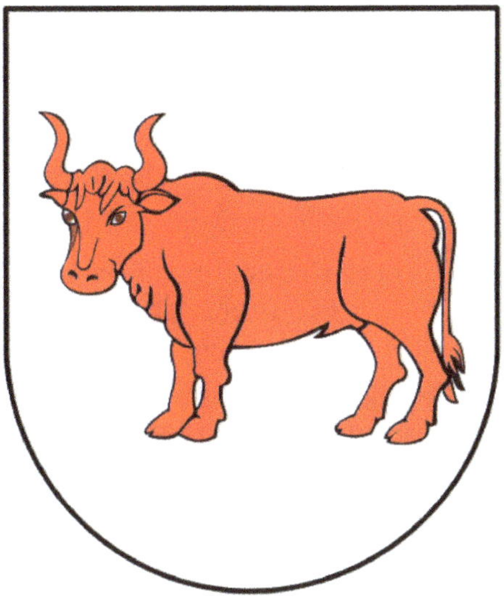

Arms of Bielsk Podlaski, Poland

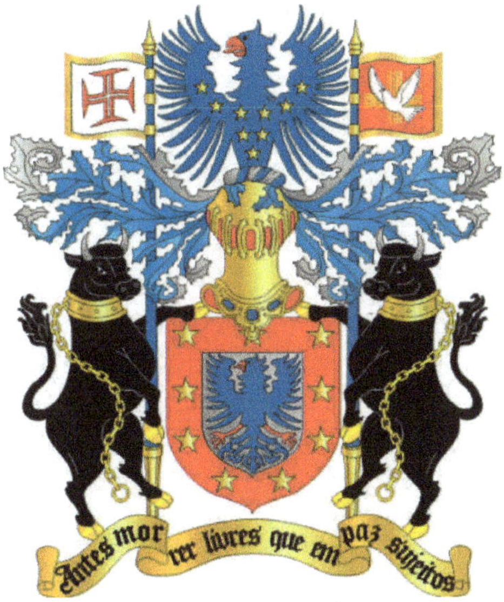

Arms of the Azores

Population

For 2013, the FAO estimated global cattle numbers at 1.47 billion. Regionally, the FAO estimate for 2013 includes: Asia 495 million; South America 348 million; Africa 305 million; Europe 122 million; North America 102 million; Central America 46 million; Oceania 42 million; and Caribbean 9 million. The following table shows the cattle population in 2009.

As of 2003, Africa had about 231 million head of cattle, raised in both traditional and non-traditional systems, but often an "integral" part of the culture and way of life.

BILIARY FEVER

Biliary fever is an illness of the liver affecting horses, dogs and cats.

This is currently the most common infectious disease of dogs in Southern Africa. It is also known as tick bite fever or "Bosluiskoors" in Afrikaans. It is caused by a tiny parasite (Babesia canis) which is introduced into the body by a tick bite. This parasite then enters and destroys red blood cells. Biliary in dogs has a lot in common with malaria in man, except that in the latter, a mosquito is the vector.

Clinical Signs of Disease

The peracute (very sudden and severe) form causes death within a few hours and treatment is of little avail. More commonly dogs suffer from the acute or subacute form. This is recognised by the dog being listless or lethargic, losing its appetite and running a temperature. If your dog is off its food, take a rectal temperature reading. If this is 39 °C or higher you should have the dog examined – do not wait until its mucous membranes become pale, white or yellow, which commonly suggests a more advanced stage of the disease. Fever is present only while the patient is actively fighting the parasite; the disease may be present with a normal (38,5 °C) or subnormal temperature. Yellow faeces and brown or red urine also suggests the presence of biliary fever.

Treatment

Treatment should only be given after a positive diagnosis has been made by means of a blood test. Usually treatment is effective, depending on several factors, but the majority will respond. In early cases simple injections are usually sufficient, but in others blood transfusions, electrolyte infusions per vein, liver tonics, blood-building, etc., may be required.

Diet

Avoid fatty foods, and give a good quality balanced dog food. A tonic and/or follow up treatment may be required if the animal does not appear to be responding to the initial treatment.

Prevention

A vaccine has been launched in South Africa at the end of 2008. Nobivac Piro, has been proven effective when combined with twice yearly booster shots. Rely on reducing the dog's tick population by regular use of approved tick control measures that may be recommended by a veterinarian.

BLADDER STONE

Bladder stones or uroliths are a common occurrence in animals, especially in domestic animals such as dogs and cats. Occurrence in other species, including tortoises, have been reported as well. The stones form in the urinary bladder in varying size and numbers secondary to infection, dietary influences, and genetics. Stones can form in any part of the urinary tract in dogs and cats, but unlike in humans, stones of the kidney are less common and do not often cause significant disease, although they can contribute to pyelonephritis and chronic renal failure. Types of stones include struvite, calcium oxalate, urate, cystine, calcium phosphate, and silicate. Struvite and calcium oxalate stones are by far the most common.

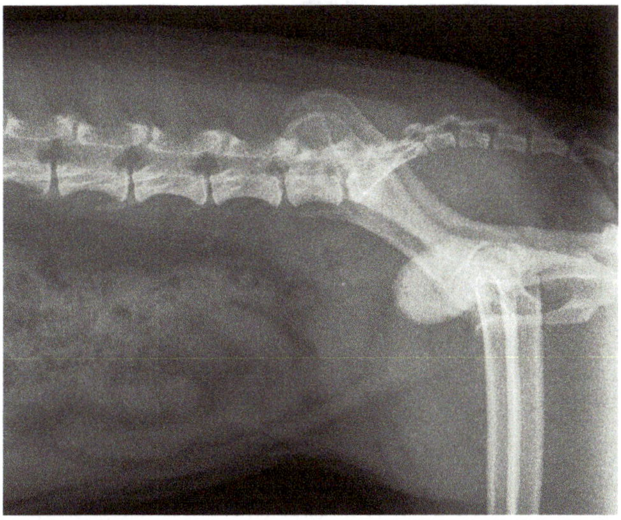

X-ray of a single, large bladder stone in a dog with a bladder located more to the rear than is usual

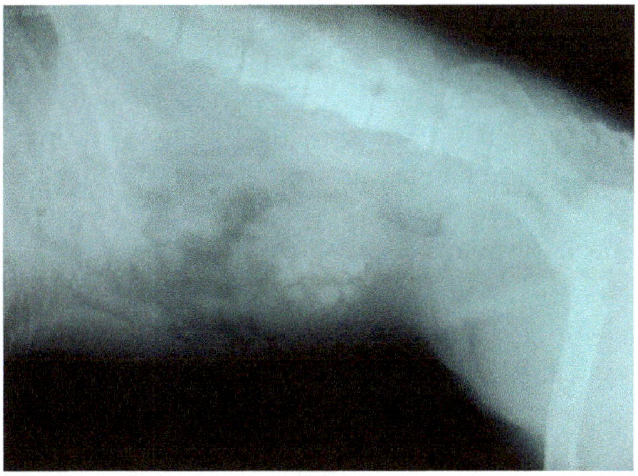

X-ray of bladder stones in a dog

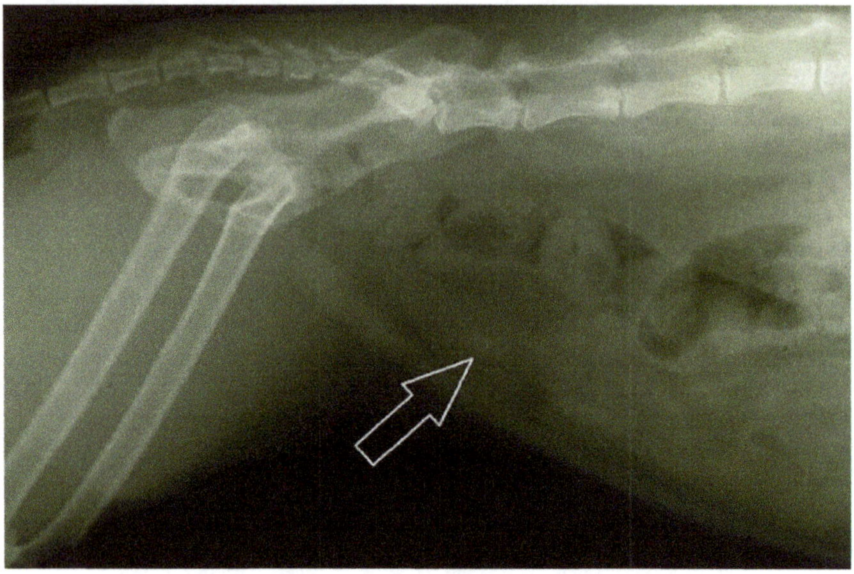

X-ray of a struvite bladder stone in a cat

Signs and Symptoms

Bladder stones may cause blood in the urine (hematuria) (giving the appearance that the animal is urinating blood) but sometimes there may be no signs at all. Painful urination or straining to urinate are other signs. Urinary tract infections are commonly associated with bladder stones. Smaller stones may become lodged in the urethra, especially in male animals, causing urinary tract obstruction and the inability to urinate. This condition causes acute renal failure, hyperkalemia, septicemia, and death within a few days.

Mechanism

Oversaturation of urine with crystals is by the far the biggest factor in 99% of animals in all of Europe. Stone formation. This oversaturation can be caused by increased excretion of crystals by the kidneys, water reabsorption by the renal tubules resulting in concentration of the urine, and changes in urine pH that influence crystallization. Other contributing factors include diet, frequency of urination, genetics, current medications, and the presence of a urinary tract infection.

The stones form around a nidus, which can consist of white blood cells, bacteria, and organic matrix mixed with crystals, or crystals alone. The nidus makes up about two to ten percent of the mass of the stone. It is possible for the nidus to be made of a different type of crystal than the rest of the stone, also known as epitaxial growth.

Diagnosis

When symptoms indicate bladder stones, the first step is usually to take an x-ray. Most types of stones will appear readily in an x-ray, urate and occasionally cystine stones being the most common exceptions. Stones smaller than three millimeters may not be visible. Ultrasonography is also useful for identifying bladder stones. Crystals identified in a urinalysis may help identify the stones, but analysis of the stones is necessary for identification of the complete chemical composition.

Struvite Stones

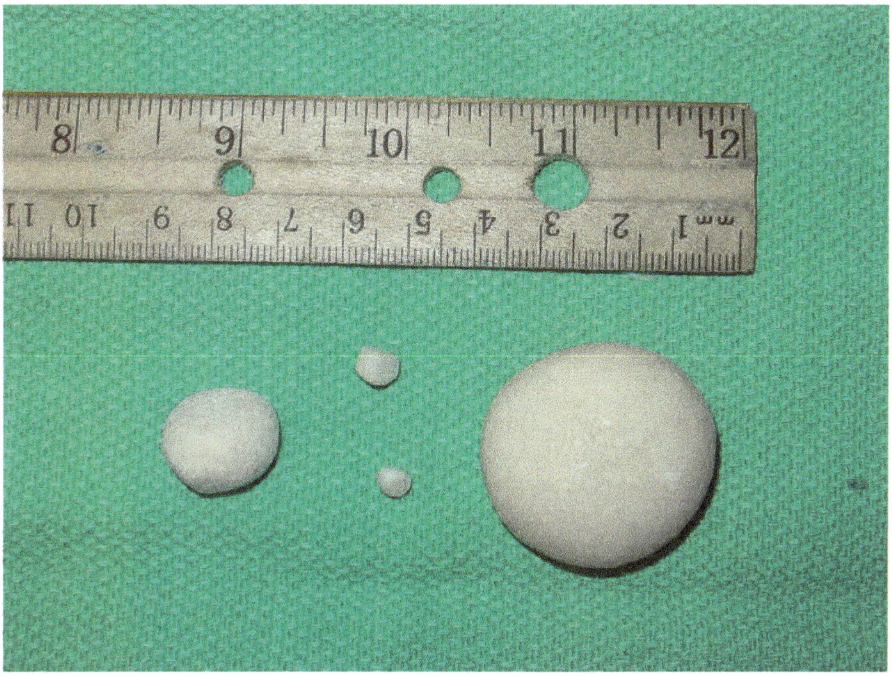

Struvite stones

Struvite stones are also known as magnesium ammonium phosphate stones due to their chemical composition - $MgNH_4PO_4 \cdot 6H_20$. Often there is a small amount of calcium phosphate present. They form at a neutral to alkaline pH of the urine. Bacterial infections contribute to their formation by increasing the pH of the urine through the urease enzyme in dogs. More than 90 percent of dogs with struvite stones have an associated urease-producing bacterial infection in the urinary tract, but in cats struvite stones usually form in sterile urine. The appearance of the stones vary from large solitary stones to multiple smaller stones. They can assume the shape of the bladder or urethra.

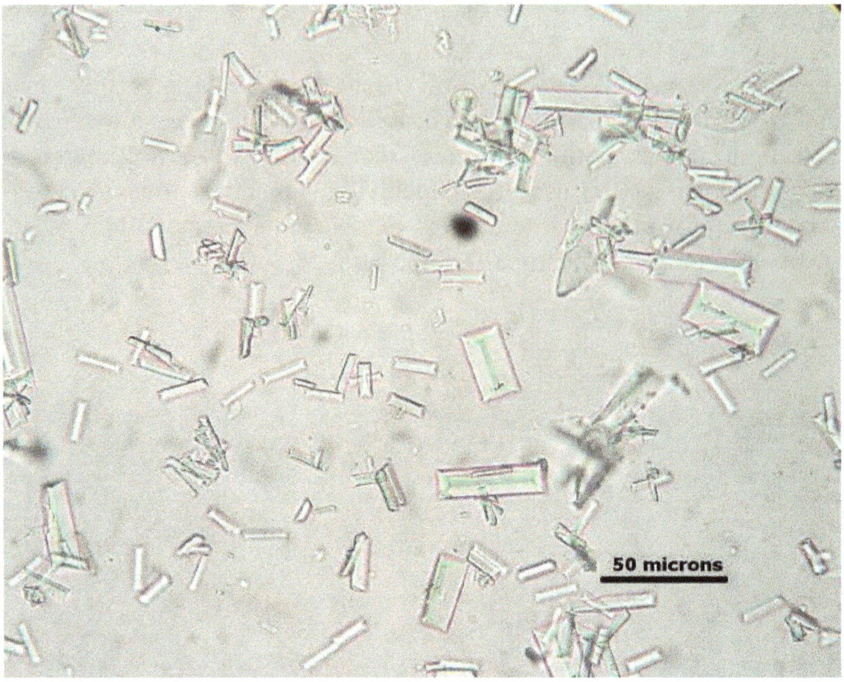

Struvite crystals

Dissolution of the struvite stones depends on acidification of the urine through diet or urinary acidifiers. Special diets for dissolution also have reduced protein, phosphorus, and magnesium, as well as increased salt to increase water consumption and dilute the urine. The diet needs to be fed exclusively, but it can only be fed for a few months total due to potential side effects. Contraindications to this diet include heart failure, liver failure, kidney failure, pancreatitis, hypertension (high blood pressure), and hypoalbuminemia (low serum albumin). Prevention of struvite stones is with a similar diet with milder restrictions.

Certain dog breeds are predisposed to struvite stones, including Miniature Schnauzers, Bichon Frises, and Cocker Spaniels. They are the most commonly reported bladder stone in female dogs and in ferrets (pregnant ferrets may be especially predisposed). For frequency in cats, see below.

Calcium Oxalate Stones

Calcium oxalate stones form in an acidic to neutral urine. Two types naturally occur, calcium oxalate monohydrate, or whewellite ($CaC_2O_4{\cdot}H_2O$), and calcium oxalate dihydrate, or weddellite ($CaC_2O_4{\cdot}2H_2O$). Their appearance can be rough, smooth, spiculated (needle-like), or jackstone. Calcium oxalate stones form more readily in animals with hypercalcaemia, which can caused by Addison's disease or certain types of cancer. Hypercalcaemia results in hypercalciuria, which can also be caused by Cushing's syndrome or hyperparathyroidism.

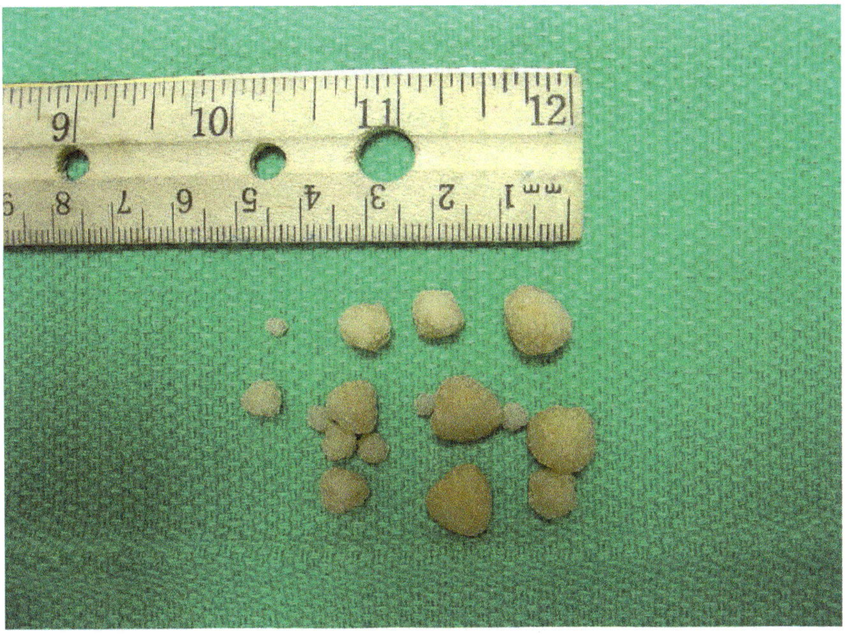

Calcium oxalate stones

There is no recommended diet to dissolve calcium oxalate stones. For prevention a diet low in protein and oxalates and high in magnesium, phosphorus, and calcium is recommended. Increased dietary magnesium and phosphorus decreases the amount of calcium in the urine, and increased dietary calcium reduces absorption of oxalates from the intestines. Potassium citrate has been recommended as a preventative for calcium oxalate stone formation because it forms a soluble complex with oxalates and promotes the formation of alkaline urine.

Dog breeds possible prone to calcium oxalate stones include Miniature Schnauzers, Lhasa Apsos, Yorkshire Terriers, Miniature Poodles, Shih Tzus, and Bichon Frises. They are the most common stone in male dogs. Calcium oxalate stones are also common in domestic rabbits. Rabbits are prone to hypercalciuria due to intestinal absorption of calcium not being dependent on vitamin D and a high fractional urinary excretion of calcium. The urine will appear thick and creamy or sometimes sandy. Small stones and sand can be removed using urohydropropulsion. Prevention is through reducing calcium intake by feeding more hay and less commercial rabbit pellets, and by not using mineral supplements.

Frequency of Struvite and Calcium Oxalate Stones in Cats

The Minnesota Urolith Center at the University of Minnesota College of Veterinary Medicine has done detailed analysis of uroliths from animals since 1981 and has noted changing trends in feline uroliths. In 1981, struvite stones were the most common type in cats, making up 78 percent of submitted samples, with only 2 percent comprising calcium oxalate stones. In the mid 1980s there was a substantial increase in the number of calcium oxalate samples, and between 1994 and 2002, 55 percent of feline stones were calcium oxalate and 33 percent were struvite. This may have been caused by the use of dissolution diets for struvite stones in cats and modification of other diets to prevent struvite crystal formation. These modifications predisposed to calcium oxalate crystal formation. However, in 2004, struvite stones once again surpassed calcium oxalate stones 44.9 percent to 44.3 percent, and in 2006, 50 percent of stones were struvite and 39 percent were calcium oxalate. This may have been due to the increased use of diets designed to prevent calcium oxalate crystal formation, which because of increased magnesium in the diet and decreased acidity of the urine help promote struvite crystal formation.

Urethral plugs in cats are usually composed of struvite crystals and organic matter.

Urate Stones

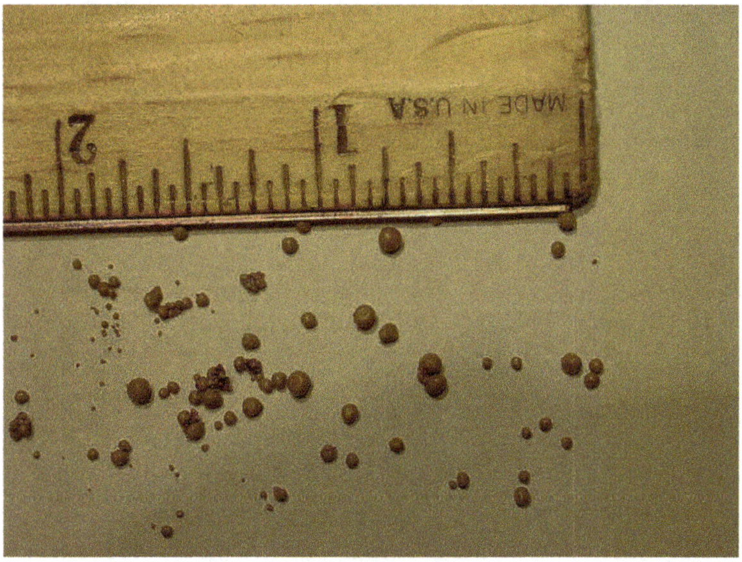

Urate stones

Urate ($C_5H_4N_4O_3$) stones, usually ammonium urate ($NH_4 \cdot C_5H_4N_4O_3$) or sodium urate monohydrate ($Na \cdot C_5H_4N_4O_3 \times H_2O$), form in an acidic to neutral urine. They are usually small, yellow-brown, smooth stones. Urate stones form due to an increased excretion of uric acid in the urine. Dalmatians (especially males) and to a lesser extent Bulldogs are genetically predisposed to the formation of urate stones because of an altered metabolism of purines. Dalmatians have a decreased rate of urate hepatic transport, leading to only about 30 to 40 percent conversion of urate to allantoin, compared with greater than 90 percent conversion in other breeds. Dogs with portosystemic shunts or endstage liver disease also have increased uric acid excretion in the urine due to reduced conversion of uric acid to allantoin and ammonia to urea. Urate stones make up about six percent of all stones in the cat.

Urate stones can be dissolved using a diet with reduced purines that alkalinizes and dilutes the urine. Allopurinol is used in dogs with altered purine metabolism to prevent the formation of uric acid. Feeding a diet high in purines while simultaneously administering allopurinol can result in the formation of xanthine ($C_5H_4N_4O_2$) stones.

Cystine Stones

Cystine ($(SCH_2CHNH_2COOH)_2$) stones form in an acidic to neutral urine. They are usually smooth and round. They are caused by increased urine excretion of cystine (a relatively insoluble amino acid) in dogs with a defect in renal tubule reabsorption of cystine. Dietary reduction of protein and alkalinization of the urine may help prevent formation. Medications such as D-penicillamine and 2-MPG contain thiol, which forms a soluble complex with cystine in the urine. Dog breeds possibly predisposed to formation of cystine stones include Bulldogs, Dachshunds, Basset Hounds, Chihuahuas, Yorkshire Terriers, Irish Terriers, and Newfoundlands. In Newfoundlands, cystinuria is inherited as an autosomal recessive trait, but in the other breeds it is a sex linked trait and found primarily in male dogs.

Calcium Phosphate Stones

Calcium phosphate, also known as hydroxyapatite ($Ca_{10}(PO_4)_6(OH)_2$), stones form in neutral to alkaline urine. They are usually smooth and round. Calcium phosphate is usually a component of struvite or calcium oxalate stones and is infrequently a pure stone. They form more readily with hypercalcaemia. Dog breeds possibly predisposed to calcium phosphate stone formation include Yorkshire Terriers, Miniature Schnauzers, and Cocker Spaniels.

Silicate Stones

Silicate (SiO_2) stones form in acidic to neutral urine. They are usually jackstone in appearance. There is possibly an increased incidence associated with dogs on diets that have a large amount of corn gluten or soybean hulls. Dog breeds possibly predisposed include German Shepherd Dogs, Golden Retrievers, Labrador Retrievers, and Miniature Schnauzers.

Treatment

Reasons for treatment of bladder stones include recurring symptoms and risk of urinary tract obstruction. Some stones can be dissolved using dietary modifications and/or medications. Small stones in female dogs may possibly be removed by urohydropropulsion, a nonsurgical procedure. Urohydropropulsion is performed under sedation by filling the bladder with saline through a catheter, holding the dog vertically, and squeezing the bladder to expel the stones through the urethra. Bladder stones can be removed surgically by a cystotomy, opening of the bladder. Stones lodged in the urethra can often be flushed into the bladder and removed, but sometimes a urethrotomy is necessary. In male dogs with recurrent urinary tract obstruction a scrotal urethrostomy creates a permanent opening in the urethra proximal to the area where most stones lodge, behind the os penis. In male cats, stones lodge where the urethra narrows in the penis. Recurrent cases can be treated surgically with a perineal urethrostomy, which removes the penis and creates a new opening for the urethra.

To prevent recurrence of stones, special diets can be used for each type of stone. Increasing water consumption by the animal dilutes the urine, which prevents oversaturation of the urine with crystals.

BLAIN

Blain was an animal disease of unknown etiology that was well known in the eighteenth- and nineteenth centuries. It is unclear whether it is still extant, or what modern disease it corresponds to.

According to Ephraim Chambers' eighteenth-century Cyclopaedia, or an Universal Dictionary of Arts and Sciences, blain was "a distemper" (in the archaic eighteenth-century sense of the word, meaning "disease") occurring in animals, consisting in a "Bladder growing on the Root of the Tongue against the Wind-Pipe", which "at length swelling, stops the Wind". It was thought to occur "by great chafing, and heating of the Stomach".

Blain is also mentioned in Cattle: Their Breeds, Management, and Diseases, published in 1836, where it is also identified as "gloss-anthrax". W. C. Spooner's 1888 book The History, Structure, Economy and Diseases of the Sheep also identifies blain as being the same as gloss-anthrax.

Modern scholarship suggests that "gloss-anthrax" was not the same disease as modern-day anthrax, but instead could have been foot-and-mouth disease, or a viral infection with a secondary Fusobacterium necrophorum infection. It has also been suggested that it may have been due to a variant strain of true anthrax that is no longer in existence. Other sources also report epizootics known as "blain" or "black-blain" in the 13th and 14th centuries, but it is not clear if the disease involved was the same as "gloss-anthrax".

HIP DISLOCATION

Dislocation of hip (coxofemoral luxation) may occur **in domestic animals**.

It is a not rare condition, usually unilateral, in:

- cattle, among others, after calving.
- dogs, resulting from trauma or as a complication of hip dysplasia.

The same illness also exists in human medicine.

Symptoms

In dogs, it occurs mainly in an upwards and forwards direction. Hence, the affected leg is shortened, and the greater trochanter prominent.

In cattle, it occurs mainly craniodorsally or caudoventrally, but other directions are possible. A typical stance is seen in craniodorsal luxations, with a shortened limb, and a protrusion of greater trochanter.

Treatment

Attempts in reduction in cattle are generally not successful. Affected animals, at least not too heavy ones, can live with the disease for a long time because of the formation of a sort of pseudo-joint in the hip.

Dogs with hip dysplasia and unilateral dislocation can live if the other leg is not too severely hit. Then there is a severe muscular atrophy of the thigh. Compensation occurs with musculation of the shoulders.

EPILEPSY

Seizures are caused by abnormal bursts of electrical activity in the brain. They can start and stop very abruptly and last any amount of time from a few seconds to a few minutes. Epilepsy can occur in animals other than humans. Canine epilepsy is often genetic but epilepsy in cats and other pets is rarer, likely because there is no hereditary component to epilepsy in these animals.

Characteristics

Epilepsy is most commonly recognised by involuntary movements of the head and limbs, however other characteristics include salivation, lack of bodily functions and anxiety. Animals often lose consciousness and are not aware of their surroundings.

Handling Seizures

Watching an animal or person have a seizure can be quite frightening. There is not much that can be done during a seizure except to ensure that you remain calm and do not leave the animal alone. If your pet is having a seizure it is important to make sure they are laying down on the floor away from any water, stairs or other animals. When an animal has a seizure, do not try to grab their tongue or clear their mouth as there is a high chance you will be bitten; contrary to popular myth, neither humans nor animals can "swallow their tongue" during a seizure so it is safest to stay well away from their mouth during one. Timing seizures is also crucial; if a seizure lasts for more than 5 minutes or your pet is having multiple seizures per day then a veterinary doctor should be contacted. Take notes of seizures - what time they occur, how often and any other specific information which can be passed onto the vet or emergency animal clinic.

Canine Epilepsy

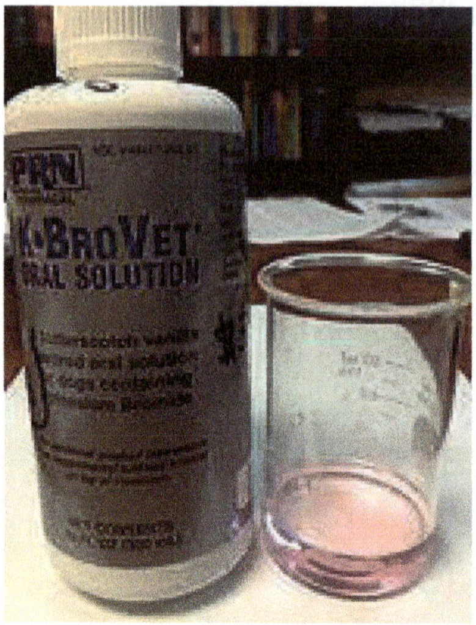

A bottle of PRN Pharmaceutical Company (Pensacola, FL) ***K•BroVet*** veterinary pharmaceutical potassium bromide oral solution (250 mg / mL). The product is intended to be used in dogs, primarily as an antiepileptic (to stop seizures).

In dogs, epilepsy is often an inherited condition. The incidence of epilepsy/seizures in the general dog population is estimated to be between 0.5% and 5.7%. In certain breeds, {{such as the Belgian Shepherd varieties}}, the incidence may be much higher.

Diagnosis

There are three types of epilepsy in dogs: reactive, secondary, and primary. Reactive epileptic seizures are caused by metabolic issues, such as low blood sugar or kidney or liver failure. Epilepsy attributed to brain tumor, stroke or other trauma is known as secondary or symptomatic epilepsy.

There is no known cause for primary or idiopathic epilepsy, which is only diagnosed by eliminating other possible causes for the seizures. Dogs with idiopathic epilepsy experience their first seizure between the ages of one and three. However, the age at diagnosis is only one factor in diagnosing canine epilepsy, as one study found cause for seizures in one-third of dogs between the ages of one and three, indicating secondary or reactive rather than primary epilepsy.

A veterinarian's initial work-up for a dog presenting with a history of seizures may include a physical and neurological exam, a complete blood count, serum chemistry profile, urinalysis, bile tests, and thyroid function tests. These tests verify seizures and may determine cause for reactive or secondary epilepsy. Veterinarians may also request that dog owners keep a "seizure log" documenting the timing, length, severity, and recovery of each seizure, as well as dietary or environmental changes.

Treatment

Many antiepileptic drugs are used for the management of canine epilepsy. Oral phenobarbital, in particular, and imepitoin are considered to be the most effective antiepileptic drugs and usually used as 'first line' treatment. Other anti-epileptics such as zonisamide, primidone, gabapentin, pregabalin, sodium valproate, felbamate and topiramate may also be effective and used in various combinations. A crucial part of the treatment of pets with epilepsy is owner education to ensure compliance and successful management.

Feline Epilepsy

Seizures in Feline patients are caused by various onsets. As with dogs, Felines can have reactive, primary (idiopathic) or secondary seizures. Idiopathic seizures are not as common in cats as in dogs however a recent study conducted showed that of 91 feline seizures, 25% were suspected to have Idiopathic epilepsy. In the same group of 91 cats, 50% were secondary seizures and 20% reactive.

classifications

Idiopathic epilepsy does not have a classification due to the fact there are no known causes of these seizures, however both reactive and symptomatic secondary epilepsy can be placed into classifications.

Symptomatic

Neoplasia

meningiomas, Lymphomas and glial cell brain tumours are the most common cancers in cats and are all common causes of seizures.

Vascular Disease

Vascular disease refers to any condition that effects the flow of blood to the brain and can potentially result in seizure disorders. common vascular diseases in felines include, feline ischemic encephalopathy, polycythemia and hypertension.

Inflammatory/ Infectious

Any inflammatory or infectious disease that reaches the brain can result in inducing seizures. the most common inflammatory or infectious diseases which cause seizures in cats include, feline infectious peritonitis, toxoplasmosis and cryptococcus.

Reactive Seizure Disorders

Many diseases that occur as a result from illness in parts of the body other than the brain can cause felines to have seizures, especially in older cats. Some of the common metabolic causes of seizures in felines include, Hepatic Encephalopathy, Renal Encephalopathy, Hypoglycaemia and Hypothyroidism.

IMPACTION

Impaction is bowel obstruction that can occur in various kinds of animals when they consume something that they cannot digest. For example, in reptiles, common causes of impaction are rocks and sand, which might be accidentally consumed when the reptile attacks its prey. In livestock, rough fodder such as straw can risk impaction. Once the substance is ingested it will block the digestive tract and, if untreated, cause death.

Symptoms

Some symptoms include a lack of appetite or lethargy. On many reptiles a large blue seemingly bruised spot will be visible in the abdomen; however, this only shows through if the skin on the species is clear enough to see the lower internal organs.

Treatment

Common treatments involve placing the reptile in a lukewarm bath and gently rubbing the area under the impaction to help the passing of the consumed substance, place both thumbs on the back at the middle, put the first two fingers under the belly and rub gently in a circular way until the beaded dragon puffs up, when the lizard puffs up it will go the loo. If this fails, the animal must have an enema.

MYOPIA

Some animals suffer from shortsightedness and have poor eyesight. In domestic animals, myopia, with or without astigmatism, occurs frequently.

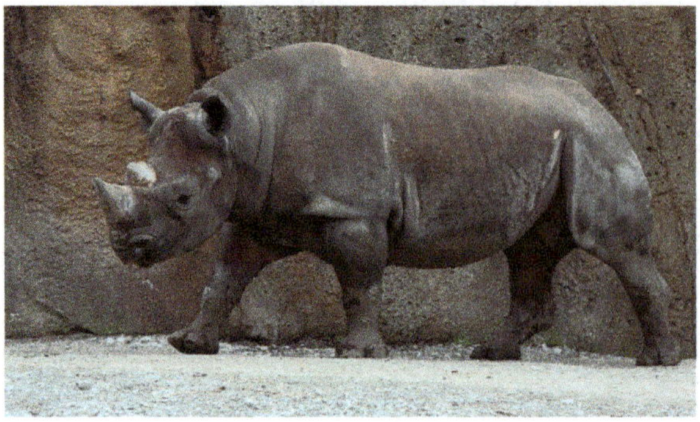

A rhinoceros, known for its poor eyesight

In Rhinoceroses

Whereas the rhinoceros may suffer from less-than-adequate eyesight, it generally survives by concentrating with its superior hearing and sense of smell. Some reports, however state that it can see better when focussing with one eye, particularly when walking, posturing, and combatting.

Research

Myopia, with or without astigmatism, is the most common eye condition in horses. Several types of occlusion myopia have been recorded in tree shrews, macaques, cats and rats, deciphered from several animal-inducing myopia models. Preliminary laboratory investigations using retinoscopy of 240 dogs found myopic problems with varying degrees of refraction errors depending on the breed. In cases involving German Shepherds, Rottweilers and Miniature horses, the refraction errors were indicative of myopia. Nuclear sclerosis of the crystalline lens was noticed in older dogs.

Experiments into newborn macaque monkeys have revealed that surgically fusing the eyelid for one year results in eye deterioration as the eye has not had a chance to grow and develop. Keeping monkeys in the dark for a similar period, however, does not lead to myopia. In 1996, Maurice and Mushin conducted tests on rabbits by raising their body temperatures and intraocular pressures (IOP) and noted that while younger rabbits were prone to developing myopia, older rabbits were not. Some tests have revealed that myopia in some animals can be improved with eye drops containing zinc, by increasing the activity of superoxide dismutase (SOD).

The rhesus monkey's vision amplitude reduction is noticeable in its second decade of life; however the condition does not impede normal functioning. Older rhesus monkeys have more difficulty accommodating this reduction in vision amplitude, encountering difficulty in focussing on objects at close range, even objects on the ground within an arm's length.

In Zoo Animals and Pets

In Central Park Zoo, New York, several myopic animals have been reported, including a 39-year-old elephant, a Cape buffalo, and some monkeys. Young elephants and other animals are said to be myopia free. Pet dogs with progressive myopia have been reported.

PHOTOSENSITIVITY

Photosensitivity is an abnormal skin reaction to direct sunlight exposure. It is unrelated to a sunburn. These reactions are due to photosensitization, the accumulation of photosensitive compounds beneath the skin. In some cases, the photodynamic substances come from ingested plants or drugs, after being metabolized or not. In other cases, the photodynamic substances may be produced in the body itself due to inborn errors in pigment metabolism, especially those involving the heme synthesis. Photosensitivity reactions are usually seen in herbivorous or omnivorous animals, though such reactions are not uncommon among carnivores.

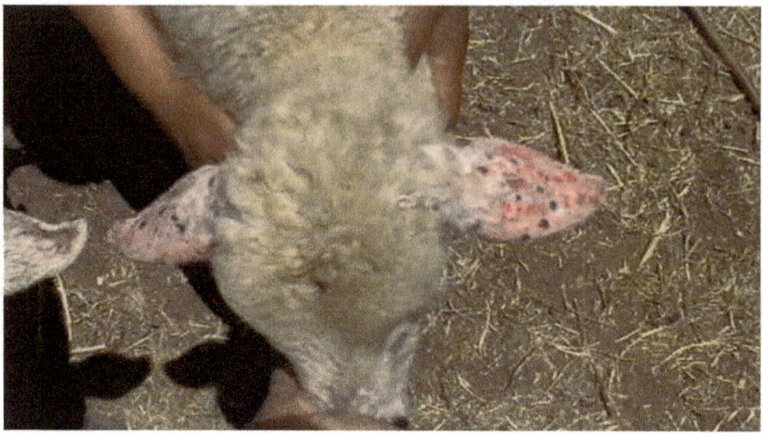

Photosensitization to Hypericum tomentosum in a lamb: healing lesions on the upper face of ears

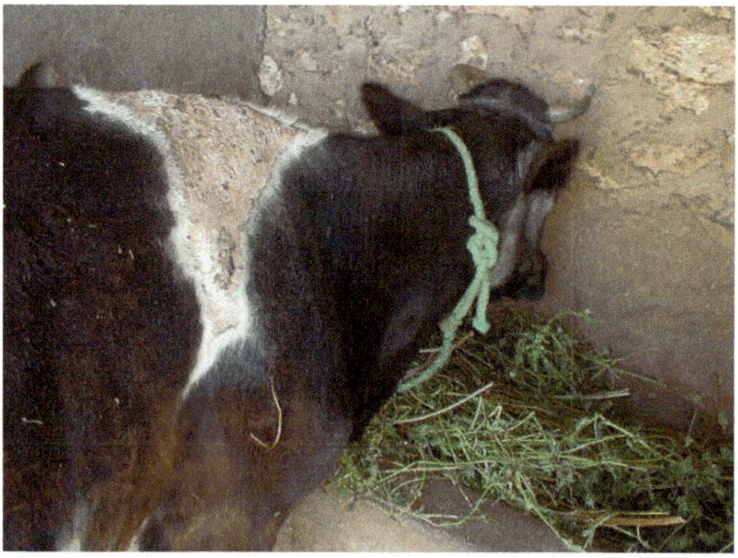

Photosensitization in a Friesian cow (unknown aetiology): lesions limited to white skin.

Effects of Photosensitivity

Photosensitivity reactions are characterized by severe inflammation of the skin with depigmentation and ulceration. In some cases (Type I), pigments are excreted through urine or deposited in hard tissues such as bones and teeth, causing discolouration. Affected animals should be protected from direct sunlight until the photodynamic compounds have been completely eliminated from the body or the appropriate treatments have been given.

Biological Mechanism of Photosensitivity Reactions

Photodynamic compounds are activated by sunlight, which excites them to a higher energy state. They immediately release the excess energy and transfer it to the surrounding acceptor molecules, such as enzymes or free radicals. These molecules are thus activated and cause the skin reaction.

Classification of Photosensitivity Reactions

Photosensitivity reactions are classified by origin into four types: Type I, Type II, Type III and Type IV.

Type I Photosensitivity

Type I Photosensitivity occurs when the photodynamic compounds need not undergo metabolism to be activated and so may accumulate under the skin directly following ingestion. Examples of plants producing Type I Photosensitivity include Buckwheat and St John's wort (Hypericum perforatum). Certain drugs such as phenothiazine or its derivatives may also lead to photosensitivity reactions, commonly in sheep. Phenothiazine is converted by the body into the photodynamic compound phenothiazine sulfoxide.

Type II Photosensitivity

Type II Photosensitivity is caused by inborn errors in the metabolism of certain biological pigments. In the absence of some key metabolic enzymes, the products of intermediary metabolism accumulate. They are either eliminated through the urine and body fluids or are deposited in some body tissue, such as bone and teeth. A common condition seen in animals is congenital porphyria due to the accumulation of Uroporphyrin, which is deposited in the teeth and bones, giving them a pink discolouration, or excreted through the urine, exhibiting a pinkish fluorescence under ultraviolet light.

Type III Photosensitivity

Type III (aka hepatic photosensitivity) is the most common type of photosensitivity reaction seen in animals. In this type, the photodynamic substance is phylloerythrin, a derivative of chlorophyll produced in the body. Normally, phylloerythrin is secreted into the intestine by the biliary system and excreted through the feces. In Type III Photosensitivity, damage to the biliary transport mechanism prevents the excretion of phylloerythrin, allowing the photodynamic substance to enter the circulatory system and accumulate under the skin. This condition is exacerbated by the presence of hepatic parasites.

Type IV Photosensitivity

Type IV Photosensitivity occurs following the ingestion of certain plants, such as alfalfa. The reason is obscure or idiopathic.

Treatment

Affected animals should be transferred to shade. To overcome shock, corticosteroid therapy and fluid infusions may be tried. Antihistamines are also useful.

REFERENCES

1. Muller, George H.; Scott, Danny W.; Kirk, Robert Warren; Miller, William Howard (2001). Muller and Kirk's Small Animal Dermatology. Elsevier Health Sciences. p. 887. ISBN 978-0-7216-7618-0. Retrieved 31 October 2012.
2. Burns, Tony; Breathnach, Stephen; Cox, Neil; Griffiths, Christopher (26 April 2010). Rook's Textbook of Dermatology, 4 Volume Set, Print and Online Package. John Wiley & Sons. p. 2. ISBN 978-1-4051-6169-5. Retrieved 31 October 2012.
3. Oglesbee, Barbara L. (26 July 2011). Blackwell's Five-Minute Veterinary Consult: Small Mammal. John Wiley & Sons. p. 52. ISBN 978-0-8138-2018-7. Retrieved 31 October 2012.
4. Dvorak, Glenda; Spickler, Anna Rovid; Roth, James A. (1 January 2008). Handbook for Zoonotic Diseases of Companion Animals. CFSPH Iowa State University. p. 117. ISBN 978-0-9745525-6-9. Retrieved 31 October 2012.
5. Levy, Janey (31 August 2006). Alopecia Areata. The Rosen Publishing Group. p. 46. ISBN 978-1-4042-0693-9. Retrieved 31 October 2012.
6. Giant tortoise cheats death Archived July 26, 2011, at the Wayback Machine. ("Evening Express", Aberdeen, 31/01/2009)
7. Ettinger, Stephen J.; Feldman, Edward C. (1995). Textbook of Veterinary Internal Medicine (4th ed.). W.B. Saunders Company. ISBN 0-7216-6795-3.
8. "Urolithiasis: Overview". The Merck Veterinary Manual. 2006. Retrieved 2007-04-14.
9. Buffington, Tony (2004). "Nutrition and Urolithiasis". Proceedings of the 29th World Congress of the World Small Animal Veterinary Association. Retrieved 2006-07-16.
10. Hoskins, Johnny D. (November 2006). "Feline Urolithiasis". DVM. Advanstar Communications: 6S–7S.
11. "Canine Urolithiasis". The Merck Veterinary Manual. 2006. Retrieved 2007-04-14.
12. Zoran, Debra L. (2006). Role of Diet in Feline and Canine Urolithiasis.
13. Hillyer, Elizabeth V.; Quesenberry, Katherin E. (1997). Ferrets, Rabbits, and Rodents: Clinical Medicine and Surgery (1st ed.). W.B. Saunders Company. ISBN 0-7216-4023-0.

14. Osborne, Carl A.; Lulich, Jody P. (February 2007). "Changing trends in composition of feline uroliths and urethral plugs". DVM. Advanstar Communications: 38–40.
15. Escolar E, Bellanato J (2003). "Analysis of feline urinary calculi and urethral plugs by infrared spectroscopy and scanning electron microscopy". Vet Rec. 152 (20): 625–8. doi:10.1136/vr.152.20.625. PMID 12790167.
16. Albasan H, Lulich J, Osborne C, Lekcharoensuk C (2005). "Evaluation of the association between sex and risk of forming urate uroliths in Dalmatians". J Am Vet Med Assoc. 227 (4): 565–9. doi:10.2460/javma.2005.227.565. PMID 16117063.
17. "Feline Urolithiasis and Feline Lower Urinary Tract Disease". The Merck Veterinary Manual. 2006. Retrieved 2007-04-14.

CHAPTER 2

Veterinary Medicine

Chapter Contents

- **Introduction**
- **Practice**
- **Animal Bite**
- **Antimicrobial Resistance**
- **Organisms**
- **Antibiotic Use in Livestock**
- **Mallein**
- **Traditional Chinese Veterinary Medicine**
- **History of Veterinary Medicine in the Philippines**
- **History of Veterinary Medicine in Pennsylvania**

Veterinary medicine is the medical science concerned with the diagnosis, treatment, and prevention of diseases in animals. Aside from diagnosing and treating sick and injured animals, veterinarians prevent the transmission of animal diseases to people, and advise owners on the proper care of animals. Veterinarians work to ensure a safe food supply by maintaining the health of agricultural animals and by inspecting food processing industries. Veterinarians are also involved in the preservation of wildlife. Veterinary school is usually 4 years and requires a prior college degree in the US and Canada the degree graduation is a DMV (Doctor of Veterinary Medicine).

INTRODUCTION

Veterinary acupuncture is the practice of performing acupuncture on animals.

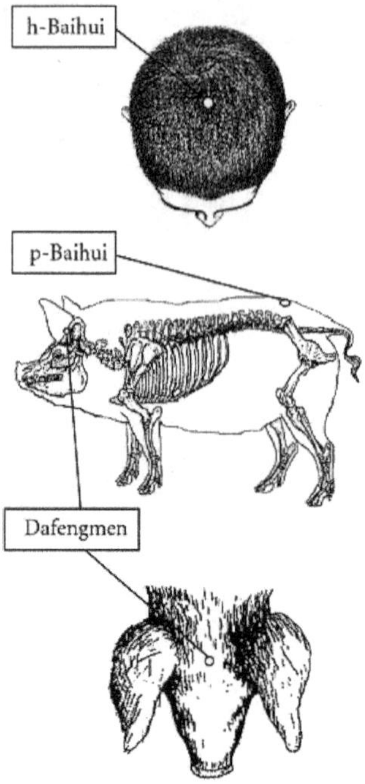

According to traditional chinese medicine, the Baihui acupuncture point in humans, which is the midpoint of a line connecting both ears, is anatomically similar to the Dafengmen point in pigs

Traditional Chinese veterinary medicine (TCVM) has been practiced on animals for thousands of years. For nearly 3,000 years, from the Zhou dynasty and the reign of Emperor Mu around 930 B.C., up until the Yuan dynasty of the 14th century, Chinese medicine was used sparingly on large animals. Much of the focus was on the treatment of horses since they were so essential to the military. In more modern times it has been used increasingly on pet animals. Acupuncture is one of the five branches of TCVM.

In historical Asian culture, people known as "horse priests" commonly used acupuncture. The flow of information from the East to the West regarding animal treatment, including acupuncture, is thought to have started from Mesopotamia around 300 BC. Acupuncture remained a major interest in veterinary medicine for centuries. Its use for dogs was first described in the Tang Dynasty.

In the 20th century, animal acupuncture was first introduced in the United States in 1971 by two acupuncturists of the National Acupuncture Association, Gene Bruno and John Ottaviano. In the process of treating thousands of small animals and several hundred horses, Bruno and Ottaviano trained veterinarians who later founded the International Veterinary Acupuncture Society (IVAS). The demand for veterinary acupuncture has steadily increased since the 1990s.

PRACTICE

Acupuncture is used mainly for functional problems such as those involving noninfectious inflammation, paralysis, or pain. For small animals, acupuncture has been used for treating arthritis, hip dysplasia, lick granuloma, feline asthma, diarrhea, and certain reproductive problems. For larger animals, acupuncture has been used for treating downer cow syndrome, facial nerve paralysis, allergic dermatitis, respiratory problems, nonsurgical colic, and certain reproductive disorders. Acupuncture has also been used on competitive animals, such as those involved in racing and showing. Veterinary acupuncture has also recently been used on more exotic animals, such as an alligator with scoliosis, though this is still quite rare.

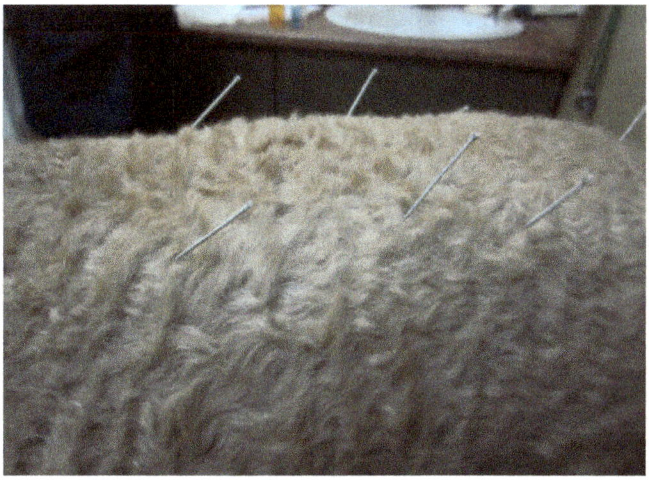

Veterinary acupuncture in dog

Mechanism

Research on the mechanism of acupuncture began as early as 1976 with the introduction of the endorphin hypothesis and the gate control theory of pain, which accounts for the inhibition of nociceptive information via interneurons. Stimulation of nerve fibres contributes to the release of cytokines and inflammatory mediators around the needle as part of a neuromodulatory process resulting from the needling effect on connective tissue and fibroblasts. In response to needle stimulation, neuropeptides are released into the local blood flow. These neuropeptides include calcitonin gene-related peptide (CGRP), nerve growth factor, substance P, and vasoactive intestinal peptide.

In recent years, research has been prompted by the introduction of neuroimaging techniques such as functional magnetic resonance imaging (fMRI) and positron emission tomography (PET), both of which have further elucidated the relation between acupuncture stimulation and activation of neural structures. In addition, deactivation of the limbic system by acupuncture stimulation has been reported in human studies, possibly accounting for its sedative effect in horses. A diverse array of neurotransmitters and receptors contribute to acupuncture analgesia including opioids, glutamate and NMDA receptors, serotonin and cholecystokinins. The autonomic neuromodulatory signaling of tissue cytokines affects both somatic and viseral structures to restore the balance between the parasympathetic nervous system and the sympathetic nervous system. In equine populations, clinical responses may occur within minutes to hours after treatment.

Efficacy

In 2001, a review found insufficient evidence to support equine acupuncture. The review found uniformly negative results in the highest quality studies. In 2006, a systematic review of veterinary acupuncture found "no compelling evidence to recommend or reject acupuncture for any condition in domestic animals", citing trials with, on average, low methodological quality or trials that are in need of independent replication. In 2009, a review on canine arthritis found "weak or no evidence in support of" various treatments, including acupuncture.

Recent (i.e. post-2011) reviews in both veterinary text books and scientific journals indicate that acupuncture can be used for therapeutic or homeostatic effects in animals, especially in the three areas of pain management, geriatric medicine and sports medicine. Conditions that have the best responses to veterinary acupuncture are considered to be pain, immune-related dysfunction and visceral dysfunction.

In 2015, the American Animal Hospital Association (AAHA) and American Association of Feline Practitioners (AAFP) issued joint guidelines for the management of pain in cats and dogs. The guidelines stated, "There is a solid and still growing body of evidence for the use of acupuncture for the treatment of pain in veterinary medicine to the extent that it is now an accepted treatment modality for painful animals."

Related Methods

Acupuncture refers to the use of dry needles; however, there are several related methods which do not use these, or may use a modified type of needle or stimulator.

- Electroacupuncture: Electrical stimulation at an acupuncture point. This may by given on or through the surface of the skin. Various combinations of acupuncture points can be selected to induce electropuncture analgesia in animals. Generally, analgesia is achieved near to the sites of electropuncture.

A study on the use of electroacupuncture on dogs after back surgery reported ambiguous results. In the study, the post-operation dogs were assigned a pain score eight times within a 72-hour time-frame. Though significantly lower pain scores were found in the treatment group at 36 hours, the scores did not differ from the control group at any other time.

- Aquapuncture: Injection of a drug or a liquid (e.g. vitamin B12) at acupuncture points.
- Acupressure: Application of pressure at acupuncture points.
- Moxibustion: Using a burning herbal stick to stimulate and warm acupuncture points.
- Lasers: Lasers can sometimes be used to stimulate acupunture points.

- Implantation: Gold or silver beads (or other stimulants) are sometimes implanted at acupuncture points.

Organizations

The International Veterinary Acupuncture Society (IVAS) was founded in the US in 1974 and the first certification exam was held in 1975 when there were only 80 members of the society. IVAS has grown worldwide and in 2015 the membership exceeds 1,800. The Association of British Veterinary Acupuncturists was formed in 1987. In 2014, American Veterinary Medical Association (AVMA) admitted the American Academy of Veterinary Acupuncture (AAVA) as a "Constituent Allied Veterinary Organization". The American Board of Animal Acupuncture (ABAA) is the only certification agency for licensed acupuncturists practicing animal acupuncture in the US.

ANIMAL BITE

An animal bite is a wound, usually lacerations, caused by the teeth. An animal bite usually results in a break in the skin but also includes contusions from the excessive pressure on body tissue from the bite. The contusions can occur without a break in the skin. Bites can be provoked or unprovoked. Other bite attacks may be apparently unprovoked. Biting is a physical action not only describing an attack but it is a normal response in an animal as it eats, carries objects, softens and prepares food for its young, removes ectoparasites from its body surface, removes plant seeds attached to its fur or hair, scratching itself, and grooming other animals. Animal bites often result in serious infections and mortality. Animal bites not only include injuries from the teeth of reptiles, mammals, but fish, and amphibians. Arthropods can also bite and leave injuries.

Signs and Symptoms

Bite wounds can cause a number of signs and symptoms

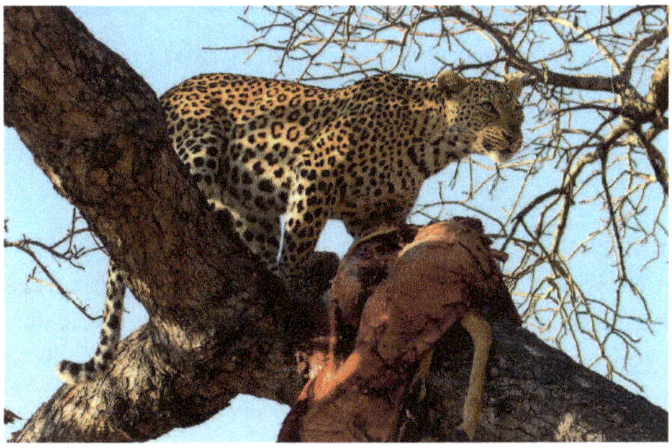

Impala killed and skinned by leopard bites

- Generalized tissue damage due to tearing and scratching
- Serious hemorrhage if major blood vessels are pierced
- Infection by bacteria or other pathogens, including rabies
- Introduction of venom into the wound by venomous animals such as some snakes
- Introduction of other irritants into the wound, causing inflammation and itching

Classification

Bites are usually classified by the type of creature causing the wound. Many different creatures are known to bite humans.

Vertebrates

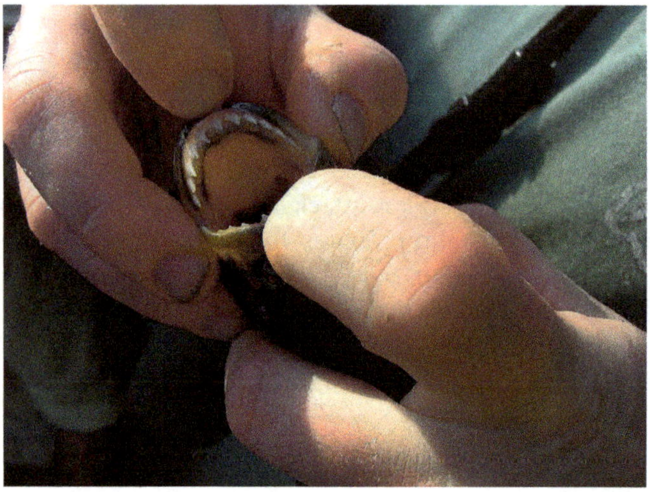

Jaw of the piranha with biting equipment displayed

- Companion animals, including dogs, cats, ferrets, and parrots, may bite humans.
- Wildlife may sometimes bite humans. The bites of various mammals such as bats, skunks, wolves, raccoons, etc. may transmit rabies, which is almost always fatal if left untreated.

Involuntary biting injuries due to closed-fist injuries from fists striking teeth (referred to as reverse bite injuries) are a common consequence of fist fights. These have been termed “fight bites”. Injuries in which the knuckle joints or tendons of the hand are bitten into tend to be the most serious.

Teething infants are known to bite objects to relieve pressure on their growing teeth, and may inadvertently bite people’s hands or arms while doing so. Young children may also bite people out of anger or misbehaviour, although this is usually corrected early in the child’s life.

Arthropods

The bites of arthropods have some of the most serious health consequences known. Mosquito bites transmit serious disease and result in millions of deaths and illnesses in the world. Ticks also transmit many diseases such as Lyme disease.

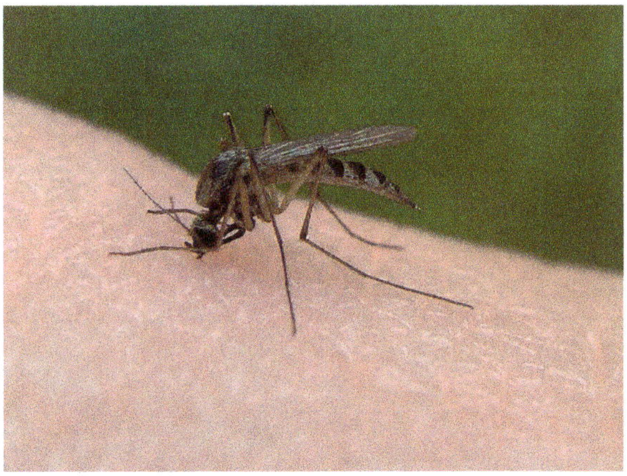

A mosquito bite

- Spider bite
- Insect bites and stings
- Flea bites are responsible for the transmission of plague.
- Mosquito bites are responsible for the transmission of dengue fever and malaria.
- Leech bite

Mechanism

Trauma

One of the first consequences of a bite is the trauma inflicted upon tissue. Some animals involved in inflicting bites are also receiving them during the confrontation. Trauma includes scratching of the skin surface, tooth loss, puncture wounds, superficial and deep lacerations, amputations, and the ripping off of skin and hair. If major blood vessels are damaged, severe blood loss can occur.

Infection

Pathogen organisms can be introduced into the bite. Some of the pathogens can originate from the mouth of the 'biter', the substrate onto which the injured person or animal can fall or from the naturally occurring microorganisms that are present on the skin or hair of the animal. The advent of antibiotics improved the outcome of bite wound infections.

Rabies

Animal bites, most commonly dogs and bats, transmit rabies to humans. Rabies from other animals is rare. If the animal is caught alive or dead with its head preserved, the head can be analyzed to detect the disease. Signs of rabies include foaming at the mouth, growling, self-mutilation, jerky behavior, red eyes, and hydrophobia.

If the animal cannot be captured, preventative rabies treatment is recommended in many places. Certain places, such as Hawaii, Australia, and the United Kingdom, are known not to have native rabies.

Treatment

The first step in treatment includes washing the bite wound. If there is a low risk of infection the wound may be sutured. Debridement and drainage bite wounds was practiced in the pre-antibiotic era, but still had a high infection rate.

Antibiotics

Antibiotics to prevent infection are recommended for dog and cat bites of the hand, and human bites if they are more than superficial. They are also recommended in those who have poor immune function. Evidence for antibiotics to prevent infection in bites in other areas is not clear.

The first choice is amoxicillin with clavulanic acid, and if the person is penicillin-allergic, doxycycline and metronidazole. The antistaphylococcal penicillins (e.g., cloxacillin, nafcillin, flucloxacillin) and the macrolides (e.g., erythromycin, clarithromycin) are not used for empirical therapy, because they do not cover *Pasteurella* species.

Rabies prevention is generally available in North America and the Northern European states.

Tetanus toxoid treatment is recommended in those whose vaccinations are not up to date and have a bite that punctures the skin. Tetanus immune globulin is indicated in people with more than 10 years since prior vaccination. Tetanus boosters (Td) should be given every ten years.

Epidemiology

Human bites are the third most frequent type of bite after dog and cat bites. Dog bites are commonplace, with children the most commonly bitten and the face the most common target. About 4.7 million dog bites are reported annually in the United States. The US estimated annual count of animal bites is 250,000 human bites, 1 to 2 million dog bites, 400,000 cat bites, and 45,000 bites from snakes. Bites from skunks, horses, squirrels, rats, rabbits, pigs, and monkeys may be up to 1% of bite injuries. Pet ferrets attacks that were unprovoked have caused serious facial injuries. Non-domesticated animals though assumed to be more common especially as a cause of rabies infection, make up less than one% of reported bite wounds. When a person is bitten, it is more likely to occur on the right arm, most likely due to defensive reactions when the person uses their dominant arm. Estimates are that three quarters of bites are located on the arms or legs of humans. Bites to the face of humans constitute only 10% of the total. Two thirds of bite injuries in humans are suffered by children aged ten and younger.

Up to three fourths of dog bites happen to those younger than 20 years-old. In the United States, the costs associated with dog bites are estimated to be more than $1 billion annually. The age groups that suffer most from dog bites are children 5 to 9 years-old. Often, bites go unreported and no medical treatment given - these bites go unreported. As many as one% of pediatric emergency room visits are for treatment for animal bites. This is more frequent during the summer months. Up to five% of children receiving emergency care for dog bites are then admitted to the hospital. Bites typically occur in the late afternoon and early evening. Girls are bitten more frequently by cats than they are by dogs. Boys are bitten by dogs two times more often than girls are bitten by dogs.

The bites of humans are recorded during the biblical area. Reports of secondary infection occurring after a human bite in children have been noted in the United States since at least 1910. Morbidity and mortality rates improved with the use of antibiotics.

ANTIMICROBIAL RESISTANCE

Antimicrobial resistance (AMR) is the ability of a microbe to resist the effects of medication previously used to treat them. This broader term also covers antibiotic resistance, which applies to bacteria and antibiotics. Resistance arises through one of three ways: natural resistance in certain types of bacteria; genetic mutation; or by one species acquiring resistance from another. Resistance can appear spontaneously because of random mutations; or more commonly following gradual buildup over time, and because of misuse of antibiotics or antimicrobials. Resistant microbes are increasingly difficult to treat, requiring alternative medications or higher doses—which may be more costly or more toxic. Microbes resistant to multiple antimicrobials are called multidrug resistant (MDR); or sometimes superbugs. Antimicrobial resistance is on the rise with millions of deaths every year. A few infections are now completely untreatable because of resistance. All classes of microbes develop resistance (fungi, antifungal resistance; viruses, antiviral resistance; protozoa, antiprotozoal resistance; bacteria, antibiotic resistance).

Antibiotics should only be used when needed as prescribed by health professionals. The prescriber should closely adhere to the five rights of drug administration: the right patient, the right drug, the right dose, the right route, and the right time. Narrow-spectrum antibiotics are preferred over broad-spectrum antibiotics when possible, as effectively and accurately targeting specific organisms is less likely to cause resistance. Cultures should be taken before treatment when indicated and treatment potentially changed based on the susceptibility report. For people who take these medications at home, education about proper use is essential. Health care providers can minimize spread of resistant infections by use of proper sanitation: including handwashing and disinfecting between patients; and should encourage the same of the patient, visitors, and family members.

Rising drug resistance can be attributed to three causes use of antibiotics: in the human population; in the animal population; and spread of resistant strains between human or non-human sources. Antibiotics increase selective pressure in bacterial populations, causing vulnerable bacteria to die—this increases the%age of resistant bacteria which continue growing. With resistance to antibiotics becoming more common there is greater need for alternative treatments. Calls for new antibiotic therapies have been issued, but new drug-development is becoming rarer. There are multiple national and international monitoring programs for drug-resistant threats. Examples of drug-resistant bacteria included in this program are: methicillin-resistant Staphylococcus aureus (MRSA), vancomycin-resistant S. aureus (VRSA), extended spectrum beta-lactamase (ESBL), vancomycin-resistant Enterococcus (VRE), multidrug-resistant A. baumannii (MRAB).

A World Health Organization (WHO) report released April 2014 stated, "this serious threat is no longer a prediction for the future, it is happening right now in every region of the world and has the potential to affect anyone, of any age, in any country. Antibiotic resistance—when bacteria change so antibiotics no longer work in people who need them to treat infections—is now a major threat to public health." Increasing public calls for global collective action to address the threat include proposals for international treaties on antimicrobial resistance. Worldwide antibiotic resistance is not fully mapped, but poorer countries with weak healthcare systems are more affected. According to the Centers for Disease Control and Prevention: "Each year in the United States, at least 2 million people become infected with bacteria that are resistant to antibiotics and at least 23,000 people die each year as a direct result of these infections."

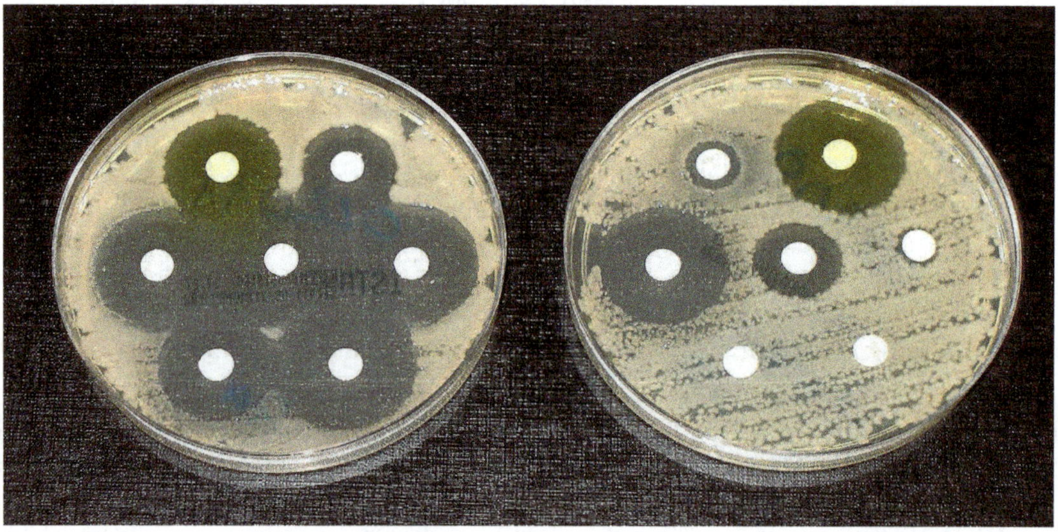

Antibiotic resistance tests: Bacteria are streaked on dishes with white antibiotic impregnated disks. Clear rings, such as those on the left, show that bacteria have not grown—indicating that the bacteria are not resistant. Those on the right are fully susceptible to only three of the seven antibiotics tested.

Definition

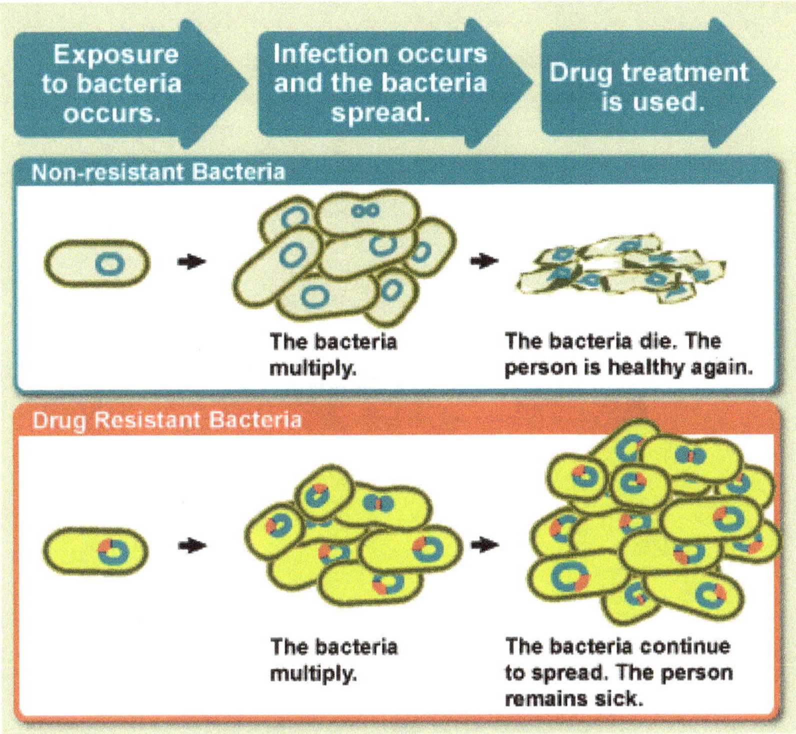

Diagram showing the difference between non-resistant bacteria and drug resistant bacteria. Non-resistant bacteria multiply, and upon drug treatment, the bacteria die. Drug resistant bacteria multiply as well, but upon drug treatment, the bacteria continue to spread.

The WHO defines antimicrobial resistance as a microorganism's resistance to an antimicrobial drug that was once able to treat an infection by that microorganism. A person cannot become resistant to antibiotics. Resistance is a property of the microbe, not a person or other organism infected by a microbe.

Causes

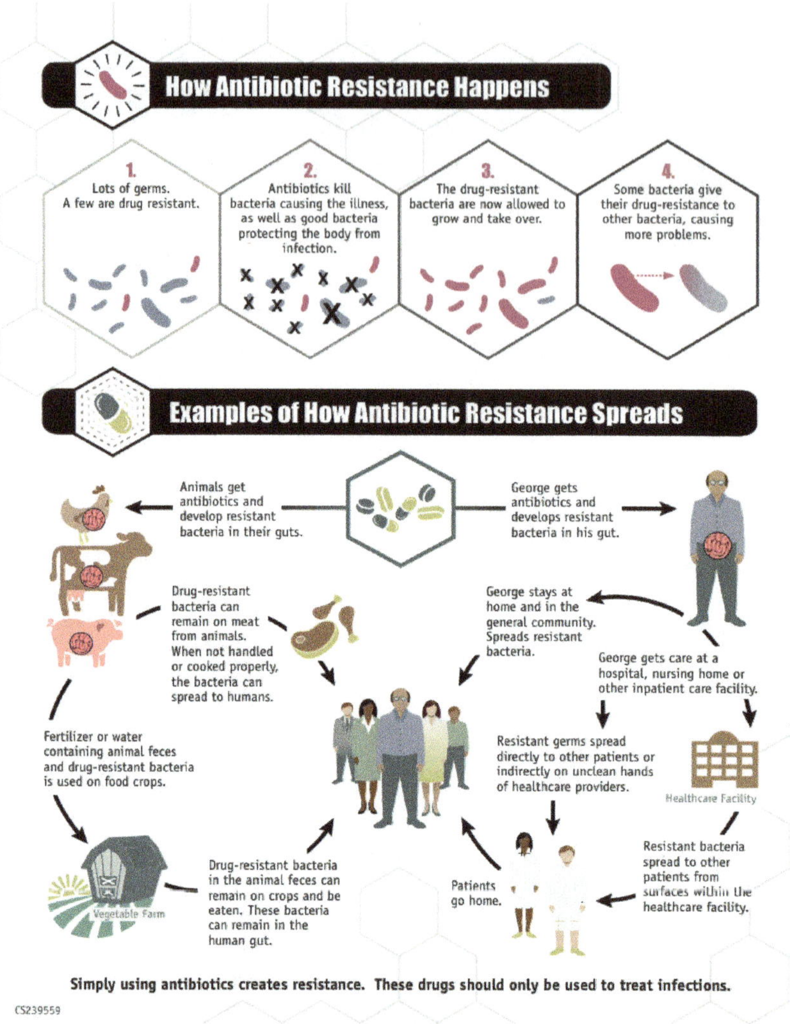

How antibiotic resistance evolves and spreads

Bacteria with resistance to antibiotics predate medical use of antibiotics by humans; however, widespread antibiotic use has made more bacteria resistant through the process of evolutionary pressure.

Reasons for the widespread use of antibiotics include:

- increasing global availability over time since the 1950s
- uncontrolled sale in many low or middle income countries, where they can be obtained over the counter without a prescription, potentially resulting in antibiotics being used when not indicated.[1060] This may result in emergence of resistance in any remaining bacteria.

Antibiotic use in livestock feed at low doses for growth promotion is an accepted practice in many industrialized countries and is known to lead to increased levels of resistance. Releasing large quantities of antibiotics into the environment during pharmaceutical manufacturing through inadequate wastewater treatment increases the risk that antibiotic-resistant strains will develop and spread. It is uncertain whether antibacterials in soaps and other products contribute to antibiotic resistance, but they are discouraged for other reasons.

Human Medicine

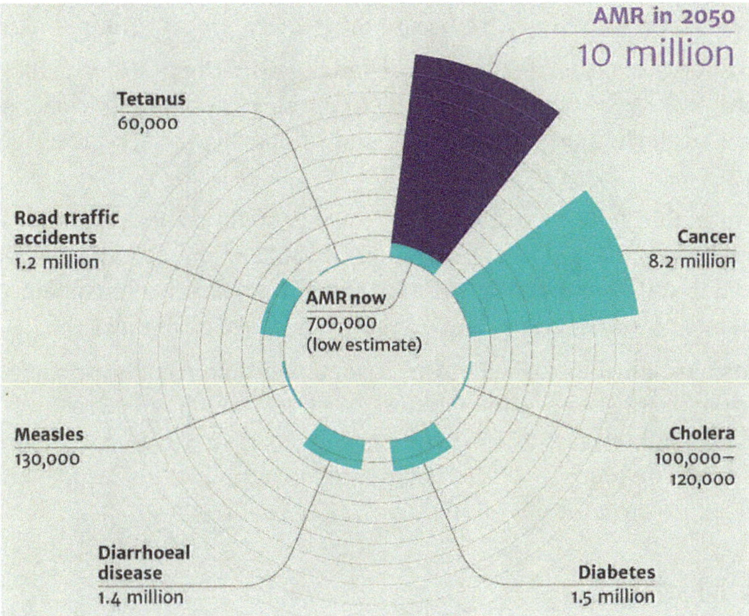

Deaths attributable to antimicrobial resistance every year compared to other major causes of death.

Increasing bacterial resistance is linked with the volume of antibiotic prescribed, as well as missing doses when taking antibiotics.Inappropriate prescribing of antibiotics has been attributed to a number of causes, including people insisting on antibiotics, physicians prescribing them as they feel they do not have time to explain why they are not necessary, and physicians not knowing when to prescribe antibiotics or being overly cautious for medical and/or legal reasons.

Up to half of antibiotics used in humans are unnecessary and inappropriate. For example, a third of people believe that antibiotics are effective for the common cold, and the common cold is the most common reason antibiotics are prescribed even though antibiotics are useless against viruses. A single regimen of antibiotics even in compliant individuals leads to a greater risk of resistant organisms to that antibiotic in the person for a month to possibly a year.

Antibiotic resistance increases with duration of treatment; therefore, as long as an effective minimum is kept, shorter courses of antibiotics are likely to decrease rates of resistance, reduce cost, and have better outcomes with fewer complications. Short course regimens exist for community-acquired pneumonia spontaneous bacterial peritonitis, suspected lung infections in intense care wards, so-called acute abdomen, middle ear infections, sinusitis and throat infections, and penetrating gut injuries. In some situations a short course may not cure the infection as well as a long course. A BMJ editorial recommended that antibiotics can often be safely stopped 72 hours after symptoms resolve. Because individuals may feel better before the infection is eradicated, doctors must provide instructions to them so they know when it is safe to stop taking a prescription. Some researchers advocate doctors' using a very short course of antibiotics, reevaluating the patient after a few days, and stopping treatment if there are no clinical signs of infection.

Certain antibiotic classes result in resistance more than others. Increased rates of MRSA infections are seen when using glycopeptides, cephalosporins, and quinolones. Cephalosporins, and particularly quinolones and clindamycin, are more likely to produce colonisation with *Clostridium difficile*.

Factors within the intensive care unit setting such as mechanical ventilation and multiple underlying diseases also appear to contribute to bacterial resistance. Poor hand hygiene by hospital staff has been associated with the spread of resistant organisms, and an increase in hand washing compliance results in decreased rates.

Improper use of antibiotics can often be attributed to the presence of structural violence in particular regions. Socioeconomic factors such as race and poverty affect accessibility of and adherence to drug therapy. The efficacy of treatment programs for drug-resistant strains depends on whether or not programmatic improvements take into account the effects of structural violence.

Veterinary Medicine

The World Health Organization concluded that inappropriate use of antibiotics in animal husbandry is an underlying contributor to the emergence and spread of antibiotic-resistant germs, and that the use of antibiotics as growth promoters in animal feeds should be restricted. The World Organisation for Animal Health has added to the Terrestrial Animal Health Code a series of guidelines with recommendations to its members for the creation and harmonization of national antimicrobial resistance surveillance and monitoring programs, monitoring of the quantities of antibiotics used in animal husbandry, and recommendations to ensure the proper and prudent use of antibiotic substances. Another guideline is to implement methodologies that help to establish associated risk factors and assess the risk of antibiotic resistance.

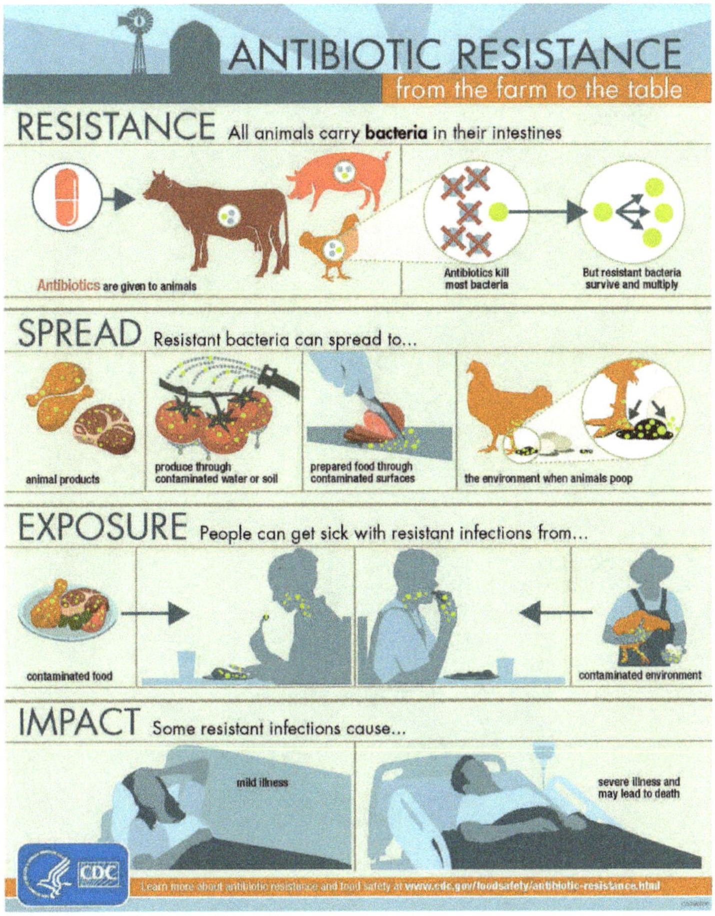

All animals carry bacteria in their intestines. Antibiotics are given to animals. Antibiotics kill most bacteria. But resistant bacteria survive and multiply.

United States

Eighty% of antibiotics sold in the United States are used on livestock. The majority of these antibiotics are given to animals that are otherwise healthy. Rather, it is normal practice to mix antibiotics with livestock food to promote healthier living conditions and to encourage animal growth. The use of antibiotics in animals is to a large degree involved in the emergence of antibiotic-resistant microorganisms. Antibiotics are used in food with the intention of not only preventing, controlling, and treating diseases, but also to promote growth. Antibiotic use in animals can be classified into therapeutic, prophylactic, metaphylactic, and growth promotion uses of antibiotics. All four patterns select for bacterial resistance, since antibiotic resistance is a natural evolutionary process, but the non-therapeutic uses expose larger number of animals, and therefore of bacteria, for more extended periods, and at lower doses. They therefore greatly increase the cross-section for the evolution of resistance.

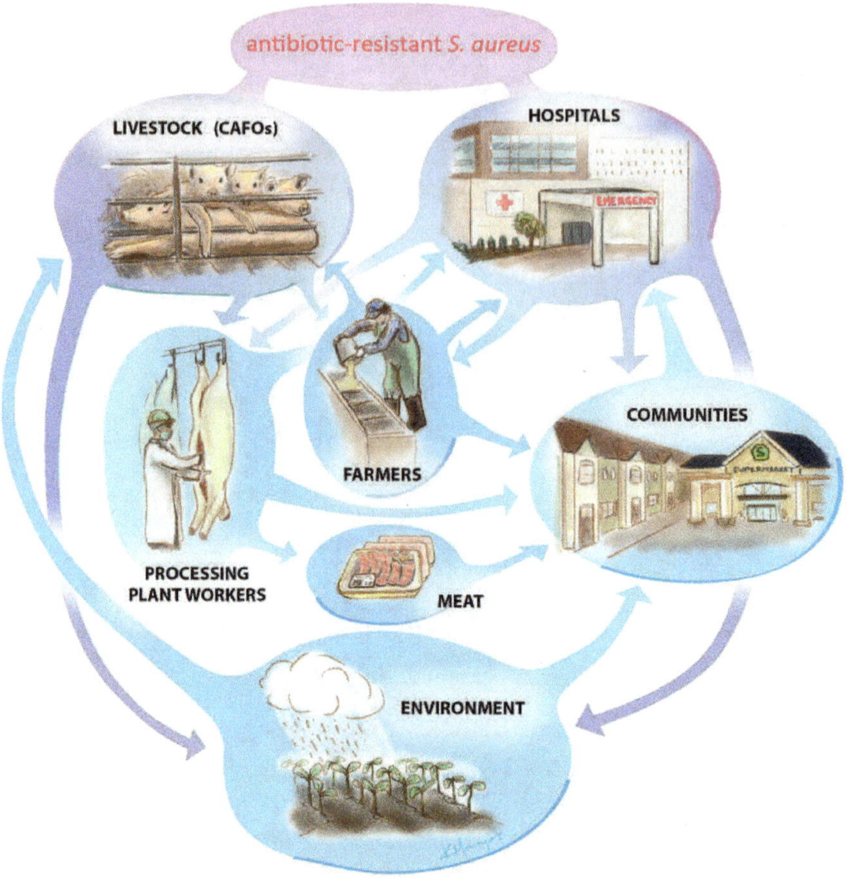

The origins of antibiotic-resistant *Staphylococcus aureus* (CAFO: concentrated animal feeding operations)

Since the last third of the 20th century, antibiotics have been used extensively in animal husbandry. In 2013, 80% of antibiotics used in the US were used in animals and only 20% in humans; in 1997 half were used in humans and half in animals. Some antibiotics are not used and not considered significant for use in humans, because they either lack efficacy or purpose in humans, such as ionophores in ruminants, or because the drug has gone out of use in humans. Others are used in both animals and humans, including penicillin and some forms of tetracycline. Historically, regulation of antibiotic use in food animals has been limited to limiting drug residues in meat, egg, and milk products, rather than by direct concern over the development of antibiotic resistance. This mirrors the primary concerns in human medicine, where, in general, researchers and doctors were more concerned about effective but non-toxic doses of drugs rather than antibiotic resistance.

In 2001, the Union of Concerned Scientists estimated that greater than 70% of the antibiotics used in the U.S. are given to food animals (for example, chickens, pigs, and cattle), in the absence of disease. The amounts given are termed «sub-therapeutic», i.e., insufficient to combat disease. Despite no diagnosis of disease, the administration of these drugs (most of which are not significant to human medicine) results in decreased mortality and morbidity and increased growth in the animals so treated. It is theorized that sub-therapeutic dosages kills some, but not all, of the bacterial organisms in the animal — likely leaving those that are naturally antibiotic-resistant. Studies have shown, however, that, in essence, the overall population levels of bacteria are unchanged; only the mix of bacteria is affected. The actual mechanism by which sub-therapeutic antibiotic feed additives serve as growth promoters is thus unclear. Some people have speculated that animals and fowl may have sub-clinical infections, which would be cured by low levels of antibiotics in feed, thereby allowing the creatures to thrive. No convincing evidence has been advanced for this theory, and the bacterial load in an animal is essentially unchanged by use of antibiotic feed additives. The mechanism of growth promotion is therefore probably something other than «killing off the bad bugs».

Antibiotics are used in U.S. animal feed to promote animal productivity. In particular, poultry feed and water is a common route of administration of drugs, because of higher overall costs when drugs are administered by handling animals individually.

In research studies, occasional animal-to-human spread of antibiotic-resistant organisms has been demonstrated. Resistant bacteria can be transmitted from animals to humans in three ways: by consuming animal products (milk, meat, eggs, etc.), from close or direct contact with animals or other humans, or through the environment. In the first pathway, food preservation methods can help eliminate, decrease, or prevent the growth of bacteria in some food classes. Evidence for the transfer of macrolide-resistant microorganisms from animals to humans has been scant, and most evidence shows that pathogens of concern in human populations originated in humans and are maintained there, with rare cases of transference to humans.

Natural Occurrence

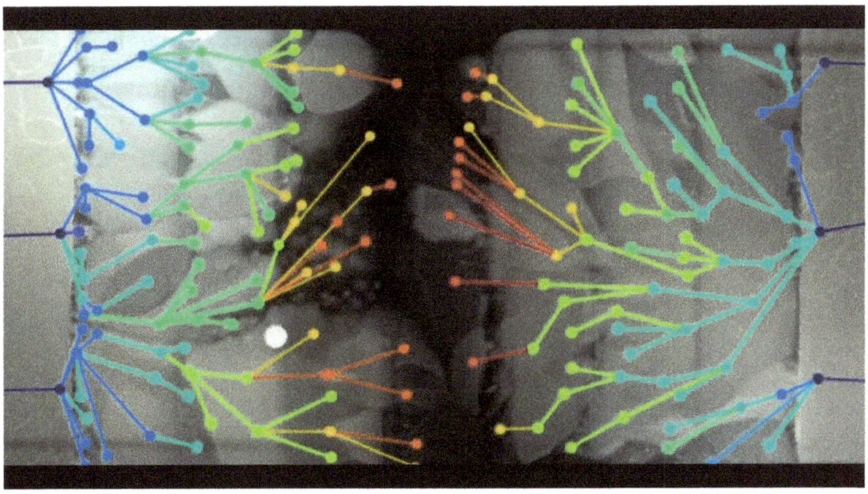

The Evolution of Bacteria on a “Mega-Plate” Petri Dish

Naturally occurring antibiotic resistance is common. Genes for resistance to antibiotics, like antibiotics themselves, are ancient. The genes that confer resistance are known as the environmental resistome. These genes may be transferred from non-disease-causing bacteria to those that do cause disease, leading to clinically significant antibiotic resistance. In 1952 it was shown that penicillin-resistant bacteria existed before penicillin treatment; and also preexistent bacterial resistance to streptomycin. In 1962, the presence of penicillinase was detected in dormant endospores of *Bacillus licheniformis*, revived from dried soil on the roots of plants, preserved since 1689 in the British Museum. Six strains of *Clostridium*, found in the bowels of William Braine and John Hartnell (members of the Franklin Expedition) showed resistance to cefoxitin and clindamycin. Penicillinase may have emerged as a defense mechanism for bacteria in their habitats, such as the case of penicillinase-rich *Staphylococcus aureus*, living with penicillin-producing *Trichophyton*; however, this may be circumstantial.Search for a penicillinase ancestor has focused on the class of proteins that must be *a priori* capable of specific combination with penicillin. The resistance to cefoxitin and clindamycin in turn was attributed to Braine›s and Hartnell›s contact with microorganisms that naturally produce them or random mutation in the chromosomes of *Clostridium* strains. There is evidence that heavy metals and other pollutants may select for antibiotic-resistant bacteria, generating a constant source of them in small numbers.

Environmental

Antibiotic resistance is a growing problem among humans and wildlife in terrestrial or aquatic environments. In this respect, the spread and contamination of the environment, especially through "hot spots" such as hospital wastewater and untreated urban wastewater, is a growing and serious public health problem. Antibiotics have been polluting the environment since their introduction through human waste (medication, farming), animals, and the pharmaceutical industry. Along with antibiotic waste, resistant bacteria follow, thus introducing antibiotic-resistant bacteria into the environment. As bacteria replicate quickly, the resistant bacteria that enter the environment replicate their resistance genes as they continue to divide. In addition, bacteria carrying resistance genes have the ability to spread those genes to other species via horizontal gene transfer. Therefore, even if the specific antibiotic is no longer introduced into the environment, antibiotic-resistance genes will persist through the bacteria that have since replicated without continuous exposure. Antibiotic resistance is widespread in marine vertebrates, and they may be important reservoirs of antibiotic-resistant bacteria in the marine environment.

Prevention

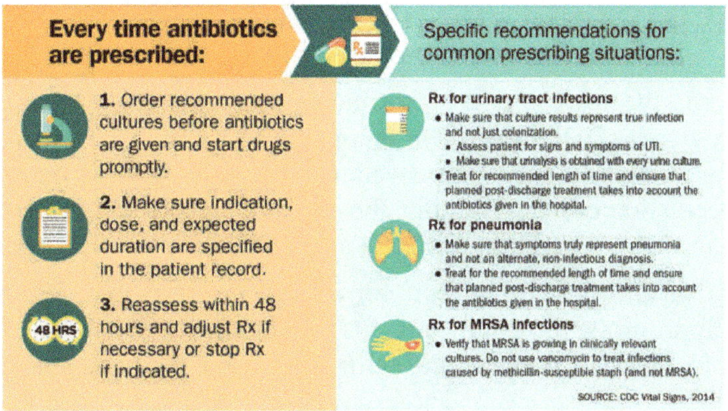

Mission Critical: Preventing Antibiotic Resistance (CDC report, 2014)

World Health Organization

In 2014, the WHO stated:

- People can help tackle resistance by:
    - using antibiotics only when prescribed by a doctor;
    - completing the full prescription, even if they feel better;
    - never sharing antibiotics with others or using leftover prescriptions.
- Health workers and pharmacists can help tackle resistance by:
    - enhancing infection prevention and control;
    - only prescribing and dispensing antibiotics when they are truly needed;
    - prescribing and dispensing the right antibiotic(s) to treat the illness.
- Policymakers can help tackle resistance by:
    - strengthening resistance tracking and laboratory capacity;
    - regulating and promoting appropriate use of medicines.
- Policymakers and industry can help tackle resistance by:
    - fostering innovation and research and development of new tools;
    - promoting cooperation and information sharing among all stakeholders.

Duration of Antibiotics

Antibiotic treatment duration should be based on the infection and other health problems a person may have. For many infections once a person has improved there is little evidence that stopping treatment causes more resistance. Some therefore feel that stopping early may be reasonable in some cases. Other infections, however, do require long courses regardless of whether a person feels better.

Antibiotic usage

The Netherlands has the lowest rate of antibiotic prescribing in the OECD, at a rate of 11.4 defined daily doses (DDD) per 1,000 people per day in 2011. Germany and Sweden also have lower prescribing rates, with Sweden's rate having been declining since 2007. By contrast, Greece, France and Belgium have high prescribing rates of more than 28 DDD. It is unclear if rapid viral testing affects antibiotic use in children.

About a third of antibiotic prescriptions written in outpatient settings in the United States were not appropriate in 2010 and 2011. Doctors in the U.S. wrote 506 annual antibiotic scripts for every 1,000 people, with 353 being medically necessary.

Monitoring

ResistanceOpen, an online global map of antimicrobial resistance developed by HealthMap, displays aggregated data on antimicrobial resistance from publicly available and user submitted data. The website can display data for a 25-mile radius from a location. Users may submit data from antibiograms for individual hospitals or laboratories. European data is from the EARS-Net (European Antimicrobial Resistance Surveillance Network), part of the ECDC. ResistanceMap, by the Center for Disease Dynamics, Economics & Policy, also provides data on antimicrobial resistance on a global level.

Strategies

Excessive antibiotic use has become one of the top contributors to the development of antibiotic resistance. Since the beginning of the antibiotic era, antibiotics have been used to treat a wide range of disease. Overuse of antibiotics has become the primary cause of rising levels of antibiotic resistance. The main problem is that doctors are willing to prescribe antibiotics to ill-informed individuals who believe that antibiotics can cure nearly all illnesses, including viral infections like the common cold. In an analysis of drug prescriptions, 36% of individuals with a cold or an upper respiratory infection (both viral in origin) were given prescriptions for antibiotics. These prescriptions accomplished nothing other than increasing the risk of further evolution of antibiotic resistant bacteria.

In a recent years, antimicrobial stewardship teams in hospitals have encouraged optimal use of antimicrobials. The goals of antimicrobial stewardship are to help practitioners pick the right drug at the right dose and duration of therapy while preventing misuse and minimizing the development of resistance.

There have been increasing public calls for global collective action to address the threat, including a proposal for international treaty on antimicrobial resistance. Further detail and attention is still needed in order to recognize and measure trends in resistance on the international level; the idea of a global tracking system has been suggested but implementation has yet to occur. A system of this nature would provide insight to areas of high resistance as well as information necessary for evaluation of programs and other changes made to fight or reverse antibiotic resistance.

On March 27, 2015, the White House released a comprehensive plan to address the increasing need for agencies to combat the rise of antibiotic-resistant bacteria. The Task Force for Combating Antibiotic-Resistant Bacteria developed *The National Action Plan for Combating Antibiotic-Resistant Bacteria* with the intent of providing a roadmap to guide the US in the antibiotic resistance challenge and with hopes of saving many lives. This plan outlines steps taken by the Federal government over the next five years needed in order to prevent and contain outbreaks of antibiotic-resistant infections; maintain the efficacy of antibiotics already on the market; and to help to develop future diagnostics, antibiotics, and vaccines.

The Action Plan was developed around five goals with focuses on strengthening health care, public health veterinary medicine, agriculture, food safety and research, and manufacturing. These goals, as listed by the White House, are as follows:

- Slow the Emergence of Resistant Bacteria and Prevent the Spread of Resistant Infections
- Strengthen National One-Health Surveillance Efforts to Combat Resistance
- Advance Development and use of Rapid and Innovative Diagnostic Tests for Identification and Characterization of Resistant Bacteria
- Accelerate Basic and Applied Research and Development for New Antibiotics, Other Therapeutics, and Vaccines
- Improve International Collaboration and Capacities for Antibiotic Resistance Prevention, Surveillance, Control and Antibiotic Research and Development

By following are goals set to meet by 2020:

- Establishment of antimicrobial programs within acute care hospital settings
- Reduction of inappropriate antibiotic prescription and use by at least 50% in outpatient settings and 20% inpatient settings
- Establishment of State Antibiotic Resistance (AR) Prevention Programs in all 50 states
- Elimination of the use of medically important antibiotics for growth promotion in food-producing animals.

The World Health Organization has promoted the first World Antibiotic Awareness Week running from 16–22 November 2015. The aim of the week is to increase global awareness of antibiotic resistance. It also wants to promote the correct usage of antibiotics across all fields in order to prevent further instances of antibiotic resistance.

Vaccines

Microorganisms do not develop resistance to vaccines because a vaccine enhances the body's immune system, whereas an antibiotic operates separately from the body's normal defenses. Furthermore, if the use of vaccines increase, there is evidence that antibiotic resistant strains of pathogens will decrease; the need for antibiotics will naturally decrease as vaccines prevent infection before it occurs. However, new strains that escape immunity induced by vaccines may evolve; for example, an updated influenza vaccine is needed each year.

While theoretically promising, antistaphylococcal vaccines have shown limited efficacy, because of immunological variation between *Staphylococcus* species, and the limited duration of effectiveness of the antibodies produced. Development and testing of more effective vaccines is underway.

Alternating Therapy

Alternating therapy is a proposed method in which two or three antibiotics are taken in a rotation versus taking just one antibiotic such that bacteria resistant to one antibiotic are killed when the next antibiotic is taken. Studies have found that this method reduces the rate at which antibiotic resistant bacteria emerge in vitro relative to a single drug for the entire duration.

Development of New Drugs

Since the discovery of antibiotics, research and development (R&D) efforts have provided new drugs in time to treat bacteria that became resistant to older antibiotics, but in the 2000s there has been concern that development has slowed enough that seriously ill people may run out of treatment options. Another concern is that doctors may become reluctant to perform routine surgeries because of the increased risk of harmful infection. Backup treatments can have serious side-effects; for example, treatment of multi-drug-resistant tuberculosis can cause deafness or psychological disability. The potential crisis at hand is the result of a marked decrease in industry R&D. Poor financial investment in antibiotic research has exacerbated the situation. The pharmaceutical industry has little incentive to invest in antibiotics because of the high risk and because the potential financial returns are less likely to cover the cost of development than for other pharmaceuticals. In 2011, Pfizer, one of the last major pharmaceutical companies developing new antibiotics, shut down its primary research effort, citing poor shareholder returns relative to drugs for chronic illnesses. However, small and medium-sized pharmaceutical companies are still active in antibiotic drug research.

In the United States, drug companies and the administration of President Barack Obama have been proposing changing the standards by which the FDA approves antibiotics targeted at resistant organisms. On 12 December 2013, the Antibiotic Development to Advance Patient Treatment (ADAPT) Act of 2013 was introduced in the U.S. Congress. The ADAPT Act aims to fast-track the drug development in order to combat the growing public health threat of 'superbugs'. Under this Act, the FDA can approve antibiotics and antifungals needed for life-threatening infections based on data from smaller clinical trials. The Centers for Disease Control and Prevention (CDC) will reinforce the monitoring of the use of antibiotics that treat serious and life-threatening infections and the emerging resistance, and make the data publicly available. The FDA antibiotics labeling process, 'Susceptibility Test Interpretive Criteria for Microbial Organisms' or 'breakpoints' is also streamlined to allow the most up-to-date and cutting-edge data available to healthcare professionals under the new Act.

On 18 September 2014 Obama signed an executive order to implement the recommendations proposed in a report by the President's Council of Advisors on Science and Technology (PCAST) which outlines strategies to stream-line clinical trials and speed up the R&D of new antibiotics. Among the proposals:

- Create a 'robust, standing national clinical trials network for antibiotic testing' which will promptly enroll patients once identified to be suffering from dangerous bacterial infections. The network will allow testing multiple new agents from different companies simultaneously for their safety and efficacy.
- Establish a 'Special Medical Use (SMU)' pathway for FDA to approve new antimicrobial agents for use in limited patient populations, shorten the approval timeline for new drug so patients with severe infections could benefit as quickly as possible.
- Provide economic incentives, especially for development of new classes of antibiotics, to offset the steep R&D costs which drive away the industry to develop antibiotics.

The executive order also included a $20 million prize to encourage the development of diagnostic tests to identify highly resistant bacterial infections.

The U.S. National Institutes of Health plans to fund a new research network on the issue up to $62 million from 2013 to 2019. Using authority created by the Pandemic and All Hazards Preparedness Act of 2006, the Biomedical Advanced Research and Development Authority in the U.S. Department of Health and Human Services announced that it will spend between $40 million and $200 million in funding for R&D on new antibiotic drugs under development by GlaxoSmithKline.

One major cause of antibiotic resistance is the increased pumping activity of microbial ABC transporters, which diminishes the effective drug concentration inside the microbial cell. ABC transporter inhibitors that can be used in combination with current antimicrobials are being tested in clinical trials and are available for therapeutic regimens.

Animal Use

Europe

In 1997, European Union health ministers voted to ban avoparcin and four additional antibiotics used to promote animal growth in 1999. In 2006 a ban on the use of antibiotics in European feed, with the exception of two antibiotics in poultry feeds, became effective. In Scandinavia, there is evidence that the ban has led to a lower prevalence of antibiotic resistance in (nonhazardous) animal bacterial populations. As of 2004, several European countries established a decline of antimicrobial resistance in humans through limiting the usage antimicrobials in agriculture and food industries without jeopardizing animal health or economic cost.

United States

The United States Department of Agriculture (USDA) and the Food and Drug Administration (FDA) collect data on antibiotic use in humans and in a more limited fashion in animals. The FDA first determined in 1977 that there is evidence of emergence of antibiotic-resistant bacterial strains in livestock. The long-established practice of permitting OTC sales of antibiotics (including penicillin and other drugs) to lay animal owners for administration to their own animals nonetheless continued in all states. In 2000, the FDA announced their intention to revoke approval of fluoroquinolone use in poultry production because of substantial evidence linking it to the emergence of fluoroquinolone-resistant *Campylobacter* infections in humans. Legal challenges from the food animal and pharmaceutical industries delayed the final decision to do so until 2006. Fluroquinolones have been banned from extra-label use in food animals in the USA since 2007. However, they remain widely used in companion and exotic animals.

During 2007, two federal bills (S. 549 and H.R. 962) aimed at phasing out «nontherapeutic» antibiotics in U.S. food animal production. The Senate bill, introduced by Sen. Edward «Ted» Kennedy, died. The House bill, introduced by Rep. Louise Slaughter, died after being referred to Committee.

In March 2012, the United States District Court for the Southern District of New York, ruling in an action brought by the Natural Resources Defense Council and others, ordered the FDA to revoke approvals for the use of antibiotics in livestock that violated FDA regulations. On April 11, 2012 the FDA announced a voluntary program to phase out unsupervised use of drugs as feed additives and convert approved over-the-counter uses for antibiotics to prescription use only, requiring veterinarian supervision of their use and a prescription. In December 2013, the FDA announced the commencement of these steps to phase out the use of antibiotics for the purposes of promoting livestock growth.

Growing U.S. consumer concern about using antibiotics in animal feed has led to greater availability of «antibiotic-free» animal products. For example, chicken producer Perdue removed all human antibiotics from its feed and launched products labeled "antibiotic free" under the Harvestland brand in 2007. Consumer response was positive, and in 2014 Perdue also phased out ionophores from its hatchery and began using the "antibiotic free" labels on its Harvestland, Simply Smart, and Perfect Portions products.

Mechanisms

The four main mechanisms by which microorganisms exhibit resistance to antimicrobials are:

- Drug inactivation or modification: for example, enzymatic deactivation of *penicillin* G in some penicillin-resistant bacteria through the production of β-lactamases. Most commonly, the protective enzymes produced by the bacterial cell will add an acetyl or phosphate group to a specific site on the antibiotic, which will reduce its ability to bind to the bacterial ribosomes and disrupt protein synthesis.

- Alteration of target site: for example, alteration of PBP—the binding target site of penicillins—in MRSA and other penicillin-resistant bacteria. Another protective mechanism found among bacterial species is ribosomal protection proteins. These proteins protect the bacterial cell from antibiotics that target the cell's ribosomes to inhibit protein synthesis. The mechanism involves the binding of the ribosomal protection proteins to the ribosomes of the bacterial cell, which in turn changes its conformational shape. This allows the ribosomes to continue synthesizing proteins essential to the cell while preventing antibiotics from binding to the ribosome to inhibit protein synthesis.

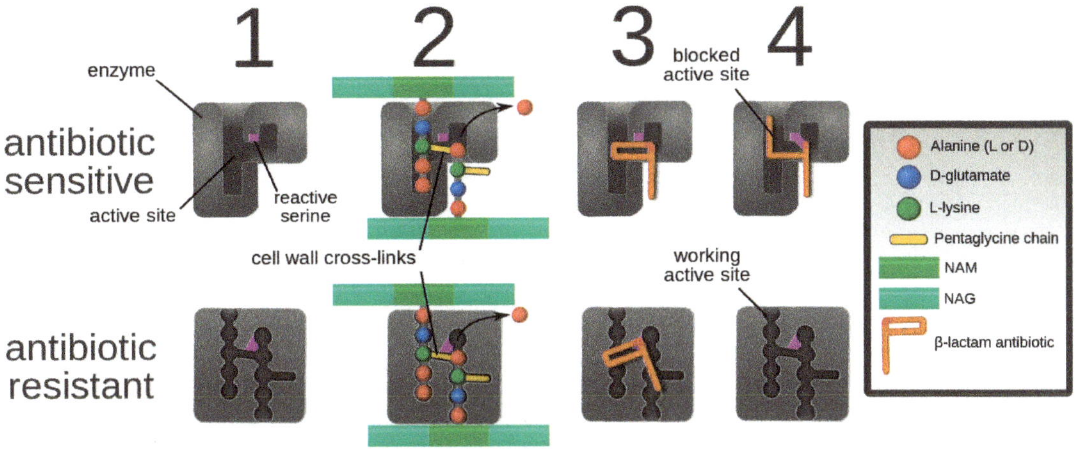

Diagram depicting antibiotic resistance through alteration of the antibiotic's target site, modeled after MRSA's resistance to penicillin. Beta-lactam antibiotics permanently inactivate PBP enzymes, which are essential for bacterial life, by permanently binding to their active sites. MRSA, however, expresses a PBP that does not allow the antibiotic into its active site.

- Alteration of metabolic pathway: for example, some sulfonamide-resistant bacteria do not require para-aminobenzoic acid (PABA), an important precursor for the synthesis of folic acid and nucleic acids in bacteria inhibited by sulfonamides, instead, like mammalian cells, they turn to using preformed folic acid.
- Reduced drug accumulation: by decreasing drug permeability or increasing active efflux (pumping out) of the drugs across the cell surface These specialized pumps can be found within the cellular membrane of certain bacterial species and are used to pump antibiotics out of the cell before they are able to do any damage. These efflux pumps are often activated by a specific substrate associated with an antibiotic.

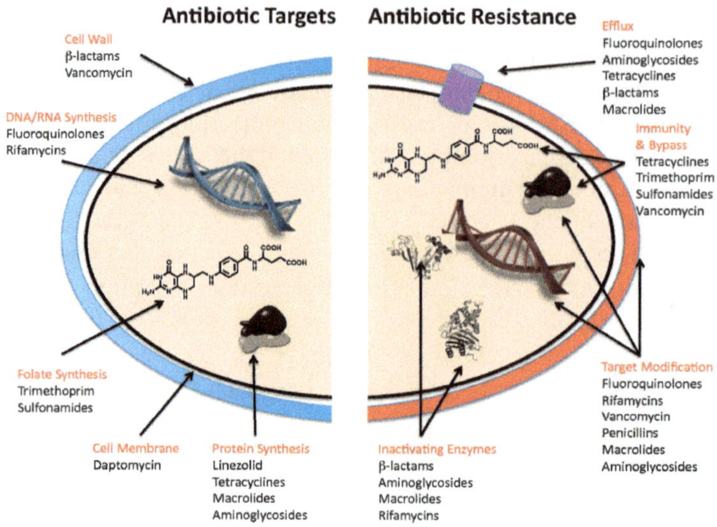

A number of mechanisms used by common antibiotics to deal with bacteria and ways by which bacteria become resistant to them.

Antibiotic resistance can be a result of horizontal gene transfer, and also of unlinked point mutations in the pathogen genome at a rate of about 1 in 10^8 per chromosomal replication. Mutations are rare but the fact that bacteria reproduce at such a high rate allows for the effect to be significant. A mutation may produce a change in the binding site of the antibiotic, which may allow the site to continue proper functioning in the presence of the antibiotic or prevent the binding of the antibiotic to the site altogether. Research has shown the bacterial protein LexA may play a key role in the acquisition of bacterial mutations giving resistance to quinolones and rifampicin. DNA damage induces the SOS gene repressor LexA to undergo autoproteolytic activity. This includes the transcription of genes encoding Pol II, Pol IV, and Pol V, which are three nonessential DNA polymerases that are required for mutation in response to DNA damage. The antibiotic action against the pathogen can be seen as an environmental pressure. Those bacteria with a mutation that allows them to survive live to reproduce. They then pass this trait to their offspring, which leads to the evolution of a fully resistant colony. Although these chromosomal mutations may seem to benefit the bacteria by providing antibiotic resistance, they also confer a cost of fitness. For example, a ribosomal mutation may protect a bacterial cell by changing the binding site of an antibiotic but it will also slow the process of protein synthesis. Additionally, a particular study specifically compared the overall fitness of antibiotic resistant strains of Escherichia coli and Salmonella typhimurium to their drug-sensitive revertants. They observed a reduced overall fitness in the antibiotic resistant strains, especially in growth rate.

There are three known mechanisms of fluoroquinolone resistance. Some types of efflux pumps can act to decrease intracellular quinolone concentration. In Gram-negative bacteria, plasmid-mediated resistance genes produce proteins that can bind to DNA gyrase, protecting it from the action of quinolones. Finally, mutations at key sites in DNA gyrase or topoisomerase IV can decrease their binding affinity to quinolones, decreasing the drug›s effectiveness.

Antibiotic resistance can also be introduced artificially into a microorganism through laboratory protocols, sometimes used as a selectable marker to examine the mechanisms of gene transfer or to identify individuals that absorbed a piece of DNA that included the resistance gene and another gene of interest. A recent study demonstrated that the extent of horizontal gene transfer among *Staphylococcus* is much greater than previously expected—and encompasses genes with functions beyond antibiotic resistance and virulence, and beyond genes residing within the mobile genetic elements.

For a long time, it has been thought that, for a microorganism to become resistant to an antibiotic, it must be in a large population. However, recent findings show that there is no necessity of large populations of bacteria for the appearance of antibiotic resistance. We know now that small populations of E.coli in an antibiotic gradient can become resistant. Any heterogeneous environment with respect to nutrient and antibiotic gradients may facilitate the development of antibiotic resistance in small bacterial populations and this is also true for the human body. Researchers hypothesize that the mechanism of resistance development is based on four SNP mutations in the genome of E.coli produced by the gradient of antibiotic. These mutations confer the bacteria emergence of antibiotic resistance.

MCR-1

In November, 2015, a Chinese team first described MCR-1 gene after finding the gene in pigs and pork. It became a matter of concern when it was discovered that it could be transferred to other organisms. MCR-1 was later discovered in Malaysia, England, China, Europe, and the United States.

NDM-1

NDM-1 is an enzyme that makes bacteria resistant to a broad range of beta-lactam antibiotics.

NDM-1 was first detected in a *Klebsiella pneumoniae* isolate from a Swedish patient of Indian origin in 2008. It was later detected in bacteria in India, Pakistan, the United Kingdom, the United States, Canada and Japan.

According to A *Lancet* study, NDM-1 (New Delhi Metallo-beta-lactamase-1) originated in India, The study came to a conclusion that Indian hospitals are unsafe for treatment as Nosocomial-infections are common and with the new super-bugs on rise in India, It can be dangerous.

ORGANISMS

Bacteria

Staphylococcus Aureus

Staphylococcus aureus (colloquially known as "Staph aureus" or a "Staph infection") is one of the major resistant pathogens. Found on the mucous membranes and the human skin of around a third of the population, it is extremely adaptable to antibiotic pressure. It was one of the earlier bacteria in which penicillin resistance was found—in 1947, just four years after the drug started being mass-produced. Methicillin was then the antibiotic of choice, but has since been replaced by oxacillin because of significant kidney toxicity. Methicillin-resistant *Staphylococcus aureus* (MRSA) was first detected in Britain in 1961, and is now "quite common" in hospitals. MRSA was responsible for 37% of fatal cases of sepsis in the UK in 1999, up from 4% in 1991. Half of all *S. aureus* infections in the US are resistant to penicillin, methicillin, tetracycline and erythromycin.

This left vancomycin as the only effective agent available at the time. However, strains with intermediate (4–8 μg/ml) levels of resistance, termed glycopeptide-intermediate *Staphylococcus aureus* (GISA) or vancomycin-intermediate *Staphylococcus aureus* (VISA), began appearing in the late 1990s. The first identified case was in Japan in 1996, and strains have since been found in hospitals in England, France and the US. The first documented strain with complete (>16 μg/ml) resistance to vancomycin, termed vancomycin-resistant *Staphylococcus aureus* (VRSA) appeared in the United States in 2002. However, in 2011, a variant of vancomycin has been tested that binds to the lactate variation and also binds well to the original target, thus reinstating potent antimicrobial activity.

A new class of antibiotics, oxazolidinones, became available in the 1990s, and the first commercially available oxazolidinone, linezolid, is comparable to vancomycin in effectiveness against MRSA. Linezolid resistance in *S. aureus* was reported in 2001, but infection rates have been at consistently low levels and in the United Kingdom and Ireland, no resistance was found in staphylococci collected from bacteremia cases between 2001 and 2006.

Community-acquired MRSA (CA-MRSA) has now emerged as an epidemic that is responsible for rapidly progressive, fatal diseases, including necrotizing pneumonia, severe sepsis, and necrotizing fasciitis. MRSA is the most frequently identified antimicrobial drug-resistant pathogen in US hospitals. The epidemiology of infections caused by MRSA is rapidly changing. Since 2000, infections caused by this organism have emerged in the community. The two MRSA clones in the United States most closely associated with community outbreaks, USA400 (MW2 strain, ST1 lineage) and USA300, often contain Panton-Valentine leukocidin (PVL) genes and, more frequently, have been associated with skin and soft tissue infections. Outbreaks of CA-MRSA infections have been reported in correctional facilities, among athletic teams, among military recruits, in newborn nurseries, and among men that have sex with men. CA-MRSA infections now appear endemic in many urban regions and cause most CA-*S. aureus* infections.

Streptococcus and *Enterococcus*

Streptococcus pyogenes (Group A *Streptococcus*: GAS) infections can usually be treated with many different antibiotics. Early treatment may reduce the risk of death from invasive group A streptococcal disease. However, even the best medical care does not prevent death in every case. For those with very severe illness, supportive care in an intensive-care unit may be needed. For persons with necrotizing fasciitis, surgery often is needed to remove damaged tissue. Strains of *S. pyogenes* resistant to macrolide antibiotics have emerged; however, all strains remain uniformly susceptible to penicillin.

Resistance of *Streptococcus pneumoniae* to penicillin and other beta-lactams is increasing worldwide. The major mechanism of resistance involves the introduction of mutations in genes encoding penicillin-binding proteins. Selective pressure is thought to play an important role, and use of beta-lactam antibiotics has been implicated as a risk factor for infection and colonization. *S. pneumoniae* is responsible for pneumonia, bacteremia, otitis media, meningitis, sinusitis, peritonitis and arthritis.

Multidrug-resistant *Enterococcus faecalis* and *Enterococcus faecium* are associated with nosocomial infections. These strains include: penicillin-resistant *Enterococcus*, vancomycin-resistant *Enterococcus*, and linezolid-resistant *Enterococcus*.

Pseudomonas Aeruginosa

Pseudomonas aeruginosa is a highly prevalent opportunistic pathogen. One of the most worrisome characteristics of *P. aeruginosa* is its low antibiotic susceptibility, which is attributable to a concerted action of multidrug efflux pumps with chromosomally encoded antibiotic resistance genes (e.g., *mexAB-oprM*, *mexXY*) and the low permeability of the bacterial cellular envelopes. *Pseudomonas aeruginosa* has the ability to produce 4-hydroxy-2-alkylquinolines (HAQs) and it has been found that HAQs have prooxidant effects, and overexpressing modestly increased susceptibility to antibiotics. The study experimented with the *Pseudomonas aeruginosa* biofilms and found that a disruption of relA and spoT genes produced an inactivation of the Stringent response (SR) in cells with nutrient limitation, which provides cells be more susceptible to antibiotics.

Clostridium Difficile

Clostridium difficile is a nosocomial pathogen that causes diarrheal disease worldwide. Diarrhea caused by *C. difficile* can be life-threatening. Infections are most frequent in people who have had recent medical and/or antibiotic treatment. *C. difficile* infections commonly occur during hospitalization.

According to a 2015 CDC report, *C. difficile* caused almost 500,000 infections in the United States over a year period. Associated with these infections were an estimated 15,000 deaths. The CDC estimates that *C. difficile* infection costs could amount to $3.8 billion over a 5-year span.

C. difficile colitis is most strongly associated with fluoroquinolones, cephalosporins, carbapenems, and clindamycin.

Some research suggests the overuse of antibiotics in the raising of livestock is contributing to outbreaks of bacterial infections such as C. difficile.

Antibiotics, especially those with a broad activity spectrum (such as clindamycin) disrupt normal intestinal flora. This can lead to an overgrowth of C. difficile, which flourishes under these conditions. Pseudomembranous colitis can follow, creating generalized inflammation of the colon and the development of «pseudomembrane», a viscous collection of inflammatory cells, fibrin, and necrotic cells. Clindamycin-resistant *C. difficile* was reported as the causative agent of large outbreaks of diarrheal disease in hospitals in New York, Arizona, Florida and Massachusetts between 1989 and 1992. Geographically dispersed outbreaks of *C. difficile* strains resistant to fluoroquinolone antibiotics, such as ciprofloxacin and levofloxacin, were also reported in North America in 2005.

Carbapenem-Resistant Enterobacteriaceae

As of 2013 hard-to-treat or untreatable infections of carbapenem-resistant Enterobacteriaceae (CRE) were increasing among patients in medical facilities. CRE are resistant to nearly all available antibiotics. Almost half of hospital patients who get bloodstream CRE infections die from the infection.

Multidrug-Resistant Acinetobacter

Acinetobacter is a gram-negative bacteria that causes pneumonia or bloodstream infections in critically ill patients. Multidrug-resistant Acinetobacter have become very resistant to antibiotics.

Drug-resistant *Campylobacter*

Campylobacter causes diarrhea (often bloody), fever, and abdominal cramps. Serious complications such as temporary paralysis can also occur. Physicians rely on ciprofloxacin and azithromycin for treating patients with severe disease although *Campylobacter* is showing resistance to these antibiotics.

Salmonella and *E. Coli*

Infection with *Escherichia coli* and *Salmonella* can result from the consumption of contaminated food and water. Both of these bacteria are well known for causing nosocomial (hospital-linked) infections, and often, these strains found in hospitals are antibiotic resistant because of adaptations to wide spread antibiotic use. When both bacteria are spread, serious health conditions arise. Many people are hospitalized each year after becoming infected, with some dying as a result. Since 1993, some strains of *E. coli* have become resistant to multiple types of fluoroquinolone antibiotics.

Although mutation alone plays a huge role in the development of antibiotic resistance, a 2008 study found that high survival rates after exposure to antibiotics could not be accounted for by mutation alone. This study focused on the development of resistance in E. coli to three antibiotic drugs: ampicillin, tetracycline, and nalidixic acid. The researchers found that some antibiotic resistance in E. coli developed because of epigenetic inheritance rather than by direct inheritance of a mutated gene. This was further supported by data showing that reversion to antibiotic sensitivity was relatively common as well. This could only be explained by epigenetics. Epigenetics is a type of inheritance in which gene expression is altered rather than the genetic code itself. There are many modes by which this alteration of gene expression can occur, including methylation of DNA and histone modification; however, the important point is that both inheritance of random mutations and epigenetic markers can result in the expression of antibiotic resistance genes.

Resistance to polymyxins first appear in 2011. An easier way for this resistance to spread, a plasmid known as MCR-1 was discovered in 2015.

Acinetobacter Baumannii

On November 5, 2004, the Centers for Disease Control and Prevention (CDC) reported an increasing number of *Acinetobacter baumannii* bloodstream infections in patients at military medical facilities in which service members injured in the Iraq/Kuwait region during Operation Iraqi Freedom and in Afghanistan during Operation Enduring Freedom were treated. Most of these showed multidrug resistance (MRAB), with a few isolates resistant to all drugs tested.

Klebsiella Pneumoniae

Klebsiella pneumoniae carbapenemase (KPC)-producing bacteria are a group of emerging highly drug-resistant Gram-negative bacilli causing infections associated with significant morbidity and mortality whose incidence is rapidly increasing in a variety of clinical settings around the world. *Klebsiella pneumoniae* includes numerous mechanisms for antibiotic resistance, many of which are located on highly mobile genetic elements. Carbapenem antibiotics (heretofore often the treatment of last resort for resistant infections) are generally not effective against KPC-producing organisms.

Mycobacterium Tuberculosis

Tuberculosis is increasing across the globe, especially in developing countries, over the past few years. TB resistant to antibiotics is called MDR TB (Multidrug Resistant TB). Globally, MDR TB causes 150,000 deaths annually. The rise of the HIV/AIDS epidemic has contributed to this.

TB was considered one of the most prevalent diseases, and did not have a cure until the discovery of Streptomycin by Selman Waksman in 1943. However, the bacteria soon developed resistance. Since then, drugs such as isoniazid and rifampin have been used. M. tuberculosis develops resistance to drugs by spontaneous mutations in its genomes. Resistance to one drug is common, and this is why treatment is usually done with more than one drug. Extensively Drug-Resistant TB (XDR TB) is TB that is also resistant to the second line of drugs.

Resistance of *Mycobacterium tuberculosis* to isoniazid, rifampin, and other common treatments has become an increasingly relevant clinical challenge. (For more on Drug-Resistant TB, visit the Multi-drug-resistant tuberculosis page.) Evidence is lacking for whether these bacteria have plasmids. Also *M. tuberculosis* lack the opportunity to interact with other bacteria in order to share plasmids.

Neisseria Gonorrhoeae

Neisseria gonorrhoeae is a sexually transmitted pathogen that causes gonorrhea, a sexually transmitted disease that can result in discharge and inflammation at the urethra, cervix, pharynx, or rectum. It can cause pelvic pain, pain on urination, penile and vaginal discharge, as well as systemic symptoms. It can also cause severe reproductive complications. The bacteria was first identified in 1879, although some Biblical scholars believe that references to the disease can be found as early as Parshat Metzora of the Old Testament.

In the 1940s effective treatment with penicillin became available, but by the 1970s resistant strains predominated. Resistance to penicillin has developed through two mechanisms: chromasomally mediated resistance (CMRNG) and penicillinase-mediated resistance (PPNG). CMRNG involves step wise mutation of penA, which codes for the penicillin-binding protein (PBP-2); mtr, which encodes an efflux pump that removes penicillin from the cell; and penB, which encodes the bacterial cell wall porins. PPNG involves the acquisition of a plasmid-bornebeta-lactamase. *N. gonorrheoea* has a high affinity for horizontal gene transfer, and as a result, the existence of any strain resistant to a given drug could spread easily across strains.

Fluoroquinolones were a useful next-line treatment until resistance was achieved through efflux pumps and mutations to the gyrA gene, which encodes DNA gyrase. Third-generation cephalosporins have been used to treat gonorrhoea since 2007, but resistant strains have emerged. As of 2010, the recommended treatment is a single 250 mg intramuscular injection of ceftriaxone, sometimes in combination with azithromycin or doxycycline. However, certain strains of *N. gonorrhoeae* can be resistant to antibiotics usually that are normally used to treat it. These include: cefixime (an oral cephalosporin), ceftriaxone (an injectable cephalosporin), azithromycin, aminoglycosides, and tetracycline.

Viruses

Specific antiviral drugs are used to treat some viral infections. These drugs prevent viruses from reproducing by inhibiting essential stages of the virus's replication cycle in infected cells. Antivirals are used to treat HIV, hepatitis B, hepatitis C, influenza, herpes viruses including varicella zoster virus, cytomegalovirus and Epstein-Barr virus. With each virus, some strains have become resistant to the administered drugs.

Resistance to HIV antivirals is problematic, and even multi-drug resistant strains have evolved. Resistant strains of the HIV virus emerge rapidly if only one antiviral drug is used.Using three or more drugs together has helped to control this problem, but new drugs are needed because of the continuing emergence of drug-resistant HIV strains.

Fungi

Infections by fungi are a cause of high morbidity and mortality in immunocompromised persons, such as those with HIV/AIDS, tuberculosis or receiving chemotherapy. The fungi candida, *Cryptococcus neoformans* and *Aspergillus fumigatus* cause most of these infections and antifungal resistance occurs in all of them. Multidrug resistance in fungi is increasing because of the widespread use of antifungal drugs to treat infections in immunocompromised individuals.

Of particular note, Fluconazole-resistant Candida species have been highlighted as a growing problem by the CDC. More than 20 Candida species of Candida can cause Candidiasis infection, the most common of which is *Candida albicans*. Candida yeasts normally inhabit the skin and mucous membranes without causing infection. However, overgrowth of Candida can lead to Candidiasis. Some Candida strains are becoming resistant to first-line and second-line antifungal agents such as azoles and echinocandins.

Parasites

The protozoan parasites that cause the diseases malaria, trypanosomiasis, toxoplasmosis, cryptosporidiosis and leishmaniasis are important human pathogens.

Malarial parasites that are resistant to the drugs that are currently available to infections are common and this has led to increased efforts to develop new drugs. Resistance to recently developed drugs such as artemisinin has also been reported. The problem of drug resistance in malaria has driven efforts to develop vaccines.

Trypanosomes are parasitic protozoa that cause African trypanosomiasis and Chagas disease (American trypanosomiasis). There are no vaccines to prevent these infections so drugs such as pentamidine and suramin, benznidazole and nifurtimox and used to treat infections. These drugs are effective but infections caused by resistant parasites have been reported.

Leishmaniasis is caused by protozoa and is an important public health problem worldwide, especially in sub-tropical and tropical countries. Drug resistance has "become a major concern".

Applications

Antibiotic resistance is an important tool for genetic engineering. By constructing a plasmid that contains an antibiotic-resistance gene as well as the gene being engineered or expressed, a researcher can ensure that, when bacteria replicate, only the copies that carry the plasmid survive. This ensures that the gene being manipulated passes along when the bacteria replicates.

In general, the most commonly used antibiotics in genetic engineering are "older" antibiotics. These include:

- ampicillin
- kanamycin
- tetracycline
- chloramphenicol

In industry, the use of antibiotic resistance is disfavored, since maintaining bacterial cultures would require feeding them large quantities of antibiotics. Instead, the use of auxotrophic bacterial strains (and function-replacement plasmids) is preferred.

Society and Culture

For the fiscal year 2016 budget, President Obama has suggested to nearly double the amount of federal funding to "combat and prevent" antibiotic resistance to more than $1.2 billion.

Since the mid-1980s pharmaceutical companies have invested in medications for cancer or chronic disease that have greater potential to make money and have "de-emphasized or dropped development of antibiotics". On January 20, 2016 at the World Economic Forum in Davos, Switzerland, more than "80 pharmaceutical and diagnostic companies" from around the world called for 'transformational commercial models' at a global level to spur research and development on antibiotics and on the "enhanced use of diagnostic tests that can rapidly identify the infecting organism".

Legal Frameworks

Some global health scholars have argued that a global, legal framework is needed to prevent and control antimicrobial resistance. For instance, binding global policies could be used to create antimicrobial use standards, regulate antibiotic marketing, and strengthen global surveillance systems.Ensuring compliance of involved parties is a challenge. Global antimicrobial resistance policies could take lessons from the environmental sector by adopting strategies that have made international environmental agreements successful in the past such as: sanctions for non-compliance, assistance for implementation, majority vote decision-making rules, an independent scientific panel, and specific commitments.

ANTIBIOTIC USE IN LIVESTOCK

Antibiotic use in livestock is the use of antibiotics for any purpose in the husbandry of livestock, which includes treatment when ill (therapeutic), treatment of a batch of animals when at least one is diagnosed as ill (metaphylaxis – similar to the way bacterial meningitis is treated in children), preventative treatment against disease or prophylaxis of infection, but also the use of subtherapeutic doses in animal feed and/or water to promote growth and improve feed efficiency in intensive animal farming outside of Europe, where the last practice has been banned since 2006. This article looks at antibiotic use for growth promotion and the situation in the United States and does not cover therapy, prophylaxis or metaphlyaxis in Europe.

Antimicrobials (including antibiotics and antifungals) and other drugs can be used by veterinarians and livestock owners in countries outside Europe to increase the growth rates of livestock, poultry, and other farmed animals, although these pharmaceuticals do not always have to be administered by a veterinarian. It is important to note the use of antibiotics for growth promotion purposes has been banned in Europe since 2006.

There are also global concerns over the use of antibiotics for growth promotion or therapy purposes because of the potential for some drugs to enter the human food chain despite rigorous withdrawal measures and testing to prevent antibiotic residues in food, increasing antibiotic resistance in animals, a potential although largely unproven link to antibiotic-resistant infections in humans, and what some consider antibiotic misuse. Other drugs may be used only under strict limits, and some organizations and authorities seek to further restrict the use of some or all drugs in animals. Other authorities, such as the World Organization for Animal Health, say that "Without antibiotics there would supply problems of animal protein for the human population".

However, in 2013 the CDC finalized and released a report detailing antibiotic resistance and classified the top 18 resistant bacterium as either being urgent, serious or concerning threats (CDC). Of those organisms, three (CDIFF, CRE and Neisseria gonorrhoeae) have been classified as urgent threats and require more monitoring and prevention (CDC). In the US alone, more than 2 million people are diagnosed with antibiotic resistant infections and over 23,000 die per year due to resistant infections (CDC).

History of the Practice

In 1910 in the United States, a meat shortage resulted in protests and boycotts. After this and other shortages, the public demanded government research into stabilization of food supplies. Since the 1900s, livestock production on United States farms has had to rear larger quantities of animals over a short period of time to meet new consumer demands. Factory farming or the use of high intensity feedlots originated in the late 19th century when advances in technology and science allowed for mass production of livestock. Global agriculture production doubled four times within 1820 and 1975, feeding one billion in 1800 and up to 6.5 billion in 2002. Along with the new large animal densities came the threat of disease, therefore requiring a greater disease control of these animals. In 1950, a group of United States scientists found that adding antibiotics to animal feed increases the growth rate of livestock. American Cyanamid published research establishing the practice.

By 2001 this practice had grown so much that a report by the Union of Concerned Scientists found that nearly 90% of the total use of antimicrobials in the United States was for non-therapeutic purposes in agricultural production.

Antibiotics have an appropriate place in the humane care of illness in livestock, when they reduce the suffering of a sick animal or control the spread of the illness to nearby animals.Thus, ideas that they should *never* be used in livestock husbandry are misguided. Instead, the goal is to prevent the allowance of preventive use from being distorted into routine use, constituting overuse.

Drugs and Growth Stimulation

Certain antibiotics, when given in low, sub-therapeutic doses, are known to improve feed conversion efficiency (more output, such as muscle or milk, for a given amount of feed) and/or may promote greater growth, most likely by affecting gut flora.

Antibiotic Growth Promoters used in Livestock Production		
drug	**class**	**effect**
Bambermycin		increase feed conversion ratio and weight gain in chickens, beef cattle, swine, and turkeys.
Lasalocid	Ionophore	increase feed conversion ratio and weight gain in beef cattle.
Monensin	Ionophore	increase feed conversion ratio and weight gain in beef cattle and sheep; promotes proficient milk production in dairy cows.
Salinomycin	Ionophore	increase feed conversion ratio and weight gain.
Virginiamycin	peptide	increase feed conversion ratio and weight gain in chickens, swine, turkeys, and beef cattle.
Bacitracin	peptide	increase weight gain and feed conversion ratio in chickens, turkeys, beef cattle, and swine; promotes egg production in chickens.
Carbadox		increase feed conversion ratio and weight gain in swine.
Laidlomycin		increase feed conversion ratio and weight gain in beef cattle.
Lincomycin		increase feed conversion ratio and weight gain in chickens and swine.
Neomycin/ oxytetracyclinee		increase weight gain and feed conversion ratio in chickens, turkeys, swine, and beef cattle.
Penicillin		increase feed conversion ratio and weight gain in chickens, turkeys, and swine.
Roxarsone		increase feed conversion ratio and weight gain in chickens and turkeys.
Tylosin		increase feed conversion ratio and weight gain in chickens and swine.

Use in different Livestock

In Swine Production

The use of antibiotics to increase the growth of pigs is most studied of all livestock. This use for growth rather than disease prevention is referred to as subtherapeutic antibiotic use. Studies have shown that administering low doses of antibiotics in livestock feed improves growth rate, reduces mortality and morbidity, and improves reproductive performance. It is estimated that over one-half of the antibiotics produced and sold in the United States is used as a feed additive. Although it is still not completely understood why and how antibiotics increase the growth rate of pigs, possibilities include metabolic effects, disease control effects, and nutritional effects. While subtherapeutic use has many benefits for raising swine, there is growing concern that this practice leads to increased antibiotic resistance in bacteria. Antibiotic resistance occurs when bacteria are resistant to one or more microbial agents that are usually used to treat infection. There are three stages in the possible emergence and continuation of antibiotic resistance: genetic change, antibiotic selection, and spread of antibiotic resistance.

In Production of Other Livestock

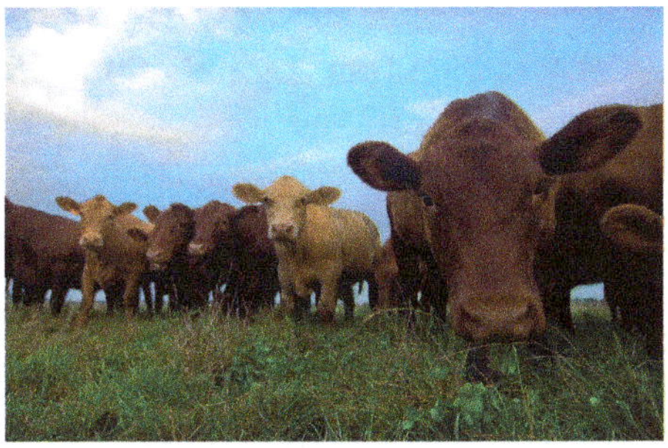

Organic beef comes from cattle who have not been fed antibiotics.

Regulatory Context

The use of drugs in food animals is regulated in nearly all countries. Historically, this has been to prevent alteration or contamination of meat, milk, eggs and other products with toxins that are harmful to humans. Treating a sick animal with drugs may lead to some of those drugs remaining in the animal when it is slaughtered or milked. Scientific experiments provide data that shows how long a drug is present in the body of an animal and what the animal's body does to the drug. Of particular concern are drugs that may be passed into milk or eggs. By the use of 'drug withdrawal periods' before slaughter or the use of milk or eggs from treated animals, veterinarians and animal owners ensure that the meat, milk and eggs is free of contamination.

These restrictions include not only poisons or drugs (such as penicillin) which may result in allergic reactions but also contaminants which may cause cancer. It is illegal in the USA to administer drugs or feed substances to animals if they have been shown to cause cancer.

One of the main restrictions is the amount that is administered to animals in the industry. These drugs should be administered to healthy livestock at a low concentration of 200 g per ton of feed. The amount distributed is also altered throughout the lifespan of livestock in order to meet specific growth needs.

Legality of the use of specific drugs in animal medicine varies according to location.

Just as in human medicine, some drugs are available over the counter and others are restricted to use only on the prescription of a veterinary physician. In the USA, the Food and Drug Administration (FDA) requires specific labels on all drugs, giving directions on the use of the drug. For animals, this includes the species, dose, reason for giving the drug (indication) and the required withdrawal period, if any. Federal law requires laypersons to use drugs only in the manner listed. Veterinarians who have examined an animal or a herd of animals may issue a replacement label, giving new directions, based on their medical knowledge. It is illegal in the USA for any layperson to administer any drug to a food animal in a way not specific to the drug label. Over-the-counter drugs which may be used by laypersons include anti-parasite drugs (including fly sprays) and antimicrobials. These drugs can be applied as sprays, creams, injections, oral pills or fluids, or as a feed additive, depending on the drug and the label.

In December 2013, the FDA updated its regulations to try to begin reducing use of antibiotics for growth enhancement. Significant lobbying comes from all directions, from those against tighter regulation to those who complain it doesn't go far enough.

Currently few policies, regulations and laws exist that promote limitation of antibiotic use on factory farms. In addition, few policies are being created that call for this decrease in antibiotic use. However, numerous state senators and members of congress showed support for the Preventing Antibiotic Resistance Act of 2015 (PARA) and the Preservation of Antibiotics for Medical Treatment Act of 2013 (PAMTA). These acts proposed amendments be made to the Federal Food, Drug and Cosmetic Act which would limit and preserve the use of antibiotics for medically necessary situations. Both of these bills died in Congress in 2015.

Administering Drugs

Drugs can be administered to animals in a variety of means, just as with humans. Among these are topical (on the skin), by injection (including intravenous, subcutaneous, subcutaneous implants, intramuscular and intraperitoneal), and orally. Oral drugs can be in pill or liquid form, or can be given by mixing with feed or drinking water. The appropriate route for treatment depends on the specific case and can vary by: illness, severity of illness, selected drug, age or condition of the animal, species of the animal, type of housing and other factors. For animals that are not regularly fed a concentrated feed or which can be handled repeatedly, a slow-release injection might be the most appropriate. Some drugs are not available or appropriate in this form and should be delivered orally. For animals that are fed regularly (rather than grazing freely) or that can not be easily handled, the most appropriate means of administering the drug may be to include the drug in feed or water. This eliminates the stress of daily (or more frequent) handling of animals, which can make the animals more ill. Poultry are most commonly medicated in this fashion, as they are easily stressed to the point of dying. Administering the drug by feed also prevents injection wounds in animals.

The timely administration of drugs is key to preventing animal suffering and economic loss to the farmer. Animals which are ill can infect other animals, and may become so ill that they can not be sold. A variety of techniques are used to monitor animals for illness so that they can be treated appropriately. Stress reduction, adequate nutrition, shelter, and quarantine of incoming stock are all important factors to promote growth and reduce illness and the need for active treatment. The age and status of an animal is also important in determining correct treatment – a young animal or pregnant animal is at greater risk and are treated more aggressively than an older animal. Specifically in calves, the period in which they begin to separate from their mothers generates stress and makes them more susceptible to catching an infection like pneumonia. Antibiotics are commonly administered in the calves' feed during this time to fight the possibility of stress-induced infections. Feed antibiotics are also used to prevent illnesses in calves caused by liver abscesses that develop during their last stages of growth.

Use by Country

European Union

The European Union (EU) in 1999 implemented an antibiotic resistance monitoring program and phase out plan for all antibiotic use by 2006. Although the European Union banned the use of antibiotics as growth agents from 2006, its use has not changed much until recently. In Germany, 1,734 tons of antimicrobial agents were used for animals in 2011 compared with 800 tons for humans. On the other hand, Sweden banned their use in 1986 and Denmark started cutting down drastically in 1994, so that its use is now 60% less. In the Netherlands, the use of antibiotics to treat diseases increased after the ban on its use for growth purposes in 2006. In 2011, the EU voted to ban the prophylactic use of antibiotics, alarmed at signs that the overuse of antibiotics is blunting their use for humans.

United States

In 2011, a total of 13.6 million kilograms of antimicrobials were sold for use in food-producing animals in the United States, which represents 80% of all antibiotics sold or distributed in the United States. Of the antibiotics given to animals fom 2009 through 2013, just above 60% distributed for food animal use are "medically-important" drugs, that are also used in humans. The rest are drug classes like ionophores which are not used in human medicine. Due to concerns about the overuse of antibiotics in food-producing animals, the U.S. Food & Drug Administration has implemented new industry guidelines that will restrict the use of medically-important drugs to uses "that are considered necessary for assuring animal health" and will require veterinary oversight. The food animal and veterinary pharmaceutical industries will need to phase out medically important antimicrobial use by January 1, 2017.

China

China produces and consumes the most antibiotics of all countries.

Antibiotic use has been measured by checking the water near factory farms in China. Measurements have also been taken from animal dung.

Half of the antibiotics manufactured in China are used in the production of livestock.

It was calculated that 38.5 million kg (or 84.9 million lbs) of antibiotics were used in China's swine and poultry production in 2012.

India

In 2012 India manufactured about a third of the total amount of antibiotics in the world.

Brazil

Brazil is the world's largest exporter of beef and the government regulates antibiotic use in the cattle production industry.

Concerns about Antibiotic Resistance

More recently, there has been increased concern about the use of anti-microbials in animals (including pets, livestock, and companion animals) contributing to the rise in antibiotic resistant infections in humans. The use of antimicrobials has been linked to the rise of resistance in every drug and species where it has been studied, including humans and livestock. However, the role of antibiotic use in food animals – in contrast to the use of antibiotics in humans – in the rise of resistant infections in humans is in dispute. The use of antimicrobials in various forms is widespread throughout animal industry, and is presented as key to preventing animal suffering and economic loss. It is linked by some activist groups to animal welfare concern, large scale commercial agriculture, international food trade, agricultural protectionist laws, environmental protection (including climate change) and other topics, which make the aims of some groups on both sides of the debate difficult to untangle.

Around 70% of all antibiotics administered are used for livestock. Most of the drugs that are given to livestock are misused and incorporated into their diets daily for the purpose of weight gain or to treat illnesses. The overuse of the antibiotic in livestock is harmful to humans because it creates an antibiotic resistant bacteria that can be transferred through several different ways such as: raw meats, consumption of meats, or it can also be airborne. Waste from food-producing animals can also contain antibiotic-resistant bacteria and is sometimes stored in lagoons. This waste is often sprayed as fertilizer and can thus contaminate crops and water with the antibiotic-resistant bacteria. Antibiotic resistance is harmful to humans because it makes them resistant to certain types of drugs for different diseases, and makes it harder for them to fight off infections.

The World Health Organization has published a list of Critically Important Antimicrobials for Human Medicine with the intent that it be used "as a reference to help formulate and prioritize risk assessment and risk management strategies for containing antimicrobial resistance due to human and non-human antimicrobial use."

Positions of Advocates for Restricting Antibiotic Use

The practice of using antibiotics for growth stimulation is problematic for these reasons:

- it is the largest use of antimicrobials worldwide
- subtherapeutic use of antibiotics results in bacterial resistance

- every important class of antibiotics are being used in this way, making every class less effective
- the bacteria being changed harm humans

Donald Kennedy, former director of the United States Food and Drug Administration, has said "There's no question that routinely administering non-therapeutic doses of antibiotics to food animals contributes to antibiotic resistance." David Aaron Kessler, another former director of the FDA, said that "We have more than enough scientific evidence to justify curbing the rampant use of antibiotics for livestock, yet the food and drug industries are not only fighting proposed legislation to reduce these practices, they also oppose collecting the data."

In 2013 the United States Centers for Disease Control and Prevention (CDC) published a white paper discussing antibiotic resistance threats in the US and calling for "improved use of antibiotics" among other measures to contain the threat to human health. The CDC asked leaders in agriculture, healthcare, and other disciplines to work together to combat the issue of increasing antibiotic resistance.

Some scientists have said that "all therapeutic antimicrobial agents should be available only by prescription for human and veterinary use."

The Pew Charitable Trusts have stated that "hundreds of scientific studies conducted over four decades demonstrate that feeding low doses of antibiotics to livestock breeds antibiotic-resistant superbugs that can infect people. The FDA, the U.S. Department of Agriculture and the Centers for Disease Control and Prevention all testified before Congress that there is a definitive link between the routine, non-therapeutic use of antibiotics in food animal production and the challenge of antibiotic resistance in humans."

Moderate Positions

The World Organisation for Animal Health has acknowledged the need to protect antibiotics but argued against a total ban on antibiotic use in animal production.

Positions of Advocates for Status Quo

In 2011 the National Pork Producers Council, an American trade association, has said "Not only is there no scientific study linking antibiotic use in food animals to antibiotic resistance in humans, as the U.S. pork industry has continually pointed out, but there isn't even adequate data to conduct a study." The statement contradicts scientific consensus, and was issued in response to a United States Government Accountability Office report that asserts "antibiotic use in food animals contributes to the emergence of resistant bacteria that may affect humans".

The National Pork Board, a Government-owned corporation of the United States, has said that "the vast majority of producers use (antibiotics) appropriately."

Effects of Restricting Antibiotic Use

When government regulation restricts use of antibiotics the negative economic impact is not often considered.

Regulation of antibiotics in livestock production would affect the business models of corporations including Tyson Foods, Cargill, and Hormel.

Difficulties with Determining Relevant Facts

It is difficult to set up a comprehensive surveillance system for measuring rates of change in antibiotic resistance. The US Government Accountability Office published a report in 2011 stating that government and commercial agencies had not been collecting sufficient data to make a decision about best practices.

Currently there is no regulatory agency in the United States that systematically collects detailed data on antibiotic use in humans and animals. It is not clear which antibiotics are prescribed for which purpose and at what time. Furthermore, the world has no surveillance infrastructure to monitor emerging antibiotic resistance threats. Because of these issues, it is difficult to quantify antibiotic resistance, to regulate antibiotic prescribing practices, and to detect and respond to rising threats.

Specific Resistance that has been Identified and Human Impact

There have been many studies that document antibiotic resistant bacteria in livestock, though the impact of the different bacteria in humans is still undergoing research. At this time, the most well-documented impact on humans is foodborne gastrointestinal illness. In most cases, these illnesses are mild and do not require antibiotics; though if the infectious bacteria is drug-resistant, research has shown that these bacteria have increased virulence (ability to cause disease), leading to prolonged illness. Furthermore, in approximately 10% of cases, the disease becomes severe, requiring more advanced treatments. These treatments can take the form of intravenous antibiotics, supportive care for blood infections, and hospital stays, leading to higher costs and greater morbidity with a trend toward higher mortality. Severe disease with this outcome is more common with drug-resistant bacteria. Though all people are susceptible, populations shown to be at higher risk for severe disease include children, the elderly, and those with chronic disease.

Over the past 20 years, the most common drug-resistant foodborne bacteria in industrialized countries have been non-typhoidal salmonella and campylobacter. Research has consistently shown the main contributing factors are bacteria sourced in livestock. One example of this was a 1998 outbreak of multidrug-resistant salmonella in Denmark linked back to two Danish swine herds. Coupled with the discovery of this link, there have been improved monitoring systems that have helped to quantify the impact. In the United States, it is estimated that there are approximately 400,000 cases and over 35,000 hospitalizations per year attributable to increasing resistant strains of salmonella and campylobacter. In terms of financial impact in the US, the treatment of non-typhoidal salmonella infections alone is now estimated to cost $365 million per year. In light of this, in its inaugural 2013 report on antibiotic resistance threats in the United States, the CDC identified resistant non-typhoidal salmonella and campylobacter as "serious threats" and called for improved surveillance and intervention in food production moving forward.

There are other bacteria as well, where research is evolving and revealing that bacterial resistance acquired through use in livestock may be contributing to disease in humans. Examples of these include Enterococcus, E. coli 0157 and Staphylococcus Aureus. In the case of foodborne illness from E.coli, though it is still not typically treated with antibiotics because of associated risk of renal failure, increasing rates of antibiotic resistant infections have been correlated with increasing virulence of the bacteria. In the case of enterococcus and staphylococcus aureus, resistant forms of both of these bacteria have resulted in greatly increasing morbidity and mortality in the US. At this point, there have been studies, though a limited number, that definitively link antibiotic use in food production to these resistance patterns in humans and further research will help to further characterize this relationship.

Mechanisms for Transfer to Humans

Humans can be exposed to antibiotic-resistant bacteria by ingesting them through the food supply. Dairy products, ground beef and poultry are the most common foods harboring these pathogens. There is evidence that a large proportion of resistant *E. coli* isolates causing blood stream infections in people are from livestock produced as food.

When manure from antibiotic-fed swine is used as fertilizer elsewhere, the manure may be contaminated with bacteria which can infect humans.

Studies have also shown that direct contact with livestock can lead to the spread of antibiotic-resistant bacteria from animals to humans.,

Action and Advocacy by Country

Legislation and activism worldwide have aimed at restricting antibiotic use in livestock.

European Union

On 1 January 2006 the European Union banned the non-medicinal use of antibiotics in livestock production.

United States

Some grocery stores have policies about voluntarily not selling meat produced by using antibiotics to stimulate growth. In 2012 in the United States advocacy organization Consumers Union organized a petition asking the store Trader Joe's to discontinue the sale of meat produced with antibiotics.

The U.S. Animal Drug User Fee Act was passed by Congress in 2008 and requires that drug manufacturers report all sales of antibiotics into the food animal production industry.

Some proposed legislation in the US has failed to be adopted. The Animal Drug and Animal Generic Drug User Fee Reauthorization Act of 2013 proposes other regulation.

In the United States the danger of emergence of antibiotic-resistant bacterial strains due to wide use of antibiotics to promote weight gain in livestock was determined by the United States Food and Drug Administration in 1977, but nothing effective was done to prevent the practice. In March, 2012 the United States District Court for the Southern

District of New York, ruling in an action brought by the Natural Resources Defense Council and others, ordered the FDA to revoke approvals for the use of antibiotics in livestock which violated FDA regulations.On 11 April 2012 the FDA announced a program to phase out unsupervised use of drugs as feed additives and, on a voluntary basis, convert approved uses for antibiotics to therapeutic use only, requiring veterinarian supervision of their use and a prescription.

In response to consumer concerns about the use of antibiotics in poultry, in 2007, Perdue removed all human antibiotics from its feed and launched the Harvestland brand, under which it sold products that met the requirements for an "antibiotic-free" label. By 2014, Perdue had also phased out ionophores (antibiotics used in animals to lower production costs by promoting growth, and preventing disease) from its hatchery and began using the "antibiotic free" labels on its Harvestland, Simply Smart and Perfect Portions products. By 2015, 52% of the company's chickens were raised without the use of any type of antibiotics.

In 1970 the FDA started recommending that antibiotic use in livestock be limited but set no actual regulations governing this recommendation. Further, in 2004 the Government Accountability Office (GAO) heavily critiqued the FDA for not collecting enough information and data on antibiotic use in factory farms. From this the GAO concluded that the FDA does not have enough information to create effective policy changes regarding antibiotic use. In response to this the FDA insisted that more research was being conducted and voluntary efforts within the industry would solve the problem of antibiotic resistance.

China

In 2012, U.S. News & World Report described the Chinese government's regulation of antibiotics in livestock production as "weak".

India

In 2011 the Indian government proposed a "National policy for containment of antimicrobial resistance". Other policies set schedules for requiring that food producing animals not be given antibiotics for a certain amount of time before their food goes to market. A study released by Centre for Science and Environment (CSE) on 30 July 2014 found antibiotic residues in chicken. This study claims that Indians are developing resistance to antibiotics — and hence falling prey to a host of otherwise curable ailments. Some of this resistance might be due to large-scale unregulated use of antibiotics in the poultry industry. CSE finds that India has not set any limits for antibiotic residues in chicken and says that India will have to implement a comprehensive set of regulations including banning of antibiotic use as growth promoters in the poultry industry. Not doing this will put lives of people at risk.

Brazil

Antibiotic resistant bacteria have been found in Brazilian cattle.

South Korea

In 1998 some researchers reported use in livestock production was a factor in the high prevalence of antibiotic resistant bacteria in Korea. In 2007 *The Korea Times* noted that Korea has relatively high usage of antibiotics in livestock production. In 2011 the Korean government banned the use of antibiotics as growth promoters in livestock.

New Zealand

In 1999 the New Zealand government issued a statement that they would not then ban the use of antibiotics in livestock production. In 2007 ABC Online reported on antibiotic use in chicken production in New Zealand.

Research into Alternatives

Increasing concern due to the emergence of antibiotic resistant bacteria has led researchers to look for alternatives to using antibiotics in livestock. Probiotics, cultures of a single bacteria strain or mixture of different strains, are being studied in livestock as a production enhancer. Prebiotics are non-digestible carbohydrates. The carbohydrates are mainly made up of oligosaccharides which are short chains of monosaccharides. The two most commonly studied prebiotics are fructooligosaccharides (FOS) and mannanoligosaccharides (MOS). FOS has been studied for use in chicken feed. MOS works as a competitive binding site, as bacteria bind to it rather than the intestine and are carried out.

Bacteriophages are able to infect most bacteria and are easily found in most environments colonized by bacteria, and have been studied as well.

In another study it was found that using probiotics, competitive exclusion, enzymes, immunomodulators and organic acids prevents the spread of bacteria and can all be used in place of antibiotics. Another research team was able to use bacteriocins, antimicrobial peptides and bacteriophages in the control of bacterial infections. While further research is needed in this field, alternative methods have been identified in effectively controlling bacterial infections in animals. All of the alternative methods listed pose no known threat to human health and all can lead the elimination of antibiotics in factory farms. With further research it is highly likely that a cost effective and health effective alternative could and will be found.

MALLEIN

The mallein test is a sensitive and specific clinical test for glanders, a common bacterial disease of equids (horses, donkeys, mules). This test is an allergic hypersensitivity test used as a diagnosis for glanders. It is caused by a bacterium called Burkholderia mallei, which is contagious for humans and other species. The occurrence of glanders must be reported to the World Organisation for Animal Health. Mallein, a protein fraction of B. mallei, is usually injected by an eye-drop. If an animal is infected, the animal will show swelling in the eye from around 48 hours of injection and may be accompanied by secretion and conjunctivitis. Mallein is non toxic to normal animals.

Mallein was discovered in 1890. Before 1934, glanders was widespread. In the early 1900s, glanders was common in Europe, the United States of America, and Canada, and has been successfully eliminated by mass testing and the slaughter and destruction of campaigns. Glanders is still present in Asia, the Middle East and South America

Limitations and Benefits

Limitations

Although Mallein is the most commonly used form of testing for glanders, cross reactions were reported between *Burkholderia mallei* and *Streptococcus equi*, which is a bacteria-caused contagious upper respiratory tract infection of equines. This resulted in false-positive reactions.

Benefits

The specificity of Mallein tests and the efficiency and potency of it are connected to the "molecular weight of protein fractions, antigenic range, and virulence".

Test Procedures and Methods

- Preparation of crude mallein
- Purification of malleo proteins
- Trichloroacetic acid (TCA) preparation
- Ammonium sulfate precipitation
- Gel filtration chromatography
- Sensitization of animals
- Potency test
- Intradermopalpebral

TRADITIONAL CHINESE VETERINARY MEDICINE

Traditional Chinese veterinary medicine (TCVM) is the ancient veterinary treatment of animals based on the same theories as traditional Chinese medicine (TCM). TCM and TCVM have developed over a period of over 3,500 years and are practiced all over the world. In Western cultures such as the U.S., TCVM has rapidly grown as an adjunct therapeutic modality for animals that do not respond favorably to typical Western veterinary treatments.

Chinese philosophical truths based on Taoism are the underpinnings that influence the practice of TCVM. The fundamental truth for health in TCVM is balance—balance within yourself, balance with others, balance with your diet, and balance with nature.

TCVM practices include four major fundamental branches: Chinese food therapy, acupuncture, herbal therapy,and Tui na ("twee-na")

Its counterpart TCM includes other such treatments as herbal medicine (中药), acupuncture, dietary therapy, and both tui-na and shiatsu massage. Qigong and Taijiquan are also closely associated with TCM.

TCVM has evolved simultaneously with the evolution of TCM. TCVM originated thousands of years ago through meticulous observation of nature, the cosmos, and the human body. Major contributing theories that apply to the practice of both TCM and TCVM include: the Yin-yang theory, the five-element theory, the human body Channel system, Zang-Fu organ physiology, six confirmations, four layers, etc.

Food Therapy

Food therapy is the art and science of combining foods based on their inherent energetic properties. Unlike Western medicine, food is an integral component of treating and preventing disease in TCVM. The Eastern world is focused on the effect food has on the body after it is eaten. Each food item is described as having energetic properties such as warming, cooling, or flavors that act on the body in certain predictable yet different ways. Various food combinations may be used to maintain and support the balance of yin and yang thereby maintaining optimal health. When disease occurs, certain food combinations may be employed to return the body to a balanced state. Food therapy is one of the five fundamental branches of TCVM and a powerful component of the TCVM treatment regime.

Acupuncture

Acupuncture is an ancient form of medicine using small filiform needles placed at predetermined points on the body. The goal of acupuncture is to move Qi—the force that makes us alive. Western medicine has no equivocal term to describe Qi. Qi flows throughout the body along meridians, or paths that interconnect the external surface of the body with the internal organs. When needles are placed in points, Qi moves freely. As Qi moves freely, the body maintains its balance, or homeostasis.

Herbal Therapy

Herbal therapy is the use of therapeutic medicines derived from plants, animals, and substances occurring in the natural environment. Herbs are used to move Qi as well as tonify Yin and Yang. Yin and yang are equal yet opposing forces that occur in all naturally occurring phenomena. For instance, Yin corresponds to nighttime, cold, or resting of the body. Yang, on the other hand, corresponds to daytime, heat, and activity of the body. Whenever Yin or Yang becomes deficient or excessive, the balance of the body is lost, and disease results. Herbs are used to restore this natural balance. The Western equivalent to Chinese herbs is pharmaceutical drugs, such as antibiotics and anti-inflammatory medicines. Both western drugs and Chinese herbs are prescribed based on a medical diagnosis. Lately, Western herbals have become popular in the United States. However, distinct differences exist between Western and Chinese herbs. Western herbs are used in a singular form to treat symptoms of disease without a medical diagnosis. Chinese herbs are often a formula or mixture of herbs prescribed according to a medical diagnosis. Generally, in treating a patient, acupuncture is used in conjunction with herbal medicine.

Tui-Na

Tui-Na is medical manipulation with the hands much like the modern versions of Western chiropractic and massage therapy. Various techniques are employed to massage the meridians and enhance the flow of Qi throughout the body. Certified Tui-Na practitioners often teach pet owners several techniques to use at home to enhance the treatment of disease.

Qi-Gong

Qi-Gong is the combination of exercise and meditation in which the flow of Qi is improved. It also is a way to balance the yin and yang of the body. This branch of Traditional Chinese Medicine does not apply to animals.

HISTORY OF VETERINARY MEDICINE IN THE PHILIPPINES

The history of veterinary medicine in the Philippines discusses the history of veterinary medicine as a profession in the Philippines. Its history in the Philippines began in 1828, while the Philippines was still a colony of Spain, progressing further during the time when the Philippines became a territory of the United States, until the establishment of the Philippines as an independent Republic in the modern-day era.

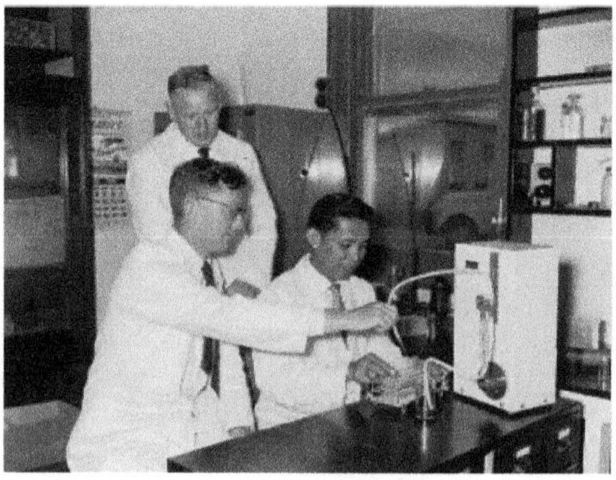

Filipino veterinary physician Dr. Alejandrino S. Quizon, Colombo Plan Fellow and a research veterinarian with the Laboratory Services Division of the Philippines Bureau of Animal Industries, was photographed in 1959 while he was nearing the end of a four-month Australian tour during which he had been studying cattle diseases. In the picture above, Dr. Quizon prepares to carry out a blood test while being assisted by two bacteriologists from the Queensland Animal Research Institute, namely Mr. G. C. Simmons, standing at rear, and Mr. C. G. Ludford, on the left.

Spanish Era (1521–1898)

Although there was a Spanish Royal Decree that was issued on May 31, 1828 assigning that there should be one veterinarian for the Philippine islands (a number later increased to two veterinarians in 1843), the highlight of the history of veterinary medicine in the Philippines was in 1888, when the need to investigate the occurrence of the Rinderpest epizootic (cattle plague) in the Philippine islands emerged. The cattle plague that affected the cow and carabao (water buffalo) population between Manila and Bulacan were caused by sick animals that were imported from Indochina and Hong Kong. The Commission assigned to perform the investigation was appointed by Don Benigno Quiroga y Ballesteros, the Director General of the Administraction Civil de Filipinas (Civil Administration of the Philippines) during that time. The Commission was composed of an army veterinarian, a pharmacist, and a medical doctor. The army veterinarian and head of the Commission was Don Gines Geis y Gotzens. The pharmacist was Don Anacleto del Rosario y Sales, who at the time was the Director of the Laboratorio Municipal de Manila (Municipal Laboratory of Manila). The physician was Don Francisco Masip, an official in-charge of public health. The 1888 cattle plague (also known as steppe murrain) prompted the need for the services of veterinarians in the Philippines, including those from the ranks (commissioned officers) of the Spanish Army. The effects of the plague lasted from 1888 through 1939, meaning it moved on from Spanish period up to the American period in the history of the Philippines. From 1901 to 1902 alone, more than 600,000 cattle and water buffaloes were killed by the disease.

American Era (1898–1946)

Veterinary Functions

American occupation of the Philippines began in 1898. During the American period in Philippine history (1898-1946), the American government established the a veterinary department in 1899, a part of the Board of Health, the office that was in-charge of public health and safety. The government of the United States sent groups of American veterinary doctors to the Philippines to function as inspectors of cattle imported through Manila, as inspectors of both locally butchered and imported beef, as caretakers of the health of animals owned by the government (including the horses of American soldiers), and as sanitary inspectors of public and private stables. In 1899, 60 civilian American veterinarians were working hand-in-hand with the United States Army's Veterinary Corps. In 1905, the veterinary department was placed under the management of the Bureau of Agriculture (known at present as the Bureau of Animal Industry).

Philippine Veterinary Medical Association

On September 7, 1907, the Philippine Veterinary Medical Association (PVMA) was established by a group composed of veterinarians from the US Army and veterinarians from the Insular Government. At the time, the acting Chief Veterinarian was Dr. C.M. Richards, and the chief of the Animal Husbandry Division was Dr. Frank C. Gearhart.

First Veterinary School

In 1908, the College of Veterinary Science of the University of the Philippines was founded. On September 1, 1910, Dr. George E. Nesom, the first president of the Philippine Veterinary Medical Association (PVMA) and who was also the first Director of the Bureau of Agriculture was appointed as the chairman of the Committee on Forage and Committee on Beef, a committee that was a component of the Board of Officers of the Civil Government of the Philippines and the United States Army.

The UP College of Veterinary Science (later became known as the UP College of Veterinary Medicine) started to offer classes in 1910. Its first dean was Archibald Ward, an American veterinarian licensed to practice in the Philippines. Two other Americans after Ward became deans of the college. The college was first housed in Pandacan, Manila, which was later transferred to the Barlett Building built in Diliman, Quezon City (the Barlett Building was named after Murray Barlett, the first president of the University of the Philippines), before the college was moved to its current location in Los Baños, Laguna. The Veterinary Teaching Hospital (VTH) stayed in Diliman, Quezon City. From 1910 to 1960, the UP College of Veterinary Science was the only school of veterinary medicine in the Philippines. Between 1910 and 1960, the college produced 450 veterinarians. Among them was Dr. Teodulio Topacio, Sr. Topacio, Sr. was one of the first four Filipinos to enroll in and graduated from the UP College of Veterinary Science.

Curriculum

The curriculum of the college for the Doctor of Veterinary Medicine (DVM) course started as a five-year education program. It became a four-year course in 1920. It became a six-year course in 1926 due to the combination of two degrees, namely the Bachelor of Science in Agriculture and the degree in Doctor of Veterinary Medicine. In 1960, the BS degree in Agriculture was removed but the course remained as a six-year program. The first two years of the 1960 program was pre-veterinary education involving studies of the liberal arts and the natural sciences, followed by a four-year intensive veterinary training studies.

Veterinary Regulation Board

As of February 11, 1913, the practice of veterinary medicine in the Philippines was being regulated by Public Act No. 2245, and resulted in the creation of the Veterinary Examining Board. The Veterinary Examining Board begun to function on November 4, 1913. The board was composed of appointees chosen by the Governor-General and was supervised administratively by the Director of Agriculture. The board was later managed by the Department of Agriculture and Commerce because of Public Act No. 4007, transferring the authority to appoint board members to its Department Secretary.

Pioneer Veterinarians

By 1914, apart from the first graduates of the UP College of Veterinary Science which included Dr. Teodulio Topacio, Sr., other Filipinos started to become active in the field of veterinary medicine in the Philippines. Some of them graduated from schools of medicine in the United States, such as Dr. Victor A. Buencamino (a graduate from the New York State College of Veterinary Medicine at Cornell University, 1911), Dr. Vicente G. Ferriols (a graduate from the Iowa State College of Agriculture and Mechanic Arts, 1912), Dr. Ventura T. Gatchalian, and Dr. Sixto N. Almeda Carlos (a graduate from The San Francisco Veterinary College, 1916). A Spaniard veterinarian residing in the Philippines, Mariano Juan Francisco Muñoz y Tomen, was also active in the Philippines in 1914. Some Filipino veterinarians stayed in the Philippines to practice their profession. Others migrated to the United States, Australia, and other countries that has a demand for their services.

Military Veterinarians

In 1916, the veterinarian members of the Veterinary Corps of the US Army assigned to the Philippines were given military ranks (they previously did not have ranks in the US Army) and thus became commissioned military officers through the efforts of Dr. William Proctor Hill, the president of PVMA from 1910 to 1911. Dr. Hill, a graduate from the Ontario Veterinary College in Canada, was an advocate for the "regulation of the practice of veterinary medicine and surgery" in the Philippines.

Filipino Veterinary Officials

From 1907 to 1917, the PVMA were managed by American officials only. In 1918, two Filipinos (Dr. Victor A. Buencamino as vice-president and Dr. Sixto N. Almeda Carlos as treasure) became officers of the PVMA. In 1919, all officers of the PVMA were Filipinos: Dr. Victor A. Buencamino became the PVMA president while Dr. Vicente G. Ferriols became the vice-president; the two other Filipino PVMA officers elected were Dr. Angel K. Gomez (as secretary) and Dr. Santiago B. Montemayor (as treasurer).

Independent Philippine-Republics era (1946-Present)

Other Veterinary Schools

The Philippines became an independent nation on July 4, 1946. In the 1970s, there were already three veterinary schools in the Philippines. Apart from the first College of Veterinary Science that was established by the University of the Philippines in 1908, the other two were the veterinary colleges of the University of Eastern Philippines and of the Araneta University.

Regulation and Ethics

During the years of the Fifth Philippine Republic (1986–present), the regulatory law called Public Act No. 2245 of 1913 was replaced by Philippine Republic Act No. 3892 on February 23, 1992. RA No. 3892 had also become known as the *An Act to Regulate the Practice of Veterinary Medicine and Surgery in the Philippines.* The Philippine

Veterinary Medical Association that was founded in 1907 became an incorporation and became known as Philippine Veterinary Medical Association, Inc. On February 23, 1992 when the PMVA, Inc. ratified the Code of Ethics that should be followed by veterinary medicine professionals in the Philippines. The first members of the Philippine veterinary medicine Board of Ethics were Dr. Santiago Y. Rotea, Dr. Faustino Turla, and Dr. Anacleto B. Coronel, with Dr. Rotea functioning as chairman of the board.

Veterinary Organizations

Several chapters of PVMA, Inc. had been established as the profession of veterinary medicine progressed during the period of modern-day Philippines. There had been a number of veterinary associations that become affiliates to PVMA, Inc. The first association to be affiliated to PVMA, Inc. was the Cebu Veterinary Medical Society, founded in November 1963 and was then headed by Dr. Nestor R. Alonzo as its president while seconded by Dr. Rosalio C. Mandin as vice-president.

From 1974 onward, there had been other independent veterinary organizations that affiliated themselves with PVMA, Inc. Among them were the City Veterinarians League (CVL, established in 1975), the Veterinary Practitioners Association of the Philippines (VPAP, established in 1972, formerly known as the Veterinary Private Practitioners Association when it was founded by private veterinary medicine practitioners), the Veterinary Women's League (VWL, established in 1973, which later became known as the Philippine Veterinary Women's Association, PVWA), the Philippine Animal Hospital Association (PAHA, established in 1978) and the Philippine Society of Veterinary Diagnosticians (PSVD, registered with PVMA, Inc. in 1981), the Veterinary Quarantine Officers of the Philippines (VQOP, established in 1986), and the Davao Veterinary Private Practitioners Association (DVPPA, established in 1984).

HISTORY OF VETERINARY MEDICINE IN PENNSYLVANIA

The history of veterinary medicine in Pennsylvania officially began with the development of the profession in the early 1800s.

Early Veterinarians in Pennsylvania

By the early 19th century, graduate veterinarians (most from London) had started to infiltrate the American cities; many of these became prominent practitioners. With the absence of veterinary schools, young men served an apprenticeship under the best of these English Veterinarians, and went on to become practitioners themselves. There were graduate medical doctors that used their knowledge to treat animals and there were some who treated "man and beast". Most of the practitioners in the outlying areas were self-taught or not taught at all. When the process of printing became available, books on horse medicine made some contribution to the knowledge of the practitioners. In 1735, Ben Franklin advertised the reprinting of Gentleman's Pocket Ferrier which described "how to use your horse on a journey and what remedies are proper for common misfortunes that may beset him on the road."

The following quote was taken from the preface of the American Ferrier by Augustus Franklin, printed in Strasburg in 1803.

"Few subjects in the common affairs of life relating to property more immediately connects itself with the interest of individuals than an efficient knowledge of a number of means to repel such a variety of diseases as are incident to horses; and, yet, few there are who have made themselves acquainted with them, not withstanding their repeated losses, to the great injury of their circumstances – in many instances – and their excruciating suffering in their poor beasts."

This sentence and the next from the same book: "Where any surgical or medical operation is necessary for your beast, I would recommend the most mild course of it."

Individuals were pressing for scientific veterinary knowledge. The memoirs of the Philadelphia Agricultural Society, published for the first thirty years of the 19th century, contained many articles on animal diseases. Richard Peters (1770–1848), was largely responsible for this trend toward veterinary medicine at the Society meetings. He was president of the Society in 1805 and was a dominant figure promoting his pet project for many years. Peters repeatedly stressed the need for veterinary school because he realized the caliber of self-styled animal doctors. He knew that the only solution to the animal disease problem was the establishment of schools to train veterinarians.

In 1806, the Philadelphia Society offered a gold medal for "the best essay and plan for promoting veterinary knowledge." In reply to the offer, Dr. Benjamin Rush (1746–1813), introduced a series of lectures to his medical students at the University of Pennsylvania, on Studying Diseases of Domestic Animals.

Peters and Rush were the great benefactors of veterinary medicine, then their friend, Dr. James Mease, was an early investigator of disease outbreaks. In 1793, he recognized rabies as being caused by the bite of a mad dog. In his appeal for improving veterinary medicine, Mease made this statement to the Philadelphia Agricultural Society on November 3, 1813: "The veterinary art is a practical application of scientific principles, to the preservation of the health of domestic animals, and to the cure of their diseases, in the same manner as the art of medicine applies to the health and preservation of man; and the science in which this art is grounded, and which it requires for its perfect exercise, comprise the natural history, anatomy, physiology, and pathology of those animals, together with such portions of the vegetable or mineral kingdoms as are connected with them, either in the way of ailment or remedy."

One of Pennsylvania's most well known veterinarians was Dr. Isaiah Michener. It is unknown how he learned veterinary medicine but he started his practice in 1836. he contributed articles to the Philadelphia and country newspapers under column titles, *The Veterinarian* and *The Observer*. He wrote: "Companies have been formed, funds obtained almost everywhere to build a theatre, construct a railroad or dig a canal ... but the paramount interest of every agriculturist, the preservation of his livestock from the ravages of disease, is almost totally neglected. When will the farmer study his own business?"

Development of the Profession

By the mid-1800s, Philadelphia and other large cities of Pennsylvania had veterinarians who were scientists and practiced medicine based on the knowledge available from wizards in that area. But the vast majority of practitioners throughout the valleys of the state were inexpert and uneducated. It was decades before trained people filtered in. it would take close to a century for the graduate veterinarians to live down some of the unprofessional habits of their predecessors. It can only be said that a few were self-educated and experienced. It has been written that the armies of Europe were aware of the value of veterinary care as early as the 3rd century, but it took the United States Army until the Civil War to reach that conclusion. It was not until 1835 that the word "veterinarian" even appeared in an Army Regulation. That regulation required inspectors to see that "veterinarians perform their duties." It took more than one hundred years after the formation of the first Regiment of Light Dragoons to really identify a "blacksmith" and a "Ferrier". The blacksmith was held in such little regard by the Continental Congress that the Congress would not allows civilians hired by the Quartermaster to have their horses shod at government expense. "A little neglect may breed mischief: for want of a nail the shoe was lost; for want of a shoe the horse was lost; and for want of a horse the rider was lost."- Benjamin Franklin, 1757.

Horses continued to play a greater role in the U.S. Army. Finally, one hundred and three years after the first regiment of dragoons, the following paragraph appeared in General Orders Number 36, 1879: "Hereafter appointments as veterinary surgeons will be confined to the graduates of established and reputable veterinary medicine schools and colleges."

A charter was obtained from the Pennsylvania Legislature for the Veterinary College of Philadelphia. This was the first charter of its kind issued in the United States, but the school never graduated a student and subsequently lost any claim to being the first veterinary school. That honor has been singularly given to the New York College of Veterinary Surgeons, chartered in 1857 at New York University. The non-graduates were highly independent and unorganized, but the graduate veterinarians had the advantage of unity of purpose. Their leaders from Philadelphia and New York has met in 1863 to organize the United States Veterinary Medical Association. A few graduates in the Philadelphia area formed the Keystone Veterinary Medical Association, the first organized veterinary group in Pennsylvania, in 1882. Later, on August 22, 1883 a group of veterinarians joined to form the Pennsylvania Veterinary Medical Association. Twenty two veterinarians assembled to hear about the continuing education and legislative activities of veterinary conventions in other states and to consider formation of an association to conduct similar work in Pennsylvania. This was not the first time that Pennsylvania veterinarians had tried to organize. The very first veterinary association was launched in Philadelphia on May 7, 1854, by Robert Jennings. Perhaps the most successful of the PVMA's educational programs is the Mid-Atlantic States Veterinary Clinic, a one-day session of "wet" demonstrations, started in York, Pennsylvania, in 1962. Alternating annually between the York Interstate Fair Grounds in Timonium, where the clinic is sponsored by the Maryland Veterinary Medical Association, the program attracts more than 400 practitioners from at least seven states.

The need for a Veterinary college in Pennsylvania was another of the issues taken up by the PVMA in its first year of existence. There were only about three hundred graduate veterinarians in the United States 1883. The importance of strong local, state and national veterinary associations was emphasized by Dr. Hoskins in a paper presented at the keystone meeting on October 11, 1892:

"The many sudden and broad changes that have characterized the doings in the world of veterinary science during the past year seem to demand at our hands stronger consideration, stronger work. It affords us an incentive that will bring to us the end of our work a rich return, when we have properly considered and disposed of the great questions that are knocking at our doors for aid in their final dispositions. It also points strongly to the need of stronger veterinary organizations. The national one must soon tend in directions and lines that will lift it entirely from the consideration of those topics which are more or less local in character..."

The keystone has the distinction of being the first veterinary association in the country to urge "a single standard of examinations in veterinary medicine." A national board was established but it was 1955 before a standard national examination was offered. The national board of veterinary medical examiners was organized by the AVMA in 1950 with its primary objective to "elevate the standard of qualification necessary to practice by means of a comprehensive examination to be made available to licensing boards in the various states."

REFERENCES

1. FDA CVM. 2012: Guidance for Industry #209: The Judicious Use of Medically Important Antimicrobial Drugs in Food-Producing Animals.
2. http://europa.eu/rapid/press-release_IP-05-1687_en.htm
3. "Antibiotic Resistance Threats in the United States" (PDF). Centers for Disease Control and Prevention. Retrieved 30 December 2016.
4. Hamaide, Sybille de la (11 January 2012) Antibiotics for livestock vital to feed world: OIE. Reuters. Paris. Retrieved 20 April 2015.
5. Centers for Disease Control and Prevention. (2016). Antibiotic/Antimicrobial Resistance. Retrieved from http://www.cdc.gov/drugresistance/ (accessed 5.5.16).
6. Ogle, Maureen (3 September 2013). "Riots, Rage and Resistance: A Brief History of How Antibiotics Arrived on the Farm". Scientific American. Retrieved 5 November 2013. This reference should be replaced with citations to a book later published by the same author
7. Ogle, Maureen. In meat we trust : an unexpected history of carnivore America. ISBN 978-0151013401.
8. Reported locally in these:
9. "To Become Vegetarians", Mansfield (O.) News, January 17, 1910, p2
10. "150,000 at Cleveland Stop the Use of Meat" Syracuse Herald-Journal, January 25, 1910, p1
11. "Boycott on Meat is Rapidly Spreading; Men Who Are Blamed For High Price",

Atlanta Constitution, January 25, 1910, p1

12. Scully, M. (2002). Dominion: the power of man, the suffering of animals, and the call to mercy. St. Martins Griffin, New York (Book).
13. Ogle cites To meet this new consumer demand for animal meat, the improved health management has since introduced about seventeen classes of antimicrobial drugs is approved for use in food animals in the United States today.
14. "They've Doubled Gains With New Drugs". Successful Farming. 48 (6): 45. June 1950.
15. "Antibiotics Now Proved in Hog and Poultry Ratios, They're the Biggest Feeding News in 40 Years!". Successful Farming. 49 (3): 33. March 1951.
16. "Hogging It!: Estimates of Antimicrobial Abuse in Livestock". Union of Concerned Scientists. 2001.
17. Swain, Marian (2015-08-01), "Excessive use of antibiotics in livestock is creating huge problems. Here's how to fix it", Vox.com. Section "Banning all antibiotics in livestock isn't the solution".
18. Christopher D. Reinhardt, MS, PhD, Last full review/revision March 2012 Merck Veterinary Manual: Antimicrobial Feed Additives
19. Allen, Heather K.; Stanton, Thad B. (2014-01-01). "Altered egos: antibiotic effects on food animal microbiomes". Annual Review of Microbiology. 68: 297–315. doi:10.1146/annurev-micro-091213-113052. ISSN 1545-3251. PMID 25002091.
20. Reinhardt, Christopher D. (2012), "Antimicrobial Feed Additives", in Aiello, Susan E.; Moses, Michael A., Merck Veterinary Manual, Merck & Co. and Merial
21. Cromwell, G. L. (2002). "Why and How Antibiotics are Used in Swine Production". Animal Biotechnology 13 (1): 7-27. http://www.tandfonline.com/doi/full/10.1081/ABIO-120005767
22. Adjiri-Awere A., Van Lunen T. A. (2005). "Subtherapeutic use of antibiotics in pork production: Risks and alternatives". Canadian Journal of Animal Science 85 (2): 117-130. http://pubs.aic.ca/doi/abs/10.4141/A04-041
23. Graham, JP; Boland, JJ; Silbergeld, E (Jan–Feb 2007). "Growth promoting antibiotics in food animal production: an economic analysis". Public Health Reports. 122 (1): 79–87. PMID 17236612.
24. Dennis, Brady (2013-12-11), "FDA finalizes voluntary rules on phasing out certain antibiotics in livestock", Washington Post.
25. Plumer, Brad (2013-12-14), "The FDA is cracking down on antibiotics at farms. Here's what you should know.", Washington Post.
26. Govtrack.us https://www.govtrack.us/congress/bills/113/hr1150
27. "Beef Procedures: Antibiotic Use". South Dakota State University. Retrieved 2016-02-21.
28. Food and Water Watch. (2015). Antibiotic Resistance 101. Retrieved from http://www.foodandwaterwatch.org/insight/antibiotic-resistance-101 (accessed 5.5.16).

29. Regulation (EC) No 1831/2003 of the European Parliament and of the Council of 22 September 2003 on additives for use in animal nutrition. OJ L 268, 18.10.2003, p. 29–43. CELEX:32003R1831
30. Koch, Julia (20 Nov 2013). "Cutting Antibiotics: Denmark Leads Way in Healthier Pig Farming". Spiegel Online International. Retrieved 2014-05-22.
31. Cogliani,, Carol; Goossens, Herman; Christina Greko (2011). "Restricting Antimicrobial Use in Food Animals: Lessons from Europe". Microbe Magazine. Retrieved 2014-05-22.
32. Gilbert, Natasha (10 Jan 2012). "Rules tighten on use of antibiotics on farms". Nature.
33. FDA (2013)Summary Report on Antimicrobials Sold or Distributed for Use in Food-Producing Animals
34. FDA (2012) Drug Use Review
35. FDA (2003)
36. FDA (2013) Guidance for Industry #213: New Animal Drugs and New Animal Drug Combination Products Administered in or on Medicated Feed or Drinking Water of Food Producing Animals: Recommendations for Drug Sponsors for Voluntarily Aligning Product Use Conditions with GFI #209
37. FDA (2016)
38. Tatlow, Didi Kirsten (18 February 2013). "Global Health Threat Seen in Overuse of Antibiotics on Chinese Pig Farms". rendezvous.blogs.nytimes.com. Retrieved 28 August 2013.
39. Wei, R.; Ge, F.; Huang, S.; Chen, M.; Wang, R. (2011). "Occurrence of veterinary antibiotics in animal wastewater and surface water around farms in Jiangsu Province, China". Chemosphere. 82 (10): 1408–1414. doi:10.1016/j.chemosphere.2010.11.067. PMID 21159362.
40. Hu, X.; Zhou, Q.; Luo, Y. (2010). "Occurrence and source analysis of typical veterinary antibiotics in manure, soil, vegetables and groundwater from organic vegetable bases, northern China". Environmental Pollution. 158 (9): 2992–2998. doi:10.1016/j.envpol.2010.05.023. PMID 20580472.
41. Zhao, L.; Dong, Y. H.; Wang, H. (2010). "Residues of veterinary antibiotics in manures from feedlot livestock in eight provinces of China". Science of the Total Environment. 408 (5): 1069–1075. doi:10.1016/j.scitotenv.2009.11.014. PMID 19954821.
42. Wu, Alex (12 January 2012). "Livestock in China Given Too Many Antibiotics". The Epoch Times. Retrieved 28 August 2013.
43. Krishnasamy V., Otte J., Silbergeld E. (2015). "Antimicrobial use in Chinese swine and broiler poultry production". Antimicrobial Resistance and Infection Control 4 (17) http://www.aricjournal.com/content/4/1/17
44. Gale, Jason; Narayan, Adi (7 May 2012). "Drug-Defying Germs From India Speed Post-Antibiotic Era – Bloomberg". bloomberg.com. Retrieved 28 August 2013.
45. Millen, D. D.; Pacheco, R. D. L.; Meyer, P. M.; Rodrigues, P. H. M.; De Beni

Arrigoni, M. (2011). "Current outlook and future perspectives of beef production in Brazil". Animal Frontiers. 1 (2): 46. doi:10.2527/af.2011-0017.

46. Food & Water Watch. 2015: Antibiotic Resistance 101: How Antibiotic Misuse on Factory Farms Can Make You Sick 1-17.
47. Prescriptions for trouble: Using antibiotics to fatten livestock. Union of concerned Scientists. Retrieved 29 Nov 15. http://www.ucsusa.org/food_and_agriculture/our-failing-food-system/industrial-agriculture/prescription-for-trouble.html#.Vls-U79hSFU
48. World Health Organization. (2012). Critically important antimicrobials for human medicine. Retrieved from http://apps.who.int/iris/bitstream/10665/77376/1/9789241504485_eng.pdf. Accessed 4/11/16.
49. Silbergeld, E. K.; Graham, J.; Price, L. B. (2008). "Industrial Food Animal Production, Antimicrobial Resistance, and Human Health". Annual Review of Public Health. 29: 151–169. doi:10.1146/annurev.publhealth.29.020907.090904. PMID 18348709.
50. McVeigh, Karen (19 September 2012). "Scientists: overuse of antibiotics in animal agriculture endangers humans". theguardian.com. Retrieved 26 August 2013.
51. Kessler, David Aaron (27 March 2013). "Antibiotics and the Meat We Eat". The New York Times. New York City: NYTC. ISSN 0362-4331. Retrieved 26 August 2013.
52. Gilchrist, M. J.; Greko, C.; Wallinga, D. B.; Beran, G. W.; Riley, D. G.; Thorne, P. S. (2006). "The Potential Role of Concentrated Animal Feeding Operations in Infectious Disease Epidemics and Antibiotic Resistance". Environmental Health Perspectives. 115 (2): 313–316. doi:10.1289/ehp.8837. PMC 1817683 . PMID 17384785.
53. The Pew Charitable Trusts (15 October 2012). "Pew Comments on Proposed Antibiotics Legislation". pewtrusts.org. Retrieved 26 August 2013.
54. de La Hamaide, Sybille (11 January 2012). "Antibiotics for livestock vital to feed world: OIE | Reuters". reuters.com. Retrieved 28 August 2013.
55. National Pork Producers Council (15 September 2011). "Nat'l Pork Producers Council Issues Statement About GAO's Report on Antibiotic Resistance". growinggeorgia.com. Retrieved 29 August 2013.
56. Philpott, Tom (21 September 2011). "Meat Industry Still Denying Antibiotic Resistance". motherjones.com. Retrieved 29 August 2013.
57. "Antibiotic Resistance and Food Animal Production: a Bibliography of Scientific Studies (1969-2012)" (PDF). The Pew Charitable Trusts. Archived from the original (PDF) on 11 August 2012.
58. "Antibiotic Resistance: Agencies Have Made Limited Progress Addressing Antibiotic Use in Animals". U.S. Government Accountability Office. 7 September 2011. Antibiotics have saved millions of lives, but antibiotic use in food animals contributes to the emergence of resistant bacteria that may affect humans.
59. Couric, Katie (10 February 2010). "Animal Antibiotic Overuse Hurting Humans?".

CBS News. New York City: CBS. Retrieved 29 August 2013.

60. Phillips, I.; Casewell, M.; Cox, T.; De Groot, B.; Friis, C.; Jones, R.; Nightingale, C.; Preston, R.; Waddell, J. (2003). "Does the use of antibiotics in food animals pose a risk to human health? A critical review of published data". Journal of Antimicrobial Chemotherapy. 53 (1): 28–52. doi:10.1093/jac/dkg483. PMID 14657094.

61. Yukhananov, Anna (11 April 2012). "U.S. seeks voluntary antibiotic limits in livestock". reuters.com. Retrieved 28 August 2013.

62. Bax, R.; Bywater, R.; Cornaglia, G.; Goossens, H.; Hunter, P.; Isham, V.; Jarlier, V.; Jones, R.; Phillips, I.; Sahm, D.; Senn, S.; Struelens, M.; Taylor, D.; White, A. (2001). "Surveillance of antimicrobial resistance-what, how and whither?". Clinical Microbiology and Infection. 7 (6): 316–325. doi:10.1046/j.1198-743x.2001.00239.x. PMID 11442565.

63. Antibiotic Resistance: Agencies Have Made Limited Progress Addressing Antibiotic Use in Animals, U.S. Government Accountability Office, 7 September 2011, retrieved 27 August 2013

64. Molbak K. Human Health Consequences of Antimicrobial Drug-Resistant Salmonella and other Foodborne Pathogens. Food Safety. 2005. 41:1613:1620

65. Molbak K, et al. An outbreak of multidrug-resistant, quinolone-resistant Salmonella enterica serotype typhimurium DT104. New England Journal of Medicine. 1999 Nov 4;341(19):1420-5.

66. Shea K.M., (2003).Antibiotic Resistance: What is the Impact of Agricultural Uses of Antibiotics on Children's Health?, PEDIATRICS, 112 253-258

67. NARMS. National Antibiotic Resistance Monitoring System: Enteric Bacteria, Human Isolates Final Report. 2013.

68. Swartz M. Human Diseases Caused by Foodborne Pathogens of Animal Origin. Clinical Infectious Diseases. 2002. 34:S111-22.

69. Bortolaia V, et al. Human health risks associated with antimicrobial-resistant enterococci and Staphylococcus aureus on poultry meat. Clinical Microbiology and Infection. 2016 Feb;22(2):130-40.

70. Wegener H. Antibiotics in animal feed and their role in resistance development. Current Opinion in Microbiology. 2003. 6:439-445.

71. DeWaal C, Vaughn Grooters S. Antibiotic Resistance in Foodborne Pathogens. Center for Science in the Public Health Interest. May 2013.

72. Vieira, A. R.; Collignon, P.; Aarestrup, F. M.; McEwen, S. A.; Hendriksen, R. S.; Hald, T.; Wegener, H. C. (2011). "Association Between Antimicrobial Resistance inEscherichia coliIsolates from Food Animals and Blood Stream Isolates from Humans in Europe: An Ecological Study". Foodborne Pathogens and Disease. 8 (12): 1295–1301. doi:10.1089/fpd.2011.0950. PMID 21883007.

73. Zhang, S. (2013). "Pig-manure fertilizer linked to human MRSA infections". Nature. doi:10.1038/nature.2013.13752.

74. Casey JA, et al. (2013). High-Density Livestock Operations, Crop Field

Application of Manure, and Risk of Community-Associated Methicillin-Resistant Staphylococcus aureus Infection in Pennsylvania. JAMA Internal Medicine. 173(21):1980-1990.

75. Chang Q, et al. (2014). Antibiotics in agriculture and the risk to human health: how worried should we be? Evolutionary Applications. 8(3): 240-247.
76. European Commission (22 December 2005). "EUROPA – PRESS RELEASES – Press release – Ban on antibiotics as growth promoters in animal feed enters into effect". europa.eu. Retrieved 26 August 2013.
77. "Meat Without Drugs". Consumers Union. Retrieved 27 August 2013., which is described in the following works
78. Gore, Al (2013). "The Reinvention of Life and Death: Antibiotics before Swine". The Future : Six Drivers of Global Change (First edition. ed.). New York: Random House. pp. 227 and citation on 475. ISBN 9780812992946.
79. Hurd, Scott (26 June 2012). "Commentary: 'Meat without Drugs' could be inhumane". Bovine Veterinarian. Retrieved 27 August 2013. All peer-reviewed scientific risk assessments have demonstrated a negligible risk of human health harm due to livestock antibiotic use.
80. Greenaway, Twilight (20 June 2012). "Your meat on drugs: Will grocery stores cut out antibiotics?". Grist. Retrieved 27 August 2013.
81. Rogers, Laura (28 December 2012). "Laura Rogers: A New Year's Resolution: Put Animals on an Antibiotics Diet". huffingtonpost.com. Retrieved 26 August 2013.
82. Wallinga, David (12 February 2013). "David Wallinga, M.D.: Animal Antibiotic Use Continues Upwards, FDA Keeps Blinders on". huffingtonpost.com. Retrieved 27 August 2013.
83. Philpott, Tom (17 Sep 2010). "UPDATED: With the food safety bill dead, time for the FDA/USDA to grow some backbone". Grist. Retrieved 27 August 2013.
84. John Gever (23 March 2012). "FDA Told to Move on Antibiotic Use in Livestock". MedPage Today. Retrieved 24 March 2012.
85. Gardiner Harris (11 April 2012). "U.S. Tightens Rules on Antibiotics Use for Livestock". The New York Times. Retrieved 12 April 2012.
86. "FDA's Strategy on Antimicrobial Resistance – Questions and Answers". U.S. Food and Drug Administration. 11 April 2012. Retrieved 12 April 2012. "Judicious use" is using an antimicrobial drug appropriately and only when necessary; Based on a thorough review of the available scientific information, FDA recommends that use of medically important antimicrobial drugs in food-producing animals be limited to situations where the use of these drugs is necessary for ensuring animal health, and their use includes veterinary oversight or consultation. FDA believes that using medically important antimicrobial drugs to increase production in food-producing animals is not a judicious use.
87. Stephanie Strom (July 31, 2015). "Perdue Sharply Cuts Antibiotic Use in Chickens and Jabs at Its Rivals". The New York Times. Retrieved August 12, 2015.

88. "Antibiotics Position Statement". Retrieved August 12, 2015.

89. GAO. 2011: Antibiotic Resistance: Agencies Have Made Limited Progress Addressing Antibiotic Use in Animals. GAO-11-801.

90. Salamon, Maureen (11 February 2013). "China's Overuse of Antibiotics in Livestock May Threaten Human Health". health.usnews.com. Retrieved 28 August 2013.

91. Thacker, Teena (13 April 2011). "Govt wants to limit use of antibiotics in animals – Indian Express". indianexpress.com. Retrieved 28 August 2013.

92. Sinha, Kounteya (25 November 2011). "New norm to curb antibiotic resistance – Times of India". indiatimes.com. Retrieved 28 August 2013.

93. Sinha, Kounteya (6 April 2012). "In a first, antibiotics bar on food-producing animals – Times of India". indiatimes.com. Retrieved 28 August 2013.

94. "Centre For Science and Environment (CSE)". Centre for Science and Environment (CSE). 30 July 2014. Retrieved 30 July 2014.

95. Pereira, M. S. V.; Siqueira-Júnior, J. P. (1995). "Antimicrobial drug resistance in Staphylococcus aureus isolated from cattle in Brazil". Letters in Applied Microbiology. 20 (6): 391–395. doi:10.1111/j.1472-765X.1995.tb01328.x. PMID 7786507.

96. Kim, Woo Joo; Park, Seung Chull (1998). "bacterial Resistance to Antimicrobial Agents: An Overview from Korea" (PDF). Yonsei Medical Journal. 39 (6): 488–494. Retrieved 29 August 2013.

97. Won-sup, Yoon (25 June 2007). "Antibiotics in Livestock Harm Human Beings". The Korea Times. Retrieved 29 August 2013.

98. Flynn, Dan (7 June 2011). "South Korea Bans Antibiotics in Animal Feed". foodsafetynews.com. Retrieved 29 August 2013.

99. staff (7 January 1999). "NZ holds off ban on animal antibiotics – National – NZ Herald News". nzherald.co.nz. Retrieved 29 August 2013.

100. Williams, Robyn; Cook, Greg (11 August 2007). "Antibiotics and intensive chicken farming in New Zealand – The Science Show". abc.net.au. Retrieved 29 August 2013.

101. Allen H. K., Trachsel J., Looft T., Casey T. A. (2014). Finding alternatives to antibiotics. Annals of the New York Academy of Sciences 1323: 91-100. PMID 24953233

102. Hume, M. E. (2011). Historic perspective: Prebiotics, probiotics, and other alternatives to antibiotics. Poultry Science 90 (11): 2663-9. PMID 22010256

103. Griggs, J. P., Jacob, J. P. (2005) Alternatives to Antibiotics for Organic Poultry ProductionPoultry Science 14: 750-756.

104. Doyle, M.E. 2001: Alternatives to Antibiotic Use for Growth Promotion in Animal Husbandry. Food Research Institute, University of Wisconsin-Madison.

105. Joerger, R.D. 2003: Alternatives to antibiotics: bacteriocins, antimicrobial peptides and bacteriophages. Poultry Science 82(4), 640-647.

106. Tan, Michael. "Vet Med at 100". Pinoy Kasi. Philippine Daily Inquirer. Retrieved 30 November 2013.
107. Carlos, Enrique T., DVM. "PHILIPPINE VETERINARY MEDICAL ASSOCIATION, PVMA CENTENNIAL YEAR 1907-2007, HISTORY". Philippine Veterinary Medical Association. Retrieved 30 November 2013.
108. "World Factbook — Philippines". CIA. Retrieved 2008-07-24.
109. "Board of Veterinary Medicine, History". Professional Regulation Commission, Republic of the Philippines. Retrieved 30 November 2013.
110. The American Veterinary Profession: its background and development / J.F. Smithcors. Ames: Iowa State University Press, 1963.
111. American Veterinary History / by Bert W. Bierer. Madison, Wis.: Carl Olson, 1980.
112. The history of the American Association of Equine Practitioners, 1954-1979 / by Wayne O. Kester. Golden, Colo.: The Association, 1980.
113. Valuing Animals: Veterinarians and their patients in modern America / Susan D. Jones. Author: Baltimore: Johns Hopkins University Press, 2003.
114. After 1883: One hundred years of organized Veterinary Medicine. Thompson, Ray. 1982.

CHAPTER 3

Veterinary Physician

Chapter Contents

Veterinary technician a health care worker who is skilled in technical aspects of veterinary medicine and works as a professional assistant to a veterinarian or to any of various types of researchers and scientists.

INTRODUCTION

A veterinary physician, colloquially called a vet, shortened from veterinarian (American English, Australian English) or veterinary surgeon (British English), is a professional who practices veterinary medicine by treating disease, disorder, and injury in animals.

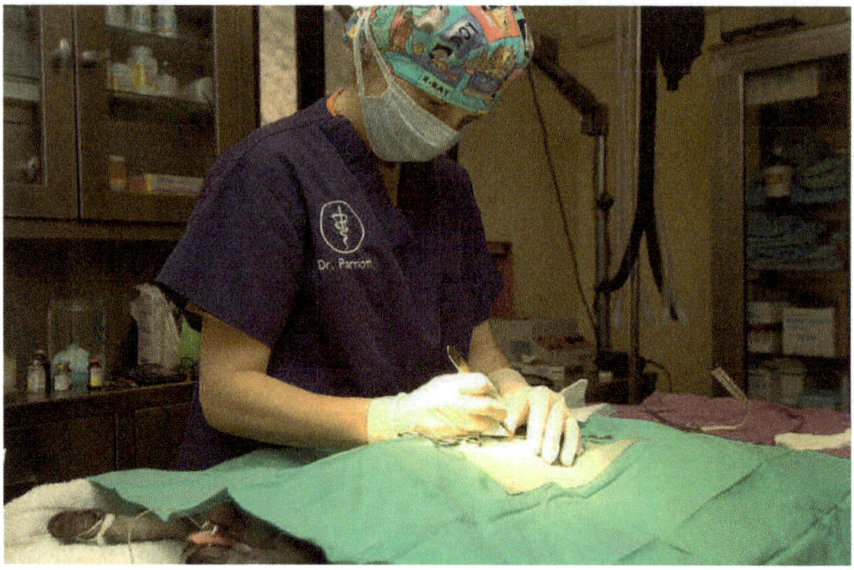

A vet conducts a routine spaying operation on a domestic cat.

DESCRIPTION

In many countries, the local nomenclature for a veterinarian is a regulated and protected term, meaning that members of the public without the prerequisite qualifications and/or licensure are not able to use the title. In many cases, the activities that may be undertaken by a veterinarian (such as treatment of illness or surgery in animals) are restricted only to those professionals who are registered as a veterinarian. For instance, in the United Kingdom, as in other jurisdictions, animal treatment may only be performed by registered veterinary physicians (with a few designated exceptions, such as paraveterinary workers), and it is illegal for any person who is not registered to call themselves a veterinarian or prescribe any treatment.

Most veterinary physicians work in clinical settings, treating animals directly. These veterinarians may be involved in a general practice, treating animals of all types; they may be specialized in a specific group of animals such as companion animals, livestock, zoo animals or equines; or may specialize in a narrow medical discipline such as surgery, dermatology or internal medicine. As with other healthcare professionals, veterinarians face ethical decisions about the care of their patients. Current debates within the profession include the ethics of certain procedures believed to be purely cosmetic or unnecessary for behavioral issues, such as declawing of cats, docking of tails, cropping of ears and debarking on dogs.

Etymology and Nomenclature

The word veterinary comes from the Latin *veterinae* meaning “working animals”. “Veterinarian” was first used in print by Thomas Browne in 1646.

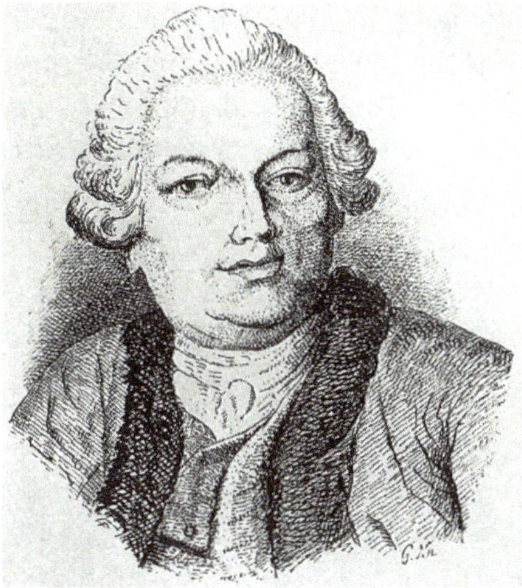

Claude Bourgelat established the earliest veterinary college in Lyon in 1761.

The first veterinary college was founded in Lyon, France in 1762 by Claude Bourgelat. According to Lupton, after observing the devastation being caused by cattle plague to the French herds, Bourgelat devoted his time to seeking out a remedy. This resulted in his founding a veterinary college in Lyon in 1761, from which establishment he dispatched students to combat the disease; in a short time, the plague was stayed and the health of stock restored, through the assistance rendered to agriculture by veterinary science and art.»

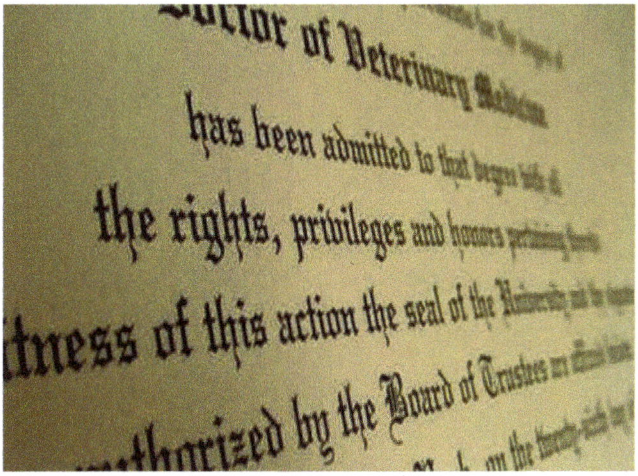
of Veterinary
has been admitted to
the rights, privileges and
of this action the seal of the
by the Board of

The Odiham Agricultural Society helped establish the veterinary profession in England.

The Odiham Agricultural Society was founded in 1783 in England to promote agriculture and industry, and played an important role in the foundation of the veterinary profession in Britain. A 1785 Society meeting resolved to "promote the study of Farriery upon rational scientific principles."

The professionalization of the veterinary trade was finally achieved in 1790, through the campaigning of Granville Penn, who persuaded the Frenchman, Benoit Vial de St. Bel to accept the professorship of the newly established Veterinary College in London. The Royal College of Veterinary Surgeons was established by royal charter in 1844.

Veterinary science came of age in the late 19th century, with notable contributions from Sir John McFadyean, credited by many as having been the founder of modern Veterinary research.

Roles and Responsibilities

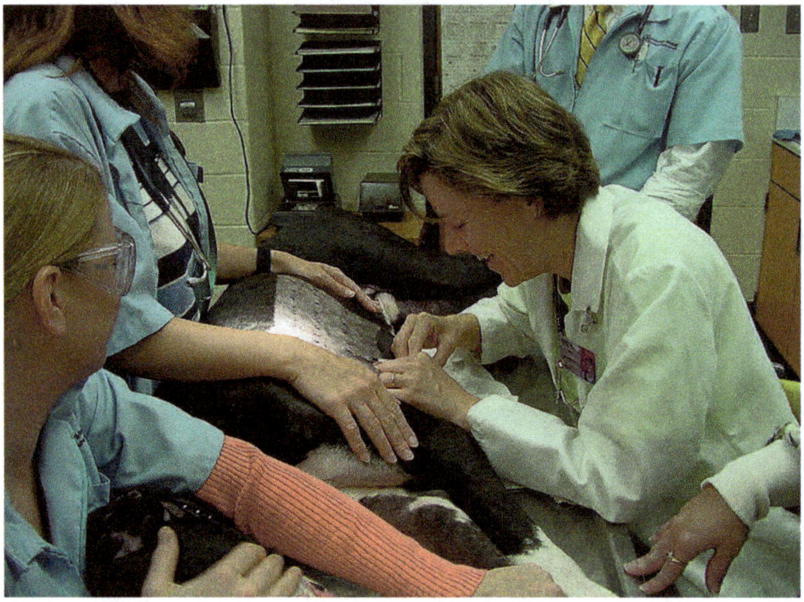

Veterinarians treat disease, disorder or injury in animals, which includes diagnosis, treatment and aftercare. The scope of practice, specialty and experience of the individual veterinarian will dictate exactly what interventions they perform, but most will perform surgery (of differing complexity).

Unlike in human medicine, veterinarians must rely primarily on clinical signs, as animals are unable to vocalize symptoms as a human would. In some cases, owners may be able to provide a medical history and the veterinarian can combine this information along with observations, and the results of pertinent diagnostic tests such as radiography, CT scans, MRI, blood tests, urinalysis and others.

Veterinarians must consider the appropriateness of euthanasia ("putting to sleep") if a condition is likely to leave the animal in pain or with a poor quality of life, or if treatment of a condition is likely to cause more harm to the patient than good, or if the patient is unlikely to survive any treatment regimen. Additionally, there are scenarios where euthanasia is considered due to the constrains of the client's finances.

As with human medicine, much veterinary work is concerned with prophylactic treatment, in order to prevent problems occurring in the future. Common interventions include vaccination against common animal illnesses, such as distemper or rabies, and dental prophylaxis to prevent or inhibit dental disease. This may also involve owner education so as to avoid future medical or behavioral issues.

Additionally veterinarians have important roles in public health and the prevention of zoonoses.

Employment

The majority of veterinarians are employed in private practice treating animals (75% of vets in the United States, according to the American Veterinary Medical Association).

Small animal veterinarians typically work in veterinary clinics, veterinary hospitals, or both. Large animal veterinarians often spend more time travelling to see their patients at the primary facilities which house them, such as zoos or farms.

Other employers include charities treating animals, colleges of veterinary medicine, research laboratories, animal food companies, and pharmaceutical companies. In many countries, the government may also be a major employer of veterinarians, such as the United States Department of Agriculture or the State Veterinary Service in the United Kingdom. State and local governments also employ veterinarians.

Focus of Practice

Veterinarians and their practices may be specialized in certain areas of veterinary medicine. Areas of focus include:

- Exotic animal veterinarian - Generally considered to include reptiles, exotic birds such as parrots and cockatoos, and small mammals such as ferrets, rabbits, chinchillas, and degus.
- Conservation medicine - The study of the relationship between animal and human health and environmental information.
- Small animal practice - Usually dogs, cats, and other companion animals/ household pets such as hamsters and gerbils. Some practices are canine-only or feline-only practices.
- Laboratory animal practice - Some veterinarians work in a university or industrial laboratory and are responsible for the care and treatment of laboratory animals of any species (often involving bovines, porcine species, felines, canines, rodents, and even exotic animals). Their responsibility is not only for the health and well being of the animals, but also for enforcing humane and ethical treatment of the animals in the facility.

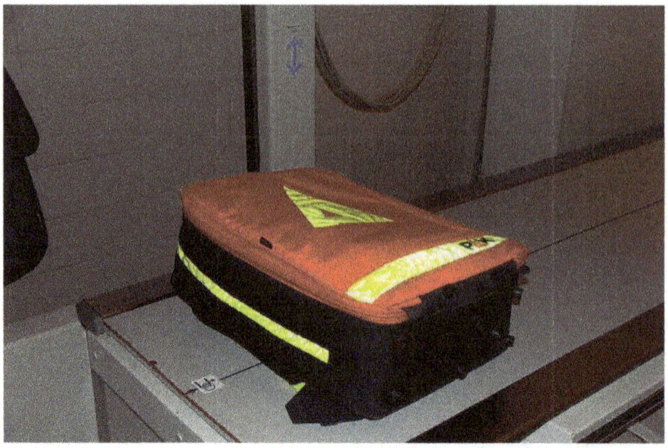

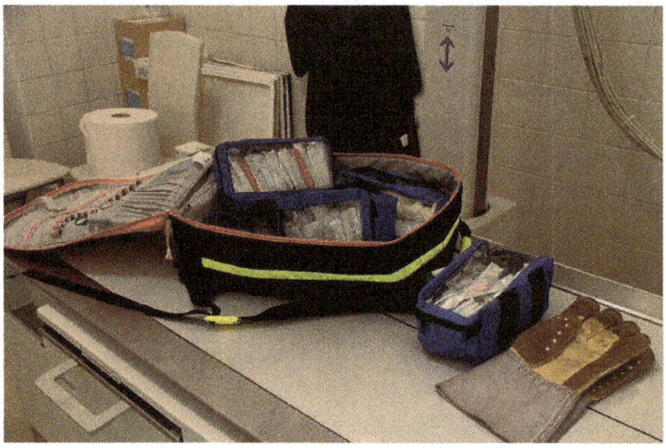

For on-call ambulance duty

- Large animal practice - Usually referring to veterinarians that work with, variously, livestock and other large farm animals, as well as equine species and large reptiles.
- Equine medicine - Some veterinarians are specialists in equine medicine. Horses are different in anatomy, physiology, pathology, pharmacology, and husbandry to other domestic species. Specialization in equine veterinary practice is something that is normally developed after qualification, even if students do have some interest before graduation.
- Food animal medicine - Some veterinarians deal exclusively or primary with animals raised for food (such as meat, milk, and eggs). Livestock practitioners may deal with ovine (sheep), bovine (cattle) and porcine (swine) species; such veterinarians deal with management of herds, nutrition, reproduction, and minor field surgery. Dairy medicine practice focuses on dairy animals. Poultry medicine practice focuses on the health of flocks of poultry; the field often involves extensive training in pathology, epidemiology, and nutrition of birds. The veterinarian treats the flock and not the individual animals.

- Food safety practice - Veterinarians are employed by both the food industry and government agencies to advise on and monitor the handling, preparation, and storage of food in ways that prevent foodborne illness.
- Wildlife medicine - A relatively recent branch of veterinary medicine, focusing on wildlife. Wildlife medicine veterinarians may work with zoologists and conservation medicine practitioners and may also be called out to treat marine species such as sea otters, dolphins, or whales after a natural disaster or oil spill.
- Aquatic medicine - mostly refers to veterinary care of fish in aquaculture (like salmon, cod, among other species), but can also include care of aquatic mammals. For certain countries with high economic income from aquaculture, this is an important part of the veterinary field (like Norway, Chile). Other countries (particularly those who are landlocked), might have little or no emphasis on aquatic medicine.

Veterinary Specialties

Veterinary specialists are in the minority compared to general practice veterinarians, and tend to be based at points of referral, such as veterinary schools or larger animal hospitals. Unlike human medicine, veterinary specialties often combine both the surgical and medical aspects of a biological system.

Veterinary specialties are accredited in North America by the AVMA through the American Board of Veterinary Specialties, in Europe by the European Board of Veterinary Specialisation and in Australasia by the Australasian Veterinary Boards Council. While some veterinarians may have areas of interest outside of recognized specialties, they are not legally specialists.

Specialties can cover general topics such as anesthesiology, dentistry, and surgery, as well as organ system focus such as cardiology or dermatology. A full list can be seen at veterinary specialties.

Mobile vs Stationary Practice

Some of the advantages of operating a mobile veterinary practice over a standard practice are the start-up and operating costs. Running a mobile practice is much less expensive than opening a brick and mortar location. A traditional physical location practice can cost upwards of $1,000,000 or more. A mobile vet can operate as low as $3000 for a box in an SUV to around $250,000 for a fully equipped custom built chassis. The advantages for the pet owner are less stress to their loved ones, less risk of disease transmission and convenience for having more than one pet all at close to the same cost as a clinic. Having to harness up or put a pet in a carrier to transport them to the clinic can be stressful to the animal. A 2015 study published in the Journal of American Veterinary Medical Association proved that blood pressure readings, pulse rates and body temperature rates were increased by 11-16% when those readings were done in the clinic versus in the home.

Salary

The mean salary for new graduates in the United States during 2010 was US$48,674, including nearly 50% going on to advanced study programs. Those not continuing their studies made US$67,359 at first, whereas veterinarians in the United Kingdom earned slightly less with new graduate wages at an average of £25,000.

The average income for private practice in the United States rose from $105,510 in 2005 to $115,447 in 2007. These increased values exceed those of public practice including uniformed services and government. In Australia, the profession wide average income was $67,000 in 2011 and this has declined compared to other professions for the past 30 years whilst graduate unemployment has doubled between 2006 and 2011.

Education and Regulation

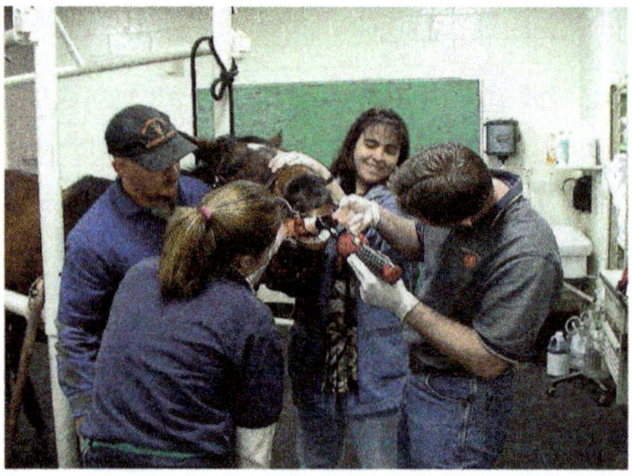

Veterinary students learning the dental treatment of a horse.

In order to practice, vets must complete both an appropriate degree in veterinary medicine, and in most cases must be registered with the relevant governing body for their jurisdiction.

Veterinary Science Degrees

Degrees in veterinary medicine culminate in the award of a veterinary science degree, although the title varies by region. For instance, in North America, graduates will receive a Doctor of Veterinary Medicine (Doctor of Veterinary Medicine or Veterinariae Medicinae Doctor; DVM or VMD), whereas in the United Kingdom or India they would be awarded a Bachelor's degree in Veterinary Science, Surgery or Medicine (BVS, BVSc, BVetMed or BVMS), and in Ireland graduates receive a Medicinae Veterinariae Baccalaureus (MVB). In continental Europe, the degree of Doctor Medicinae Veterinariae (DMV, DrMedVet, Dr. med. vet.) or Doctor Veterinariae Medicinae (DVM, DrVetMed, Dr. vet. med.) is granted.

The award of a bachelor's degree was previously commonplace in the United States, but the degree name and academic standards were upgraded to match the 'doctor' title used by graduates.

Comparatively few universities have veterinary schools that offer degrees which are accredited to qualify the graduates as registered vets. For example, there are 30 in the United States, 5 in Canada, and 8 in the United Kingdom (3 of which offer degrees accredited by the American Veterinary Medical Association (AVMA)).

Due to this scarcity of places for veterinary degrees, admission to veterinary school is competitive and requires extensive preparation. In the United States in 2007, approximately 5,750 applicants competed for the 2,650 seats in the 28 accredited veterinary schools, with an acceptance rate of 46%.

With competitive admission, many schools may place heavy emphasis and consideration on a candidate's veterinary and animal experience. Formal experience is a particular advantage to the applicant, often consisting of work with veterinarians or scientists in clinics, agribusiness, research, or some area of health science. Less formal experience is also helpful for the applicant to have, and this includes working with animals on a farm or ranch or at a stable or animal shelter and basic overall animal exposure.

In the United States, approximately 80% of admitted students are female. In the early history of veterinary medicine of the United States, most veterinarians were males. However, in the 1990s this ratio reached parity, and now it has been reversed.

Preveterinary courses should emphasize the sciences. Most veterinary schools typically require applicants to have taken one year equivalent classes in organic, inorganic chemistry, physics, general biology; and one semester of vertebrate embryology and biochemistry. Usually, the minimal mathematics requirement is college level calculus. Individual schools might require introduction to animal science, livestock judging, animal nutrition, cell biology, and genetics. However, due the limited availability of these courses, many schools have removed these requirements to widen the pool of possible applicants.

List of AVMA Accredited Veterinary Colleges

School	State/Province or City	Country
Auburn University	Alabama	United States
Tuskegee University (probationary, 2013)	Alabama	United States
Midwestern University (provisional, 2013)	Arizona	United States
University of California	California	United States
Western University of Health Sciences (minor deficiency, 2012)	California	United States
Université de Montréal	Quebec	Canada
University of Calgary	Alberta	Canada
University of Guelph	Ontario	Canada
University of Prince Edward Island	Prince Edward Island	Canada
University of Saskatchewan	Saskatchewan	Canada
Colorado State University	Colorado	United States
University of Florida	Florida	United States
Murdoch University	Western	Australia
University of Melbourne	VIC	Australia

School	State/Province or City	Country
University of Sydney	NSW	Australia
University of Queensland	QLD	Australia
James Cook University	QLD	Australia
University of London	London	England
VetAgro Sup	Marcy l'Etoile	France
University College Dublin	Dublin	Ireland
Universidad Nacional Autonoma de México	Federal District	Mexico
Massey University	Palmerston North	New Zealand
The University of Edinburgh	Edinburgh	Scotland
University of Glasgow	Glasgow	Scotland
State University of Utrecht (minor deficiency, 2014)	Utrecht	The Netherlands
Ross University	St Kitts	West Indies
St. George's University (minor deficiency, 2011)	Grenada	West Indies
University of Georgia	Georgia	United States
University of Illinois	Illinois	United States
Purdue University	Indiana	United States
Iowa State University	Iowa	United States
Kansas State University	Kansas	United States
Louisiana State University	Louisiana	United States
Tufts University	Massachusetts	United States
Michigan State University	Michigan	United States
University of Minnesota (minor deficiency, 2014)	Minnesota	United States
Mississippi State University	Mississippi	United States
University of Missouri-Columbia	Missouri	United States
Cornell University	New York	United States
North Carolina State University	North Carolina	United States
The Ohio State University	Ohio	United States
Oklahoma State University	Oklahoma	United States
Oregon State University	Oregon	United States
University of Pennsylvania	Pennsylvania	United States
University of Tennessee	Tennessee	United States
Lincoln Memorial University (provisional, 2015)	Tennessee	United States
Texas A&M University	Texas	United States
Virginia Tech	Virginia	United States
Washington State University (minor deficiency, 2010)	Washington	United States
University of Wisconsin-Madison	Wisconsin	United States

Registration and Licensing

Following academic education, most countries require a vet to be registered with the relevant governing body, and to maintain this license to practice.

Dependent on where the vet practices (or wishes to practice), they may have to complete an examination or test in order to complete this registration. For instance, in the United States, a prospective vet must receive a passing grade on a national board examination, the North America Veterinary Licensing Exam. This exam must be completed over the course of eight hours, and consists of 360 multiple-choice questions, covering all aspects of veterinary medicine, as well as visual material designed to test diagnostic skills.

Postgraduate Study

The percentage electing to undertake further study following registration in the United States has increased from 36.8% to 39.9% in 2008. About 25% of those or about 9% of graduates were accepted into traditional academic internships. (2008 -696 graduates accepted a position in advanced study, 89.2% (621) accepted an internship (private practice, 74.5%; academic, 25.3%; and other internship, 0.2%). An additional 6.0% (42) accepted a residency). Approximately 9% of veterinarians eventually board certify in one of 40 distinct specialties from 22specialty organizations recognized by the AVMA American Board of Veterinary Specialties (ABVS).

ABVS Recognized Veterinary Specialties

Anesthesiology and Analgesia	Animal Welfare	Avian Practice
Bacteriology\Mycology	Beef Cattle Practice	Behavior
Canine and Feline Practice	Canine Practice	Cardiology
Critical Care	Dairy Practice	Dentistry
Dermatology	Pharmacology	Poultry
Radiation Oncology	Radiology	Reproductive Medicine
Sports Medicine and Rehabilitation	Surgery	Swine Health Management
Toxicology	Virology	Zoological Medicine

Curriculum Comparison with Human Medicine

The first two-year curriculum in both veterinary and human medical schools are very similar in the course names, but at certain subjects relatively different in content. Generally, the more basal the field of science is (for example: biochemistry, biophysics, cell biology etc.), the more similar it is. Later on when the courses get more clinically oriented, more significant differences arise. Where some things are completely different, and other things are about the same. Considering the courses, the first two-year curriculum usually include biochemistry, physiology, histology, anatomy, pharmacology, microbiology, epidemiology, pathology and hematology.

Some veterinary school uses the same biochemistry, histology, and microbiology books as human medicine students; however, the course content is greatly supplemented to include the varied animal diseases and species specific differences. Many veterinarians were trained in pharmacology using the same text books as human physicians. As the specialty of veterinary pharmacology develop, more schools are using pharmacology textbooks written specifically for veterinarians. Veterinary physiology, anatomy, and histology is complex, as physiology often varies among species. Microbiology and virology of animals share the same foundation as human microbiology, but with grossly different disease manifestation and presentations. Epidemiology is focused on herd health and prevention of herd borne diseases, and foreign animal diseases. Pathology, like microbiology and histology, is very diverse and encompasses many species and organ systems. Most veterinary school have courses in small animal and also large animal nutrition, often taken as electives in the clinical years or as part of the core curriculum in the first two years.

The last two year curriculum of the two fields are similar only in their clinical emphasis. A veterinary student must be well prepared to be a fully functional animal physician on the day of graduation, competent in both surgery and medicine. The graduating veterinarian must be able to pass medical board examination and be prepare to enter clinical practice on the day of graduation, while most human medical doctors in the United States complete 3 to 5 years of post-doctoral residency before practicing medicine independently, usually in a very narrow and focused specialty. Many veterinarians do also complete a post-doctoral residency, but it is not nearly as common as it is in human medicine.

Impact on Human Medicine

Some veterinarians pursue post-graduate training and enter research careers and have contributed to advances in many human and veterinary medical fields, including pharmacology and epidemiology. Research veterinarians were the first to isolate oncoviruses, *Salmonella* species, *Brucella* species, and various other pathogenic agents. Veterinarians were in the forefront in the effort to suppress malaria and yellow fever in the United States. Veterinarians identified the botulism disease-causing agent, produced an anticoagulant used to treat human heart disease, and developed surgical techniques for humans, such as hip-joint replacement, limb and organ transplants.

In Popular Culture

Well-known depictions of a veterinarian at work are in James Herriot's series of books containing fictionalized stories of his career as a farm animal veterinarian in England, and the BBC's TV series *All Creatures Great and Small* based on the books.

The Three Lives of Thomasina starring Patrick McGoohan portrayed Andrew MacDhui a local veterinarian lives in a village in Scotland.

Doctor Dolittle is a series of children's books, one of which was turned into a 1967 movie. The movie was remade in 1998 with Eddie Murphy as Dr. Dolittle.

Hershel Greene from the popular series *The Walking Dead*, played by actor Scott Wilson is a veterinarian before turning his knowledge of medicine to treat human survivors and to study pathology of sick patients while in isolation during the time of the group's use of a prison as a fortified shelter.

US-based cable network Animal Planet, with animal-based programming, frequently features veterinarians. Two notable shows are *Emergency Vets* and *E-Vet Interns*, set at Alameda East Veterinary Hospital in Denver, Colorado.

The song *Grandma Got Run Over by a Reindeer*, performed by the husband and wife duo "Elmo & Patsy", is a song performed by a veterinarian, *Elmo Shropshire*, DVM.

Fictional character veterinarians in TV series and films include Steve Parker in *Neighbours*, Jim Hansen in *Providence*, and Vincent Ventresca in the horror film *Larva*.

In *Beethoven*, Dean Jones portrayed Dr. Herman Varnick, an evil veterinarian, with his associates Harvey and Vernon played by Oliver Platt and Stanley Tucci, who wanted all animals to be destroyed. They were foiled by the Newton Family and Beethoven. The Newton Family released other dogs from Dr. Varnick's captives.

Veterinary Malpractice

Most states in the US allow for malpractice lawsuit in case of death or injury to an animal from professional negligence. Usually the penalty is not greater than the value of the animal. For that reason, malpractice insurance for veterinarians is usually under $500 a year. Some states allow for punitive penalty, loss of companionship, and suffering into the award, likely increasing the cost of veterinary malpractice insurance and the cost of veterinary care. Most veterinarians carry much higher cost business, worker's compensation, and facility insurance to protect their clients and workers from injury inflicted by animals.

Criticisms

Concerns about the role of veterinary physicians in helping health threats survive and spread have been raised by several commentators, particularly with respect to pedigree dogs. Koharik Arman (2007) reached the following conclusion for example: "Veterinarians also bear some responsibility for the welfare situation of purebred dogs. In fact, the veterinary profession has facilitated the evolution of purebred dogs. 'Breeds' that would not normally be sustainable are propagated by the compliance of veterinarians to breeder wishes." This finding was echoed by Sir Patrick Bateson in his Independent Review of Dog Breeding following the broadcast of the BBC documentary *Pedigree Dogs Exposed*: "It's only the ready availability of modern veterinary medicine that has permitted some conditions...to become widespread."

VETERINARY MEDICINE IN THE UNITED KINGDOM

Veterinary medicine in the United Kingdom is the performance of veterinary medicine by licensed professionals, and strictly regulated by statute law, notably the Veterinary Surgeons Act of 1966. Veterinary medicine is led by veterinary physicians, termed 'veterinary surgeons' (with a different meaning to how it is used in some other anglophone countries, where it denotes a surgical specialist), normally referred to as 'vets'.

Vets are often assisted by registered veterinary nurses, who are able to both assist the vet and to autonomously practice a range of skills of their own, including minor surgery under direction from a responsible vet.

Other professionals are also permitted to perform some animal treatment, through exemptions in the law, and these include manipulation techniques such as physiotherapy, chiropractic and osteopathy. Other alternative medicine therapies, such as homeopathy, acupuncture, phytotherapy and aromatherapy may only be performed by a licensed veterinary surgeon.

The practice of veterinary medicine in the United Kingdom is regulated by the Royal College of Veterinary Surgeons (RCVS), who licence both veterinary surgeons and veterinary nurses.

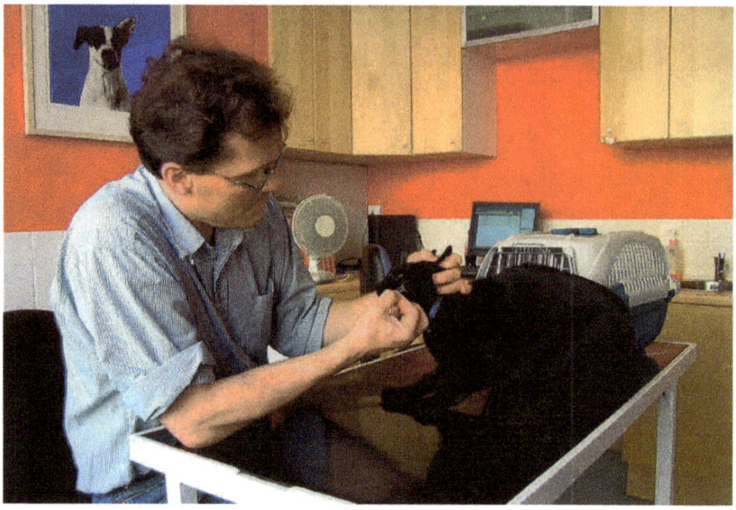

A veterinary surgeon removes stitches from a cat's face following minor surgery on an abscess.

Veterinary Surgeons

Veterinary surgeons require both a degree in veterinary science or veterinary medicine, and must hold a current registration with the RCVS in order to practice. As of 5 March 2015, the RCVS has agreed that veterinary surgeons registered with the RCVS in the UK are entitled to use the courtesy title Doctor. This makes it the third clinical degree in the UK, after Medicine and Dentistry, to allow the use of the title Dr. The origins of veterinary surgeons parallel to human surgery are reflected in human medicine where qualified surgeons also drop their Dr designation and revert to their original title. The naming convention for veterinary surgeons has been debated, with some favouring the use of the Dr title for all vets.

Education

Veterinary medicine degree courses are usually five years in length, although Cambridge University's degree takes six, and in some cases, a four-year accelerated course is available. There are a limited number of places on veterinary courses each year, with only eight British Universities offering the degree (Bristol, Cambridge, Edinburgh, Glasgow, Liverpool, Nottingham, the Royal Veterinary College, London, and Surrey).

Continuing professional development (CPD) is a mandatory and key part of career development. The RCVS recommends a minimum of 105 hours CPD over a three-year period. The RCVS Professional Development Phase (PDP) that was launched for new graduates in 2007 provides a structured approach to guide the new graduate towards the professional competences they need to develop in either small animal, equine or production animal practice.

Specialism

Vets may choose to specialise in any of a number of areas of veterinary medicine, through certificate qualifications, modular certificates or diplomas, with each speciality taking around two years to complete. Certificates cover a wide range of areas, including small animal medicine, small animal surgery, large animal medicine, welfare ethics and law, public health, cardiology and orthopaedics. A certificate is also available in advanced veterinary practice (Cert AVP).

It is important to note that there is a large and confusing array of post-nominal titles in the UK veterinary profession, which have varying levels of credibility. In particular, Certificate level qualification does not qualify a veterinary surgeon as a specialist. With further training, extensive professional experience and by publishing articles in a particular subject area, it is possible to gain Royal College of Veterinary Surgeons (RCVS) Recognised Specialist Status. The RCVS is the regulatory body for veterinary surgeons in the UK. In 2012, the ruling council of the RCVS adopted a report from the Calman Committee into specialisation in the UK veterinary profession, accepting that only those veterinary surgeons recognised by the RCVS as specialists and placed on a register held by the RCVS could be truly held up as «Specialist». Members of the public looking for an appropriately accredited specialist veterinary surgeon in the UK should therefore primarily seek those that carry the post-nominal description of «RCVS Recognisd Specialist in...» after their name. No other accolade carries authority from the appropriate regulatory body.

Some vets also undertake the training to become Official Veterinarians, (OVs), which authorises them to carry out tasks on behalf of the Department for Environment, Food and Rural Affairs, such as testing cattle for tuberculosis or issuing of documentation for the export of animals and animal products.

Employment

Most veterinary surgeons work in private practice, either in a general practice, or specialising in one type of animal (small animal, equine, zoo animal etc.). Newly qualified veterinary surgeons usually work as assistants for some time before being offered the opportunity to become a partner or a principal. Becoming a partner involves increased responsibility, the need for more business and management skills and a financial input into the practice.

Some vets are also employed by animal welfare charities who offer treatment to the public, such as Royal Society for the Prevention of Cruelty to Animals (RSPCA), the People's Dispensary for Sick Animals (PDSA) and The Blue Cross.

There are also opportunities to work for government services, including APHA (the Animal and Plant Health Agency) who are responsible for the control and eradication of major notifiable diseases, animal welfare, promotion of international trade and certain public health functions related to residues in meat and investigation of food safety incidents,and scanning surveillance, or the Veterinary Medicines Directorate (VMD) who licence veterinary medicines.

It is also possible to pursue a research and/or teaching career within universities or research bodies.

Veterinary Nurses

Veterinary Nurses are the primary paraveterinary workers in the United Kingdom and work alongside vets. Veterinary Nurses must be registered and follow a strict code of conduct. Veterinary Nurses have a scope of autonomous practice within which they can act for the animals they treat. Under schedule 3 of the Veterinary Surgeons act they can perform many complex procedures include minor surgery and monitoring anaesthesia.

Registration

All veterinary nurses must be registered with the Royal College of Veterinary Surgeons (RCVS). Registered Veterinary Nurses have dispensations in law the Veterinary Surgeons Act of 1966 amended in 2002) to undertake certain procedures to include minor surgery and anaesthesia on animals under veterinary direction. Registered Veterinary Nurses (RVNs) are bound by a code of professional conduct and are obliged to maintain their professional knowledge and skills through ongoing CPD. Those VN's listed after 2002 are automatically registered.

Education

RVNs train for the Register through either a two to three year further education diploma programme or via a qualifying foundation or honours degree which can be three to four years. All student nurses must complete a minimum of 2100 hours of work experience in general veterinary practice during their training.

RCVS badges are engraved with the nurse's personal badge number, however badges are a sign of having achieved a VN qualification and not of a person's current registered status.

Representation

UK Veterinary Nurses are represented by the British Veterinary Nursing Association (BVNA). VN's can further their formal training and gain additional postnominal letters by completing one of many specialist certificates and/or by achieving the RCVS Diploma in Advanced Veterinary Nursing (DipAVN) by following a course of study in one or more of three pathways: Small animal nursing, Equine nursing, and Veterinary nursing education. The streamlined RCVS DipAVN replaced the DipAVN(Medical) and DipAVN(Surgical) formerly administered by the BVNA up until 2005. The DipAVN is offered through Myerscough College in Lancashire since 2007 and more recently through Harper Adams University, some modules are also available from the Royal Veterinary College in conjunction with the University of London.

Animal Nursing Assistants

Lay staff, without formal qualification or status may be called animal nursing assistants (the BVNA approved term) or veterinary care assistants. These lay staff have usually undertaken some basic veterinary nurse training but are limited by law as to the procedures they may undertake on animals. They work alongside qualified vets and veterinary nurses to provide care and support to animal patients and their owners.

VETERINARY MEDICINE IN THE UNITED STATES

Veterinary medicine in the United States is the performance of veterinary medicine in the United States, normally performed by licensed professionals, and subject to provisions of statute law which vary by state. Veterinary medicine is normally led by veterinary physicians, normally termed veterinarians or vets.

Veterinarians are often assisted by paraveterinary workers including veterinary technicians and veterinary assistants, and in some cases, these para-professionals may perform work on their own.

Dependent on the jurisdiction, other professionals may be permitted to perform some animal treatment, through either specific exemptions in the law or through a lack of prohibitive legislation. This can include manipulation techniques such as physiotherapy, chiropractic and osteopathy, or animal-specific professions such as horse and cattle hoof trimmers, equine dental technicians, and technicians who specialize in cattle artificial insemination.

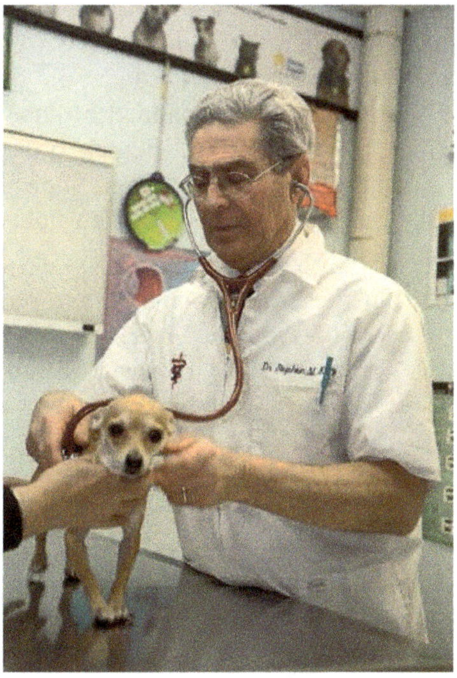

A vet examines a dog in New York

Veterinarians

Veterinarian's Oath

The Veterinarian's Oath was adopted by the American Veterinary Medical Association's House of Delegates July 1969, and amended by the AVMA Executive Board, November 1999 and December 2010.

Being admitted to the profession of veterinary medicine, I solemnly swear to use my scientific knowledge and skills for the benefit of society through the protection of animal health and welfare, the prevention and relief of animal suffering, the conservation of animal resources, the promotion of public health, and the advancement of medical knowledge.

I will practice my profession conscientiously, with dignity, and in keeping with the principles of veterinary medical ethics. I accept as a lifelong obligation the continual improvement of my professional knowledge and competence.

Qualification

In order to practice, veterinarians must obtain a degree in veterinary medicine, followed by gaining a license to practice. Previously, veterinary degrees were available as a bachelor's degree, but now all courses result in the award of a doctorate and are therefore awarded a Doctor of Veterinary Medicine (DVM) if the degree is awarded in English, or a Veterinariae Medicinae Doctoris ("Doctor of Veterinary Medicine") (VMD) if the degree is awarded in Latin.

There is a high level of competition for admission to veterinary schools; there are currently only twenty eight veterinary schools in the United States which meet the accreditation standards set by the Council on Education of the American Veterinary Medical Association (AVMA), and five in Canada. Entrance requirements vary among veterinary schools, and various pre-professional degree programs have been developed to assist undergraduates in meeting these requirements. Such "pre-vet" programs are thus similar in concept to "pre-med" programs, and are often housed in Agricultural Biology, Animal Science, or Biological Science programs.

Following qualification from the doctoral degree, the prospective veterinarian must receive a passing grade on the North America Veterinary Licensing Exam. This exam is completed over the course of eight hours, and consists of 360 multiple-choice questions. This exam covers all aspects of veterinary medicine, as well as visual material designed to test diagnostic skills.

Salary

The mean salary for new graduates in 2012 was US$67,640 including nearly 50% going on to advanced study programs.

The average income for private practice rose from $105,510 in 2005 to $115,447 in 2007. These increased values exceed those of public practice including uniformed services and government.

Veterinary Specialties

As opposed to human medicine, general practice veterinarians greatly outnumber veterinary specialists. Most veterinary specialists work at the veterinary schools, or at a referral center in large cities. As opposed to human medicine, where each organ system has its own medical and surgical specialties, veterinarians often combine both the surgical and medical aspect of an organ system into one field. The specialties in veterinary medicine often encompass several medical and surgical specialties that are found in human medicine.

Veterinary specialties are accredited in North America by the AVMA through the American Board of Veterinary Specialties. While some veterinarians may have areas of interest outside of recognized specialties, they are not legally specialists.

Veterinary Technicians

Veterinary technician logo

Veterinary technicians are the primary paraveterinary workers in the US and assist the veterinarian in the role of a nurse (and in most other anglophone countries, the equivalent role is called a veterinary nurse), providing trained support. The requirements for technicians vary by state, but in most cases, technicians are graduates of two or four year college-level programs and are legally qualified to assist veterinarians in many medical procedures.

Some states choose to license technicians, so that only people with appropriate qualifications are able to fulfill the role, but this is not the case in all jurisdictions.

Veterinary technology as an organized and credentialed career option is relatively young, only existing since the mid 20th century (although the seeds had been planted in 1908 when the Canine Nurses Institute was established in England, and as such is still struggling for recognition in many parts of the world. The first training program for technicians in the United States was established by the Air Force in 1951. The first civilian program was established ten years later in 1961 at the State University of New

York (SUNY) Agricultural and Technical College at Delhi. In 1965 Walter Collins, DVM received federal funding to develop model curricula for training technicians. He produced several guides over the next seven years, and for this work he is considered the "father of veterinary technology" in the United States).

Role and Duties

Technical skills include: venipuncture; collecting urine; performing skin scrapings; taking and processing radiographs; and performing routine lab procedures and tests in: hematology, blood chemistry, microbiology, urinalysis, and microscopy. They assist the veterinarian with physical examinations that help determine the nature of the illness or injury. Veterinary technicians also induce and maintain anesthesia, and administer medications, fluids and blood products as prescribed by the veterinarian. Tasks in patient care include: recording temperature, pulse and respiration, dressing wounds, applying splints and other protective devices, and dental procedures. They perform catheterizations – urinary, arterial, and venous; ear flushes; intravenous feedings and tube feedings. Equipment use includes operating various types of patient monitors and imaging devices to include electrocardiographic, radiographic and ultrasonographic equipment. Larger referral practices and teaching hospitals may also find veterinary technicians operating computed tomography equipment, magnetic resonance imagers, gamma cameras and other advanced medical devices. Veterinary technicians commonly assist veterinarians in surgery by providing correct equipment and instruments and by assuring that monitoring and support equipment are in good working condition. They may also maintain treatment records and inventory of all pharmaceuticals, equipment and supplies, and help with other administrative tasks within a veterinary practice such as client education. Unlike their more specialized counterparts among medical paraprofessionals, the veterinary technician is usually the only paraprofessional found in a veterinary practice and is thus often called upon to be a jack-of-all-trades.

Education and Credentialing

To become a credentialed veterinary technician, one must complete a two-year or three-year AVMA credentialled degree, most of which result in the awarding of an associate of applied science degree in veterinary technology (those completing a four-year AVMA accredited school gain a bachelor's degree are considered veterinary technologists though the distinction is rarely made with the term technician being used generally.

The education a credentialed technician receives is in-depth and crucial for medical understanding and to give proper health care. The American Veterinary Medical Association (AVMA) is responsible for accrediting schools with either Associate's degrees or Bachelor's degrees, though in some states or provinces this is not necessary. The AVMA also accredits schools that offer distance education. As a requirement of AVMA-accreditation, all distance learning programs require a significant amount of practical clinical experience before the student will be allowed to graduate.

Specialty Certification

Beyond credentialing as a veterinary technician specialty certification is also available to technicians with advanced skills. To date there are specialty recognitions in: emergency & critical care, anesthesiology, dentistry, small animal internal medicine, large animal internal medicine, cardiology, oncology, neurology, zoological medicine, equine veterinary nursing, surgery, behavior, nutrition, clinical practice (canine/feline, exotic companion animal, and production animal sub-specialties), and clinical pathology. Veterinary Technician Specialists carry the additional post-nominal letters "VTS" with their particular specialties indicated in parentheses. As veterinary technology evolves more specialty academy recognitions are anticipated.

Veterinary Assistants

Non-credentialed personnel who perform similar tasks to veterinary technicians are usually referred to as veterinary assistants though the term technician is often applied generously. In many states, a veterinary assistant cannot legally perform as many procedures as a technician. Veterinary assistants often have no formal education related to veterinary medicine or veterinary technology, however, NAVTA recently approved the designation of Approved Veterinary Assistant (AVA) for those successfully completing approved educational programs. In larger facilities with tiered hierarchies veterinary assistants typically assist veterinary technicians in their duties.

Veterinary Malpractice

Most states in the US allow for malpractice lawsuit in case of death or injury to an animal from professional negligence. Usually the penalty is not greater than the value of the animal. For that reason, malpractice insurance for veterinarians usually is well under $500 a year, compared to an average of over $15000 a year for a human doctor. Some states allow for punitive penalty, loss of companionship, and suffering into the award, likely increasing the cost of veterinary malpractice insurance and the cost of veterinary care. Most veterinarian carry much higher cost business insurance, worker's compensation, and facility insurance to protect their clients and workers from injuries inflicted by animals.

REFERENCES

1. Oxford English Dictionary, Oxford University Press.
2. Marc Mammerickx, Claude Bourgelat: avocat des vétérinaires, Bruxelles 1971
3. J.L.Lupton, "Modern Practical Farriery", 1879, in the section: "The Diseases of Cattle Sheep and Pigs" pp. 1
4. Pugh, L.P (1962). From Farriery to Veterinary Medicine 1785-1795. Heffner, Cambridge (for RCVS). pp. 8–19.
5. Cotchen, Ernest (1990). The Royal Veterinary College London, A Bicentenary History. Barracuda Books Ltd. pp. 11–13.

6. "Exacting researcher brought profession into modern age". American Veterinary Medical Association.
7. Stöhr K, Meslin FX (1997). "The role of veterinary public health in the prevention of zoonoses". Arch. Virol. Suppl. 13: 207–18. PMID 9413540.
8. "Veterinarians : Occupational Outlook Handbook : U.S. Bureau of Labor Statistics". Bls.gov. 2012-04-26. Retrieved 2013-07-05.
9. "Veterinarians". goarmy.com. Retrieved 2013-07-05.
10. Tiffany, Lynn M. "Mobile Vets are Driven to Succeed." Veterinary Practice News. 09 Jun 2011.
11. Bragg, Ryan F., et al. "Evaluation of the effects of hospital visit stress on physiologic variables in dogs." Journal of the American Veterinary Medical Association. 15 Jan 2015. Web. 26 Nov 2016
12. www.avma.org/1 year employment
13. Burns, Katie. "AVMA Survey Measures Income Trends to 2007." AVMA Journals (1 January 2009): Javma News. American Veterinary Medical Association. 2 Mar. 2009 <https://www.avma.org/News/JAVMANews/Pages/090101a.aspx>.
14. White, Tim. "How we make ends meet: economic sustainability of the veterinary profession" Australian Veterinary Journal (April 2012). 18 Apr. 2012 <http://onlinelibrary.wiley.com/doi/10.1111/j.1751-0813.2012.news_v90_i4.x/abstract>.
15. "Accredited Veterinary Colleges". AVMA. American Veterinary Medical Association. Retrieved 12 December 2015.
16. Griel, Lester C. "Advising Notes." Division of Undergraduate Studies. 7 Apr. 2008. The Pennsylvania State University. 2 Mar. 2009 <"Archived copy". Archived from the original on 27 May 2010. Retrieved 3 August 2010.>.
17. Dr. Kendon, Evan B.V.Sc "Vets And Pets" <http://www.vetschristchurch.co.nz/christchurch-pet-vet/>
18. "American Board of Veterinary Specialties". AVMA. American Veterinary Medical Association. Retrieved 12 December 2015.
19. "Market research statistics". AVMA.
20. "Recognized Veterinary Specialty Organizations". AVMA.
21. "ABVS - Recognized Veterinary Specialty Organizations". AVMA.org. American Veterinary Medical Association. Retrieved 12 December 2015.
22. "DVM Curriculum — College of Veterinary Medicine at Michigan State University". Cvm.msu.edu. 2009-12-07. Retrieved 2013-07-05.
23. "His Works". James Herriot.org. James Herriot.org. Retrieved 12 December 2015.
24. Arman, Koharik (September 2007). "A new direction for kennel club regulations and breed standards". Canadian Veterinary Journal. 48: 953–965. PMC 1950109 . PMID 17966340.
25. Bateson, Patrick (14 January 2010). "Independent Inquiry into Dog Breeding". Retrieved 16 January 2010.

26. "Professional Development Phase". Royal College of Veterinary Surgeons.
27. Pullen, Sophie; Gray, Carol (2006). Ethics, Law and the Veterinary Nurse. Philadelphia, Pennsylvania: Elsevier Limited. p. 161. ISBN 0-7506-8844-0.
28. "Veterinary qualifications: Registered veterinary nurse: RVN". Royal College of Veterinary Surgeons. Retrieved 23 May 2011.
29. "Transferring to the VN Register". Royal College of Veterinary Surgeons. Retrieved 23 May 2011.
30. "Careers". British Veterinary Nursing Association, Ltd. Retrieved 27 Feb 2009.
31. "DipAVN(Surgical/Medical)". British Veterinary Nursing Association, Ltd. Retrieved 23 May 2011.
32. "Diploma in Advanced Veterinary Nursing". Royal College of Veterinary Surgeons. Retrieved 23 May 2011.
33. http://eppws.nmsu.edu/pre-professional-program Agricultural Biology pre-professional option at the New Mexico State University.
34. http://ansci.illinois.edu/content/science-pre-veterinary-and-medical Animal Science pre-vet option at the University of Illinois.
35. "Archived copy". Archived from the original on January 7, 2014. Retrieved January 7, 2014. Biology pre-vet/pre-med option at Purdue University.
36. "General NAVLE Information". National Board of Veterinary Medical Examiners.
37. Those not continuing their studies made US$86,640, with the highest paid veterinarians earning US$149,530
38. Burns, Katie. "AVMA Survey Measures Income Trends to 2007." AVMA Journals (1 January 2009): Javma News. American Veterinary Medical Association. 2 Mar. 2009 <https://www.avma.org/News/JAVMANews/Pages/090101a.aspx>.
39. "American Board of Veterinary Specialties".
40. McCurnin, Dennis M.; Bassert, Joanna M. (2006). Clinical Textbook for Veterinary Technicians, Sixth Edition. St. Louis, Missouri: Elsevier Saunders. p. inside front cover. ISBN 0-7216-0612-1.
41. "AVMA Policy on Veterinary Technology". American Veterinary Medical Association. Retrieved 5 Dec 2012.
42. "Archived copy". Archived from the original on January 11, 2010. Retrieved January 20, 2012.

CHAPTER 4

Paraveterinary Workers

Chapter Contents

Paraveterinary workers are the members of staff that assist a veterinarian in a range of circumstances. They provide care and assistance to animals in a number of ways around the world.

INTRODUCTION

Paraveterinary workers are those people who assist a veterinary physician in the performance of their duties, or carry out animal health procedures autonomously as part of a veterinary care system. The job role varies throughout the world, and common titles include veterinary nurse, veterinary technician, veterinary assistant and veterinary technologist, and variants with the prefix of 'animal health'.

The scope of practice varies between countries, with some countries allowing suitably qualified paraveterinary workers a scope of autonomous practice, including minor surgery, whilst others restrict their workers to simple assisting of the veterinarian.

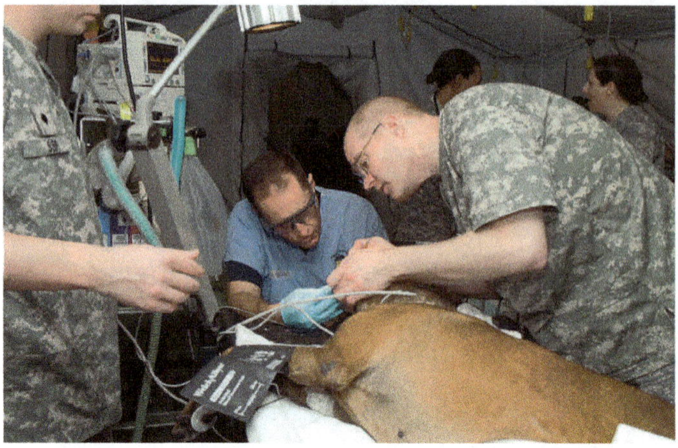

Veterinary technicians of the US Army assist in an operation on a military working dog

NOMENCLATURE

Veterinary Nurse and Technician

In the majority of anglophone countries, paraveterinary workers with a formal scope of practice, and a degree of autonomy in their role, are known as a veterinary nurses. The primary exception to this is in North America, where both the United States and Canada refer to these workers as veterinary (or animal health) technicians or technologists.

Human nursing associations have often claimed rights over the term 'nurse' and in some countries, this is protected by law. This was the case in the United Kingdom until 1984, where veterinary nurses were referred to as 'registered animal nursing auxiliaries', in line with the naming convention at the time for less qualified assistants in human nursing, called 'nursing auxiliaries'.

This is still the case in the United States, where the American Nursing Association and some state nursing associations have claimed proprietary rights to the term 'nurse'. Some veterinary technicians argue that as they spend approximately 90% of their time performing nursing tasks, they should be allowed to use the title of veterinary nurse, like their counterparts in other countries. Some argue that this is especially valid as their skill set is often greater than their human nursing counterparts, with the addition of skills such as radiology, laboratory work, pharmacy and more. Unofficially, many people (including vets and technicians) refer to these workers as veterinary nurses in conversation, as it is a succinct description of the role.

Veterinary Assistant

In most countries, a veterinary assistant is a person with fewer or no formal animal health qualifications, who has no autonomous practice, but who is designated to assist a vet and act under their direct instruction.

Training programs are often workplace-based, and no formal licence or certification is required to perform the role.

Local laws may restrict what activities a veterinary assistant may perform, as some procedures may only be legally completed by a registered practitioner, such as a vet or a veterinary nurse.

Veterinarians have had assistance from staff throughout their existence of the profession, but the first organised paraveterinary workers were the canine nurses trained by the Canine Nurses Institute in 1908, and announced in the magazine 'The Veterinary Student'. According to the founder they would "carry out directions of the veterinary surgeon, meet a genuine need on the part of the dog owners, and at the same time provide a reasonably paid occupation for young women with a real liking for animals".

In 1913, the Ruislip Dog Sanatorium was founded, and employed nurses to care for unwell dogs and in the 1920s, at least one veterinary surgery in Mayfair employed qualified human nurses to tend the animals. In the mid-1930s, the early veterinary nurses approached the Royal College of Veterinary Surgeons for official recognition, and in 1938 the Royal Veterinary College had a head nurse appointed, but the official recognition was not given until 1957, first as veterinary nurses, but changed within a year to Royal Animal Nursing Auxiliaries (RANAs) following objection from the human nursing profession.

In 1951, the first formal paraveterinary role was created by the United States Air Force who introduced veterinary technicians, and this was followed in 1961 by a civilian programme at the State University of New York (SUNY) Agricultural and Technical College. In 1965 Walter Collins, DVM received federal funding to develop model curricula for training technicians. He produced several guides over the next seven years, and for this work he is considered the "father of veterinary technology" in the United States.

In 1984, the term veterinary nurse was formally restored to paraveterinary workers in the United Kingdom.

Role and Responsibilities

The scope of practice for paraveterinary workers varies by jurisdiction, and by qualification level. In some places, more than one grade of paraveterinary worker exists. For instance, in the United Kingdom there are both veterinary nurses, who are qualified professionals with a protected title, and veterinary assistants, who do not have a single level of qualification which they must attain, and whose title is not protected. Furthermore, job roles may be divided further into roles such as Veterinary Surgical Technician, Veterinary Emergency and Critical Care Technician, Veterinary Technician Anesthesia Specialist, etc.

At the higher levels, veterinary nurses or technicians may be able to practice skills autonomously, including examinations and minor surgery on animals, without the direct supervision of a veterinarian.

Paraveterinary workers are likely to assist the vet, or perform by themselves on behalf of the vet, medical skills such as observations (e.g. taking and recording pulse, temperature, respiration etc.), wound and trauma management (e.g. cleaning and dressing wounds, applying splints etc.), physical interventions (e.g. catheterizations, ear flushes and venipuncture) and preparing and analyzing biological samples (e.g. performing skin scrapings, microbiology, urinalysis, and microscopy).

Dependant on their scope of practice and training, they may also be called upon to operate diagnostic screening equipment, including electrocardiographic, radiographic and ultrasonographic instruments, including complex machines such as computed tomography, magnetic resonance imagers and gamma cameras. In veterinary hospitals, veterinary technicians can perform complete blood counts, differential counts, and morphologic examinations of blood.

Paraveterinary workers would commonly assist veterinarians in surgery by providing correct equipment and instruments and by assuring that monitoring and support equipment are in good working condition. They may also maintain treatment records and inventory of all pharmaceuticals, equipment and supplies, and help with other administrative tasks within a veterinary practice such as client education.

Client education plays a key role of the veterinary technician's responsibilities to effectively communicate sometimes complex medical instructions in a positive and understandable way, and to facilitate the patient's care as an intermediary between the doctor, hospital and the patient. In this way, open lines of communication are established that can benefit the patient and hospital.

Education and Qualification

The level of education of a paraveterinary worker will depend on the role they are performing, and the veterinary medico-legal framework for the area in which they are working. Many areas employ veterinary assistants, who have a simple role to directly assist the vet under direction, and may hold no formal qualification or training, or have been trained on the job.

Higher level paraveterinary workers, such as veterinary nurses, veterinary technicians or veterinary technologists, who have a scope of autonomous practice which they are expected to perform without instruction, are likely to have both formal qualifications and in many jurisdictions will also require a formal registration with a monitoring body.

In countries where the role of paraveterinary workers is most advanced, the qualification required is likely to be based in higher education, such as in the United States or Canada where veterinary technicians must normally gain an associate degree at an institution recognised by the American Veterinary Medical Association or Canadian Veterinary Medical Association, and can choose to study for an extended period to gain a bachelor's degree (which in America may confer the title 'technologist', rather than 'technician'), or the United Kingdom, where veterinary nurses enter the profession through either a two-year diploma programme or through completion of a foundation degree or honours degree.

In almost all cases, regardless of the level of formalised training, a high level of practical experience is usually required prior to a student being fully qualified, which may be completed as part of their course, or during a post-qualification period. This may require maintenance of a log of all work completed, which may need to be signed by a supervising professional (such as the vet or senior member of the paraveterinary staff) to indicate competence. In some cases, such as in the United States, video records may be required of some procedures, which may then be examined by the awarding or registration body.

Many countries, including the United Kingdom, Canada, and parts of the United States, restrict some elements of practice, and may restrict use of the recognised name, to those people currently registered with an appropriate licensing body, meaning that it would be illegal for any person not on the register to represent themselves as a paraveterinary worker, or to perform some of the procedures that a licensed professional could. The precise details of these restrictions vary widely between legal areas, and neighbouring areas may have different policies, as is the case in the various states of the US.

This licensing body may have its own requirements for maintaining a registration, and those who hold the requisite academic qualification may still have to complete a further range of exams or tests to become registered. For instance, in the United States, most areas use the Veterinary Technician National Exam, and this will be used by the state licensing authority (such as a state veterinary medical association) to qualify an applicant to become a registered veterinary technician.

In some cases, those people who qualified before the introduction of formal academic qualification requirements may still be working as paraveterinary workers, and may still be entered on a required register through the use of grandfather rights. For instance, in some states of the US, people with a set number of years or hours of experience assisting a veterinarian could sit for the Veterinary Technician National Exam, however this route was phased out in 2011, and future candidates must have an academic qualification.

Specialty Certification

Beyond credentialing as a veterinary technician specialty certification is also available to technicians with advanced skills. To date there are specialty recognitions in: emergency & critical care, anesthesiology, dentistry, small animal internal medicine, large animal internal medicine, cardiology, oncology, neurology, zoological medicine, equine veterinary nursing, surgery, behavior, nutrition, clinical practice (canine/feline, exotic companion animal, and production animal sub-specialties) and clinical pathology. Veterinary Technician Specialists carry the additional post-nominal letters "VTS" with their particular specialties indicated in parentheses. As veterinary technology evolves more specialty academy recognitions are anticipated.

Global Presence

Attempts at professional solidarity resulted in the creation of the International Veterinary Nurses and Technicians Association (IVNTA) in 1993. Its members currently include Australia, Canada, Denmark, Finland, France, Germany, Ghana, Hong Kong, Ireland, Japan, Malta, Nepal, New Zealand, Norway, South Africa, Spain, Sweden, Switzerland, Thailand, Turkey, the United Kingdom, and the United States. In 2007 the Accreditation Committee for Veterinary Nurse Education (ACOVENE) was established in an attempt to standardize veterinary technology education throughout the European Union and to allow movement of veterinary nurses educated in one member nation to employment in another.

On the specialty front, the Swiss-based organization VASTA (*Veterinär Anästhesie Schule für TechnikerInnen und ArzthelferInnen -- Veterinary Anaesthesia School for Technicians and Assistants*) is a six module year-long program that is approved by the Association of Veterinary Anaesthetists (AVA), the European College of Veterinary Anaesthesia and Analgesia (ECVAA), the International Veterinary Academy of Pain Management (IVAPM), and that has applied for RACE (Registry of Approved Continuing Education) approval in the United States («Assistants» in the VASTA title refers to assistant or junior veterinarians and not to unqualified veterinary assistants). Its instructors include diplomates of the ECVAA, nurse anesthetists from the human medical field, neurologists, and veterinary physical therapists. It is currently offered in Germany, Austria, and the German-speaking regions of Switzerland. It has previously been offered in the French-speaking region of Switzerland but is currently on hiatus there due to low participation. Courses are planned for the US and the UK in 2012. Successful completion of the course results in the awarding of the post-nominal letters VAT (Veterinary Anaesthesia Technician).

VETERINARY MEDICINE

Veterinary medicine is the branch of medicine that deals with the prevention, diagnosis and treatment of disease, disorder and injury in non-human animals. The scope of veterinary medicine is wide, covering all animal species, both domesticated and wild, with a wide range of conditions which can affect different species.

Veterinary medicine is widely practiced, both with and without professional supervision. Professional care is most often led by a veterinary physician (also known as a vet, veterinary surgeon or veterinarian), but also by paraveterinary workers such as veterinary nurses or technicians. This can be augmented by other paraprofessionals with specific specialisms such as animal physiotherapy or dentistry, and species relevant roles such as farriers.

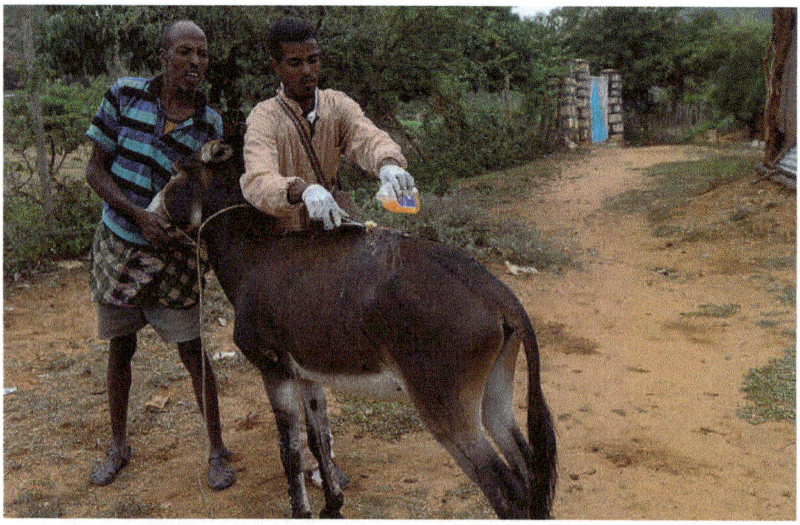

A veterinary technician in Ethiopia shows the owner of an ailing donkey how to sanitize the site of infection.

Veterinary science helps human health through the monitoring and control of zoonotic disease (infectious disease transmitted from non-human animals to humans), food safety, and indirectly through human applications from basic medical research. They also help to maintain food supply through livestock health monitoring and treatment, and mental health by keeping pets healthy and long living. Veterinary scientists often collaborate with epidemiologists, and other health or natural scientists depending on type of work. Ethically, veterinarians are usually obliged to look after animal welfare.

Premodern Era

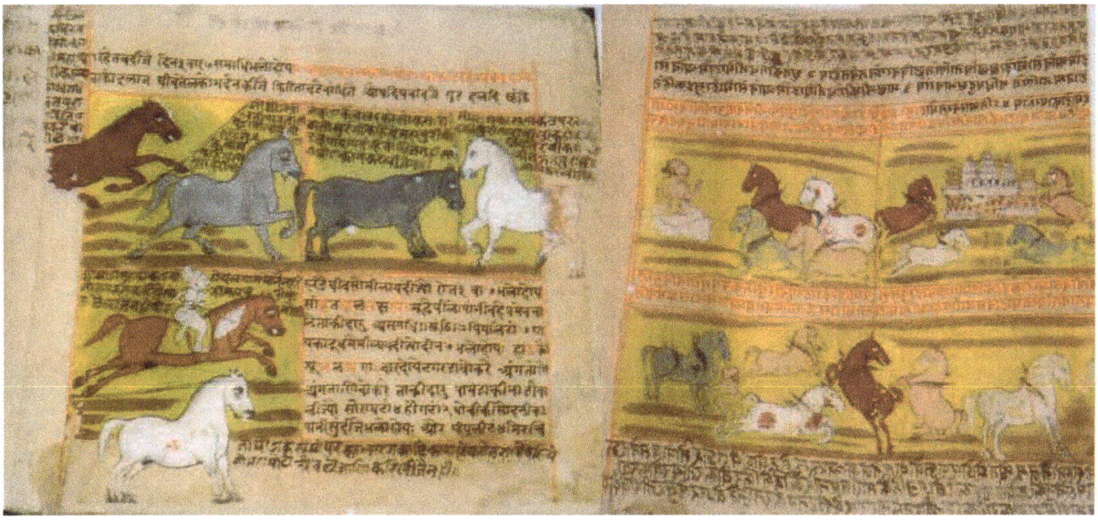

"Shalihotra" manuscript pages

The Egyptian *Papyrus of Kahun* (1900 BCE) and Vedic literature in ancient India offer one of the first written records of veterinary medicine. First Buddhist Emperor of India edicts of Asoka reads: "Everywhere King Piyadasi (Asoka) made two kinds of medicine available, medicine for people and medicine for animals. Where there were no healing herbs for people and animals, he ordered that they be bought and planted.»

The first attempts to organize and regulate the practice of treating animals tended to focus on horses because of their economic significance. In the Middle Ages from around 475 CE, farriers combined their work in horseshoeing with the more general task of «horse doctoring». In 1356, the Lord Mayor of London, concerned at the poor standard of care given to horses in the city, requested that all farriers operating within a seven-mile radius of the City of London form a «fellowship» to regulate and improve their practices. This ultimately led to the establishment of the Worshipful Company of Farriers in 1674.

Meanwhile, Carlo Ruini›s book *Anatomia del Cavallo,* (*Anatomy of the Horse*) was published in 1598. It was the first comprehensive treatise on the anatomy of a non-human species.

Establishment of Profession

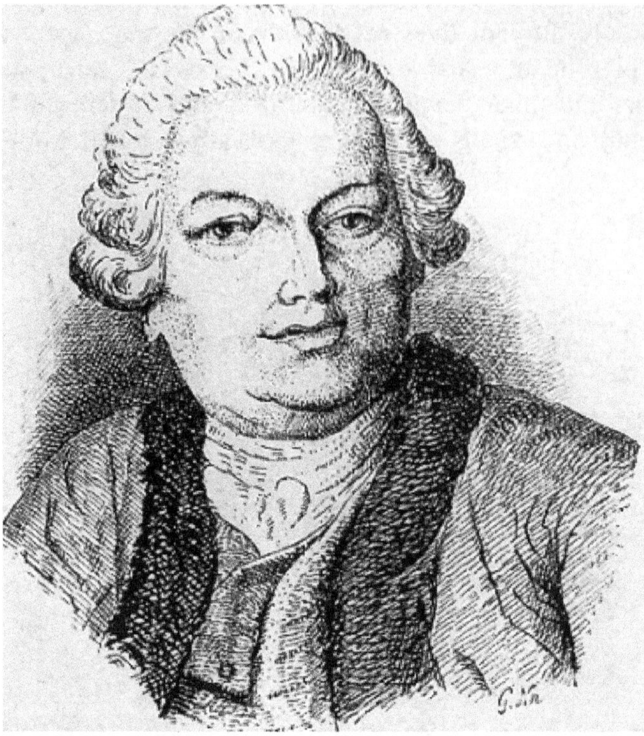

Claude Bourgelat established the earliest veterinary college in Lyon in 1762.

The first veterinary college was founded in Lyon, France in 1762 by Claude Bourgelat. According to Lupton, after observing the devastation being caused by cattle plague to the French herds, Bourgelat devoted his time to seeking out a remedy. This resulted in his founding a veterinary college in Lyon in 1761, from which establishment he dispatched students to combat the disease; in a short time, the plague was stayed and the health of stock restored, through the assistance rendered to agriculture by veterinary science and art.»

The Odiham Agricultural Society was founded in 1783 in England to promote agriculture and industry, and played an important role in the foundation of the veterinary profession in Britain. A founding member, Thomas Burgess, began to take up the cause of animal welfare and campaign for the more humane treatment of sick animals. A 1785 Society meeting resolved to «promote the study of Farriery upon rational scientific principles."

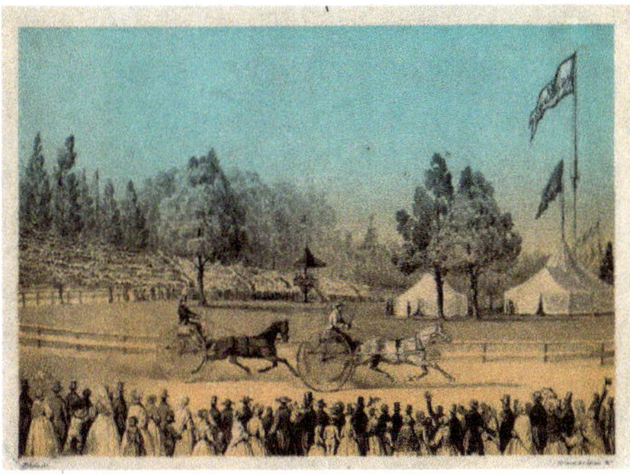

Minutes taken at the establishment of the Odiham Agricultural Society, which went on to play a pivotal role in the establishment of the veterinary profession in England.

The physician James Clark wrote a treatise entitled *Prevention of Disease* in which he argued for the professionalization of the veterinary trade, and the establishment of veterinary colleges. This was finally achieved in 1790, through the campaigning of Granville Penn, who persuaded the Frenchman, Benoit Vial de St. Bel to accept the professorship of the newly established Veterinary College in London. The Royal College of Veterinary Surgeons was established by royal charter in 1844. Veterinary science came of age in the late 19th century, with notable contributions from Sir John McFadyean, credited by many as having been the founder of modern Veterinary research.

In the United States, the first schools were established in the early 19th century in Boston, New York and Philadelphia. In 1879, Iowa Agricultural College became the first land grant college to establish a school of veterinary medicine. Suzanne Saueressig became the first accredited female veterinarian in Missouri in 1955.

Veterinary Workers

Veterinary Physicians

Veterinary care and management is usually led by a veterinary physician (usually called a vet, veterinary surgeon or veterinarian). This role is the equivalent of a doctor in human medicine, and usually involves post-graduate study and qualification.

In many countries, the local nomenclature for a vet is a protected term, meaning that people without the prerequisite qualifications and/or registration are not able to use the title, and in many cases, the activities that may be undertaken by a vet (such as animal treatment or surgery) are restricted only to those people who are registered as vet. For instance, in the United Kingdom, as in other jurisdictions, animal treatment may only be performed by registered vets (with a few designated exceptions, such as paraveterinary workers), and it is illegal for any person who is not registered to call themselves a vet or perform any treatment.

Most vets work in clinical settings, treating animals directly. These vets may be involved in a general practice, treating animals of all types; may be specialized in a specific group of animals such as companion animals, livestock, laboratory animals, zoo animals or horses; or may specialize in a narrow medical discipline such as surgery, dermatology, laboratory animal medicine, or internal medicine.

As with healthcare professionals, vets face ethical decisions about the care of their patients. Current debates within the profession include the ethics of purely cosmetic procedures on animals, such as declawing of cats, docking of tails, cropping of ears and debarking on dogs.

Paraveterinary Workers

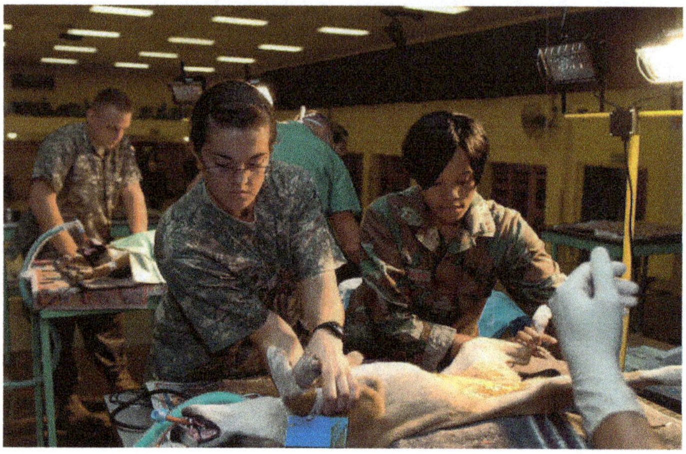

US and South African army veterinary technicians prepare a dog for spaying.

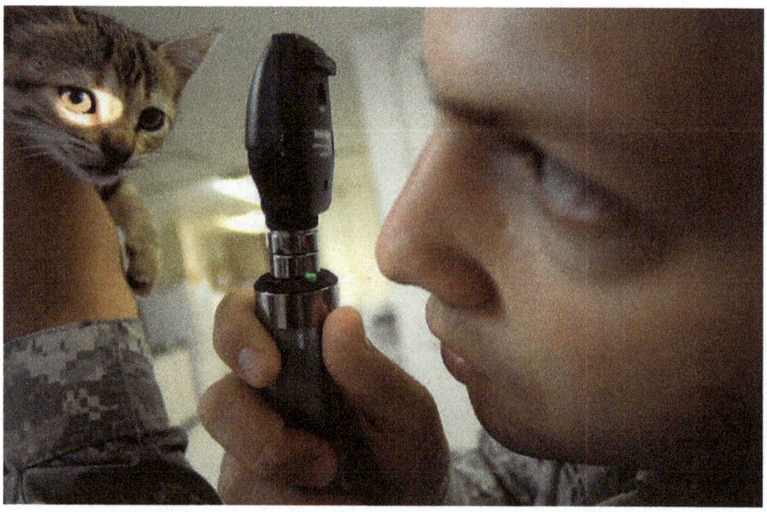

An eye exam of a kitten under way prior to the kitten's adoption.

Paraveterinary workers, including veterinary nurses, technicians and assistants, either assist vets in their work, or may work within their own scope of practice, depending on skills and qualifications, including in some cases, performing minor surgery.

The role of paraveterinary workers is less homogeneous globally than that of a vet, and qualification levels, and the associated skill mix, vary widely.

Allied Professions

A number of professions exist within the scope of veterinary medicine, but which may not necessarily be performed by vets or veterinary nurses. This includes those performing roles which are also found in human medicine, such as practitioners dealing with musculoskeletal disorders, including osteopaths, chiropractors and physiotherapists.

There are also roles which are specific to animals, but which have parallels in human society, such as animal grooming and animal massage.

Some roles are specific to a species or group of animals, such as farriers, who are involved in the shoeing of horses, and in many cases have a major role to play in ensuring the medical fitness of the horse.

Veterinary Research

Veterinary research includes research on prevention, control, diagnosis, and treatment of diseases of animals and on the basic biology, welfare, and care of animals. Veterinary research transcends species boundaries and includes the study of spontaneously occurring and experimentally induced models of both human and animal disease and research at human-animal interfaces, such as food safety, wildlife and ecosystem health, zoonotic diseases, and public policy.

Clinical Veterinary Research

As in medicine, randomized controlled trials are fundamental also in veterinary medicine to establish the effectiveness of a treatment. However, clinical veterinary research is far behind human medical research, with fewer randomized controlled trials, that have a lower quality and that are mostly focused on research animals. Possible improvement consists in creation of network for inclusion of private veterinary practices in randomized controlled trials.

REFERENCES

1. Badger (VN, Cert Ed, MBVNA), Sue. "The Good Old Days - Or Were They?". The British Veterinary Nursing Association Limited. Retrieved 5 Feb 2009.
2. Turner, Trevor; Turner, Jean. "VN Jubilee Seminar: 50 years of veterinary nursing - How did it all begin?". Royal College of Veterinary Surgeons.
3. "The Wylie Centenary Flyer" (PDF). The Wylie Veterinary Centre. October 2008.
4. McCurnin, Dennis M.; Bassert, Joanna M. (2006). Clinical Textbook for Veterinary

Technicians, Sixth Edition. St. Louis, Missouri: Elsevier Saunders. p. inside front cover. ISBN 0-7216-0612-1.

5. "Veterinary Technician Code of Ethics" (PDF). vet.purdue.edu. NAVTA. Retrieved 30 July 2016.
6. "Introduction to Veterinary Technician Salary". Vet Tech Salary. Retrieved 26 September 2014.
7. "AVMA Policy on Veterinary Technology". American Veterinary Medical Association. Retrieved 5 Feb 2009.
8. "Technologist vs Technician?". Canadian Association of Animal Health Technologists and Technicians. Retrieved 24 Jul 2011.
9. "VTNE". American Association of Veterinary State Boards. Retrieved 24 Jul 2011.
10. "Policy Update Memo April 25, 2008: Veterinary Technician National Exam (VTNE) 2010 Eligibility Requirements"(PDF). American Association of Veterinary State Boards. Retrieved 24 Jul 2011.
11. "IVNTA History". International Veterinary Nurses and Technicians Association. Retrieved 26 Feb 2009.
12. "Home". Accreditation Committee for Veterinary Nurse Education. Retrieved 18 Jun 2010.
13. "Veterinary Specialty Organizations". Archived from the original on May 1, 2006. Retrieved 2006-04-06.
14. EBVS Website Archived April 14, 2015, at the Wayback Machine.
15. ACVS Residency Program
16. ECVS Website Archived March 18, 2013, at the Wayback Machine.
17. Muir, William W.; Hubbell, John A. E. (1995). Handbook of Veterinary Anesthesia (2nd cd.). Mosby. ISBN 0-8016-7656-8.
18. Paddleford, Robert R.; Harvey, Ralph C. (1999). "Alpha2 Agonists and Antagonists". The Veterinary Clinics of North America. 29: 737–744.
19. Paddleford, Robert R. (1999). Manual of Small Animal Anesthesia (2nd ed.). W.B. Saunders Company. ISBN 0-7216-4060-5.
20. Clarke, Cathy W. (1999). "Desflurane and Sevoflurane". The Veterinary Clinics of North America. 29: 793–809.
21. N. Berger, P.H. Eeg, Veterinary Laser Surgery, Blackwell, ISBN 978-0-8138-0678-5
22. "Archived copy". Archived from the original on 2016-01-28. Retrieved 2016-03-30. Veterinary laser surgery, URL accessed March 25, 2008
23. Woolridge, Anne A.; Seahorn, Thomas L. (1999). "Proper Dental Care Is Vital For Horses". Louisiana State University Equine Veternary Research Program Newsletter. Retrieved 2006-07-29.
24. "Feline Odontoclastic Resorptive Lesions". Small Animal Dental Service. Texas A&M University Veterinary Medical Teaching Hospital. Archived from the

original on 2006-08-28. Retrieved 2006-07-29.

25. Holt, David E.; Griffin, Greg (2000). "Bite Wounds in Dogs and Cats". The Veterinary Clinics of North America. 30: 669–678.
26. Grunert E. & Luhman F., Chirurgische Versorgung von Euter- und Zitzenwunden, in Buiatrik, 2. Ed. Schaper Verlag, Hannover, 1972
27. "Archived copy". Archived from the original on 2016-05-28. Retrieved 2012-12-17.
28. Grimm, Kurt; Thurmon, John Tranquilli W.J. (2007). Lumb and Jones Veterinary Anesthesia and Analgesia. Blackwell Publishing Inc. ISBN 0-7817-5471-2.
29. "Veterinary Specialty Organizations". Retrieved 2016-06-05.
30. "ACVA History". Archived from the original on 2007-01-27. Retrieved 2007-05-07.
31. "ACVAA Directory". Retrieved 2016-06-05.
32. Dyson D.H.; Maxie M.G.; Shnurr D (1998). "Morbidity and mortality associated with anesthetic management in small animal veterinary practice in Ontario". Journal of the American Animal Hospital Association. 34 (4): 325–335. PMID 9657167.
33. "Academy of Veterinary Technician Anesthetists". Retrieved 2007-05-07.
34. Gaynor, J. S.; Dunlop, C. I.; Wagner, A.E.; et al. (January 1999). "Complications and mortality associated with anesthesia in dogs and cats". Journal of the American Animal Hospital Association. 35 (1): 13–17. doi:10.5326/15473317-35-1-13. PMID 9934922.
35. Brodbelt DC, Blissitt KJ, Hammond RA, et al. (September 2008). "The risk of death: the confidential enquiry into perioperative small animal fatalities". Vet Anaesth Analg. 35 (5): 365–73. doi:10.1111/j.1467-2995.2008.00397.x. PMID 18466167.
36. Johnston, G. M.; Eastment, J. K.; Woods, J. L. N.; et al. (2002). "The confidential enquiry into perioperative equine fatalities (CEPEF): mortality results of Phases 1 and 2.". Journal of Veterinary Anesthesia and Analgesia. 29 (4): 159–170. doi:10.1046/j.1467-2995.2002.00106.x.
37. Brodbelt David C (2009). "Perioperative mortality in small animal anaesthesia". Veterinary Journal (London). 182: 152–161.

CHAPTER 5

Animal Welfare

Chapter Contents

Animal welfare refers to the state of the animal; the treatment that an animal receives is covered by other terms such as animal care, animal husbandry, and humane treatment. ... Protecting an animal's welfare means providing for its physical and mental needs.

INTRODUCTION

Animal welfare is the well-being of animals. The standards of "good" animal welfare vary considerably between different contexts. These standards are under constant review and are debated, created and revised by animal welfare groups, legislators and academics worldwide. Animal welfare science uses various measures, such as longevity, disease, immunosuppression, behavior, physiology, and reproduction, although there is debate about which of these indicators provide the best information.

Concern for animal welfare is often based on the belief that non-human animals are sentient and that consideration should be given to their well-being or suffering, especially when they are under the care of humans. These concerns can include how animals are slaughtered for food, how they are used in scientific research, how they are kept (as pets, in zoos, farms, circuses, etc.), and how human activities affect the welfare and survival of wild species.

Animal welfare was a concern of some ancient civilizations but began to take a larger place in Western public policy in 19th-century Great Britain. In the 21st century, it is a significant focus of interest in science, ethics, and animal welfare organizations.

There are two forms of criticism of the concept of animal welfare, coming from diametrically opposite positions. One view, dating back centuries, asserts that animals are not consciously aware and hence are unable to experience poor (or good) welfare. This once-dominant argument is at odds with the predominant view of modern neuroscientists, who, notwithstanding philosophical problems with the definition of consciousness even in humans, now generally hold that animals are conscious. However, some still maintain that consciousness is a philosophical question that may never be scientifically resolved.

The other view is based on the animal rights position that animals should not be regarded as property and any use of animals by humans is unacceptable. Accordingly, some animal rights proponents argue that the perception of better animal welfare facilitates continued and increased exploitation of animals. Some authorities therefore treat animal welfare and animal rights as two opposing positions. Others see the increasing concern for animal welfare as incremental steps towards animal rights. The most widely held position in the western world is a mid-way utilitarian point-of-view; the position that it is morally acceptable for humans to use non-human animals, provided that adverse effects on animal welfare are minimized as much as possible.

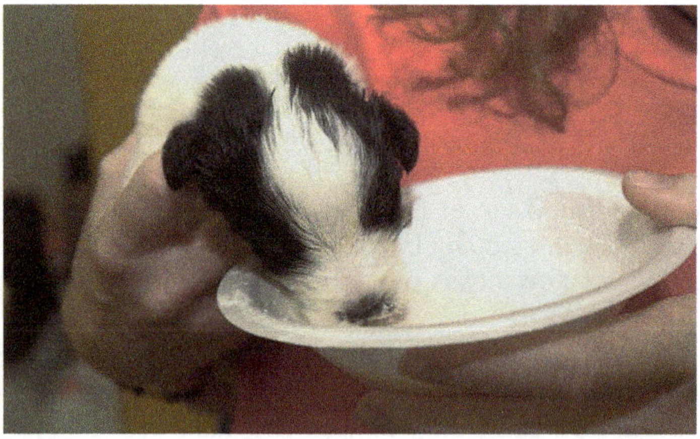

A four-week-old puppy, found alongside a road after flooding in West Virginia, United States, is fed at an Emergency Animal Rescue Service shelter in the Twin Falls State Park.

Approaches and Definitions

There are many different approaches to describing and defining animal welfare.

Conditions Provided by Humans

Providing good animal welfare is sometimes defined by a list of positive conditions which should be provided to the animal. This approach is taken by the Five Freedoms and the three principles of Professor John Webster.

The Five Freedoms are:

- Freedom from thirst and hunger – by ready access to fresh water and a diet to maintain full health and vigour
- Freedom from discomfort – by providing an appropriate environment including shelter and a comfortable resting area
- Freedom from pain, injury, and disease – by prevention or rapid diagnosis and treatment
- Freedom to express most normal behavior – by providing sufficient space, proper facilities, and company of the animal's own kind
- Freedom from fear and distress – by ensuring conditions and treatment which avoid mental suffering

John Webster defines animal welfare by advocating three positive conditions: Living a natural life, being fit and healthy, and being happy.

Production by Animals

In the past, many have seen farm animal welfare chiefly in terms of whether the animal is producing well. The argument is that an animal in poor welfare would not be producing well, however, many farmed animals will remain highly productive despite being in conditions where good welfare is almost certainly compromised, e.g., layer hens in battery cages.

Feelings of Animals

Others in the field, such as Professor Ian Duncan and Professor Marian Dawkins, focus more on the feelings of the animal. This approach indicates the belief that animals should be considered as sentient beings. Duncan wrote, "Animal welfare is to do with the feelings experienced by animals: the absence of strong negative feelings, usually called suffering, and (probably) the presence of positive feelings, usually called pleasure. In any assessment of welfare, it is these feelings that should be assessed." Dawkins wrote, "Let us not mince words: Animal welfare involves the subjective feelings of animals."

Yew-Kwang Ng defines animal welfare in terms of welfare economics: "Welfare biology is the study of living things and their environment with respect to their welfare (defined as net happiness, or enjoyment minus suffering). Despite difficulties of ascertaining and measuring welfare and relevancy to normative issues, welfare biology is a positive science."

Dictionary Definition

In the *Saunders Comprehensive Veterinary Dictionary*, animal welfare is defined as "the avoidance of abuse and exploitation of animals by humans by maintaining appropriate standards of accommodation, feeding and general care, the prevention and treatment of disease and the assurance of freedom from harassment, and unnecessary discomfort and pain."

Veterinary Profession

The American Veterinary Medical Association (AVMA) has defined animal welfare as: "An animal is in a good state of welfare if (as indicated by scientific evidence) it is healthy, comfortable, well nourished, safe, able to express innate behavior, and if it is not suffering from unpleasant states such as pain, fear, and distress." They have offered the following eight principles for developing and evaluating animal welfare policies.

- The responsible use of animals for human purposes, such as companionship, food, fiber, recreation, work, education, exhibition, and research conducted for the benefit of both humans and animals, is consistent with the Veterinarian's Oath.
- Decisions regarding animal care, use, and welfare shall be made by balancing scientific knowledge and professional judgment with consideration of ethical and societal values.
- Animals must be provided water, food, proper handling, health care, and an environment appropriate to their care and use, with thoughtful consideration for their species-typical biology and behavior.
- Animals should be cared for in ways that minimize fear, pain, stress, and suffering.
- Procedures related to animal housing, management, care, and use should be continuously evaluated, and when indicated, refined or replaced.
- Conservation and management of animal populations should be humane, socially responsible, and scientifically prudent.
- Animals shall be treated with respect and dignity throughout their lives and, when necessary, provided a humane death.
- The veterinary profession shall continually strive to improve animal health and welfare through scientific research, education, collaboration, advocacy, and the development of legislation and regulations.

Environment

Terrestrial Animal Health Code of World Organisation for Animal Health defines animal welfare as "how an animal is coping with the conditions in which it lives. An animal is in a good state of welfare if (as indicated by scientific evidence) it is healthy, comfortable, well nourished, safe, able to express innate behaviour, and if it is not suffering from unpleasant states such as pain, fear, and distress. Good animal welfare requires disease prevention and veterinary treatment, appropriate shelter, management, nutrition, humane handling and humane slaughter/killing. Animal welfare refers to the state of the animal; the treatment that an animal receives is covered by other terms such as animal care, animal husbandry, and humane treatment."

Coping

Professor Donald Broom defines the welfare of an animal as "Its state as regards its attempts to cope with its environment. This state includes how much it is having to do to cope, the extent to which it is succeeding in or failing to cope, and its associated feelings." He states that "welfare will vary over a continuum from very good to very poor and studies of welfare will be most effective if a wide range of measures is used." John Webster criticized this definition for making "no attempt to say what constitutes good or bad welfare."

Attitudes

Animal welfare often refers to a utilitarian attitude towards the well-being of nonhuman animals. It believes the animals can be exploited if the animal suffering and the costs of use is less than the benefits to humans. This attitude is also known simply as *welfarism.*

An example of welfarist thought is Hugh Fearnley-Whittingstall's meat manifesto. Point three of eight is:

Think about the animals that the meat you eat comes from. Are you at all concerned about how they have been treated? Have they lived well? Have they been fed on safe, appropriate foods? Have they been cared for by someone who respects them and enjoys contact with them? Would you like to be sure of that? Perhaps it's time to find out a bit more about where the meat you eat comes from. Or to buy from a source that reassures you about these points.

Robert Garner describes the welfarist position as the most widely held in modern society. He states that one of the best attempts to clarify this position is given by Robert Nozick:

Consider the following (too minimal) position about the treatment of animals. So that we can easily refer to it, let us label this position "utilitarianism for animals, Kantianism for people." It says: (1) maximize the total happiness of all living beings; (2) place stringent side constraints on what one may do to human beings. Human beings may not be used or sacrificed for the benefit of others; animals may be used or sacrificed for the benefit of other people or animals only if those benefits are greater than the loss inflicted.

Welfarism is often contrasted with the animal rights and animal liberation positions, which hold that animals should not be used by humans and should not be regarded as human property. However, it has been argued that both welfarism and animal liberation only make sense if it is assumed that animals have "subjective welfare".

New Welfarism

New welfarism was coined by Gary L. Francione in 1996. It is a view that the best way to prevent animal suffering is to abolish the causes of animal suffering, but advancing animal welfare is a goal to pursue in the short term. Thus, for instance, new welfarists want to phase out fur farms and animal experiments but in the short-term they try to improve conditions for the animals in these systems, so they lobby to make cages less constrictive and to reduce the numbers of animals used in laboratories.

Laws punishing cruelty to animals tend to not just be based on welfare concerns but the belief that such behavior has repercussions toward the treatment of other humans by the animal abusers. Another argument against animal cruelty is based on aesthetics. Within the context of animal research, many scientific organisations believe that improved animal welfare will provide improved scientific outcomes. If an animal in a laboratory is suffering stress or pain it could negatively affect the results of the research.

Increased affluence in many regions for the past few decades afforded consumers the disposable income to purchase products from high welfare systems. The adaptation of more economically efficient farming systems in these regions were at the expense of animal welfare and to the financial benefit of consumers, both of which were factors in driving the demand for higher welfare for farm animals. A 2006 survey concluded that a majority (63%) of EU citizens "show some willingness to change their usual place of shopping in order to be able to purchase more animal welfare-friendly products."

Interest in animal welfare continues to grow, with increasing attention being paid to it by the media, governmental and non-governmental organizations. The volume of scientific research on animal welfare has also increased significantly in some countries.

History, Principles and Practice

Systematic concern for the well-being of other animals probably arose in the Indus Valley Civilization as religious ancestors were believed to return in animal form; therefore animals must be treated with respect. This belief is exemplified in the existing religion, Jainism, and in varieties of other Indian religions. Other religions, especially those with roots in the Abrahamic religions, treat animals as the property of their owners, codifying rules for their care and slaughter intended to limit the distress, pain, and fear animals experience under human control.

Early legislation which formed the impetus for assessing animal welfare and the subsequent development of animal welfare science include the Ireland Parliament (Thomas Wentworth) "An Act against Plowing by the Tayle, and pulling the Wooll off living Sheep", 1635, and the Massachusetts Colony (Nathaniel Ward) "Off the Bruite Creatures" Liberty 92 and 93 in the "Massachusetts Body of Liberties" of 1641.

Since 1822, when Irish MP Richard Martin brought the "Cruel Treatment of Cattle Act 1822" through Parliament offering protection from cruelty to cattle, horses, and sheep, the welfare approach has had human morality and humane behaviour as its central concerns. Martin was among the founders of the world's first animal welfare organization, the Society for the Prevention of Cruelty to Animals, or SPCA, in 1824. In 1840, Queen Victoria gave the society her blessing, and it became the RSPCA. The society used members' donations to employ a growing network of inspectors, whose job was to identify abusers, gather evidence, and report them to the authorities.

In 1837 the German minister Albert Knapp founded the first German animal welfare society.

One of the first national laws to protect animals was the UK "Cruelty to Animals Act 1835" followed by the "Protection of Animals Act 1911". In the US it was many years until there was a national law to protect animals—the "Animal Welfare Act of 1966"—although there were a number of states that passed anti-cruelty laws between 1828 and 1898. In India, animals are protected by the "Prevention of Cruelty to Animals Act, 1960".

Significant progress in animal welfare did not take place until the late 20th century. In 1965, the UK government commissioned an investigation—led by Professor Roger Brambell—into the welfare of intensively farmed animals, partly in response to concerns raised in Ruth Harrison's 1964 book, *Animal Machines*. On the basis of Professor Brambell's report, the UK government set up the Farm Animal Welfare Advisory Committee in 1967, which became the Farm Animal Welfare Council in 1979. The committee's first guidelines recommended that animals require the freedoms to "stand up, lie down, turn around, groom themselves and stretch their limbs." The guidelines have since been elaborated upon to become known as the Five Freedoms.

In the UK, the "Animal Welfare Act 2006" consolidated many different forms of animal welfare legislation.

A number of animal welfare organisations are campaigning to achieve a Universal Declaration on Animal Welfare (UDAW) at the United Nations. In principle, the Universal Declaration would call on the United Nations to recognise animals as sentient beings, capable of experiencing pain and suffering, and to recognise that animal welfare is an issue of importance as part of the social development of nations worldwide. The campaign to achieve the UDAW is being co-ordinated by World Animal Protection, with a core working group including Compassion in World Farming, the RSPCA, and the Humane Society International (the international branch of HSUS).

Animal Welfare Science

Animal welfare science is an emerging field that seeks to answer questions raised by the keeping and use of animals, such as whether hens are frustrated when confined in cages,whether the psychological well-being of animals in laboratories can be maintained, and whether zoo animals are stressed by the transport required for international conservation.

ANIMAL TESTING

Animal testing, also known as animal experimentation, animal research, and in vivo testing, is the use of non-human animals in experiments that seek to control the variables that affect the behavior or biological system under study. This approach can be contrasted with field studies in which animals are observed in their natural environments. Experimental research with animals is usually conducted in universities, medical schools, pharmaceutical companies, defense establishments, and commercial facilities that provide animal-testing services to industry. The focus of animal testing varies on a continuum from pure research, done with little regard to the uses to which understanding may be put, to applied research, which may focus on answering some question of great practical importance, such as finding a cure for a disease. Examples of applied research include testing, breeding, defense research, and toxicology, including cosmetics testing. In education, animal testing is sometimes a component of biology or psychology courses. The practice is regulated to varying degrees in different countries.

Worldwide it is estimated that the number of vertebrate animals—from zebrafish to non-human primates—ranges from the tens of millions to more than 100 million used annually. In the US in 2014, official statistics indicate that 834,453 vertebrates were used in research. In the EU, these species represent 93% of animals used in research. If the same was true in the US then the total number of animals used in research is estimated to be between 12 and 25 million. One estimate of mice and rats used in the US alone in 2001 was 80 million. In the EU in 2011, 11.5 million animals were used in research. Mice, rats, fish, amphibians and reptiles together account for over 85% of research animals.

Most animals are euthanized after being used in an experiment. Sources of laboratory animals vary between countries and species; most animals are purpose-bred, while a minority are caught in the wild or supplied by dealers who obtain them from auctions and pounds.

Supporters of the use of animals in experiments, such as the British Royal Society, argue that virtually every medical achievement in the 20th century relied on the use of animals in some way. The Institute for Laboratory Animal Research of the U.S. National Academy of Sciences has argued that animal research cannot be replaced by even sophisticated computer models, which are unable to deal with the extremely complex interactions between molecules, cells, tissues, organs, organisms, and the environment. Animal rights, and some animal welfare, organizations—such as PETA and BUAV—question the need for and legitimacy of animal testing, arguing that it is cruel and poorly regulated, that medical progress is actually held back by misleading animal models that cannot reliably predict effects in humans, that some of the tests are outdated, that the costs outweigh the benefits, or that animals have the intrinsic right not to be used or harmed in experimentation.

The terms animal testing, **animal experimentation**, animal research, ***in vivo* testing**, and **vivisection** have similar denotations but different connotations. Literally, vivisection means the cutting up of a living animal, and historically referred only to experiments that involved the dissection of live animals. The term is occasionally used to refer pejoratively to any experiment using living animals; for example, the *Encyclopædia Britannica* defines "vivisection" as: "Operation on a living animal for experimental rather than healing purposes; more broadly, all experimentation on live animals", although dictionaries point out that the broader definition is "used only by people who are opposed to such work". The word has a negative connotation, implying torture, suffering, and death. The word "vivisection" is preferred by those opposed to this research, whereas scientists typically use the term "animal experimentation".

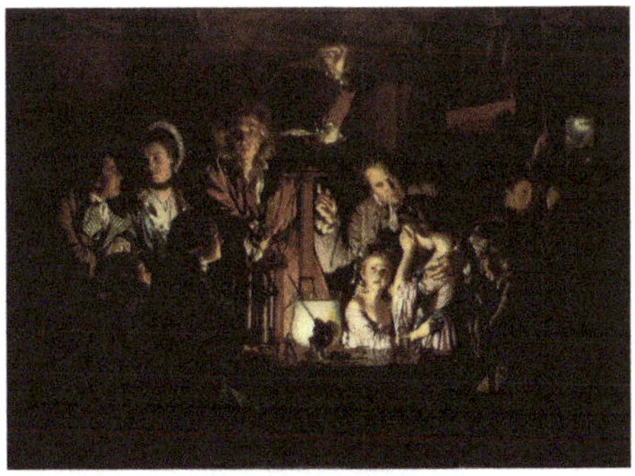

An Experiment on a Bird in an Air Pump, from 1768, by Joseph Wright

The earliest references to animal testing are found in the writings of the Greeks in the 2nd and 4th centuries BCE. Aristotle and Erasistratus were among the first to perform experiments on living animals. Galen, a physician in 2nd-century Rome, dissected pigs and goats, and is known as the father of vivisection. Avenzoar, an Arabic physician in 12th-century Moorish Spain who also practiced dissection, introduced animal testing as an experimental method of testing surgical procedures before applying them to human patients.

Animals have repeatedly been used through the history of biomedical research. The founders, in 1831, of the Dublin Zoo were members of the medical profession, interested in studying the animals both while they were alive and when they were dead. In the 1880s, Louis Pasteur convincingly demonstrated the germ theory of medicine by inducing anthrax in sheep. In the 1880s, Robert Koch infected mice and guinea pigs with anthrax and tuberculosis. In the 1890s, Ivan Pavlov famously used dogs to describe classical conditioning. In World War I, German agents infected sheep bound for Russia with anthrax, and inoculated mules and horses of the French cavalry with the equine glanders disease. Between 1917 and 1918, the Germans infected mules in Argentina bound for American forces, resulting in the death of 200 mules. Insulin was first isolated from dogs in 1922, and revolutionized the treatment of diabetes. On November 3, 1957, a Soviet dog, Laika, became the first of many animals to orbit the earth. In the 1970s, antibiotic treatments and vaccines for leprosy were developed using armadillos, then given to humans. The ability of humans to change the genetics of animals took a large step forwards in 1974 when Rudolf Jaenisch was able to produce the first transgenic mammal, by integrating DNA from the SV40 virus into the genome of mice. This genetic research progressed rapidly and, in 1996, Dolly the sheep was born, the first mammal to be cloned from an adult cell.

Toxicology testing became important in the 20th century. In the 19th century, laws regulating drugs were more relaxed. For example, in the U.S., the government could only ban a drug after a company had been prosecuted for selling products that harmed customers. However, in response to the Elixir Sulfanilamide disaster of 1937 in which the eponymous drug killed more than 100 users, the U.S. congress passed laws that required safety testing of drugs on animals before they could be marketed. Other countries enacted similar legislation. In the 1960s, in reaction to the Thalidomide tragedy, further laws were passed requiring safety testing on pregnant animals before a drug can be sold.

Historical Debate

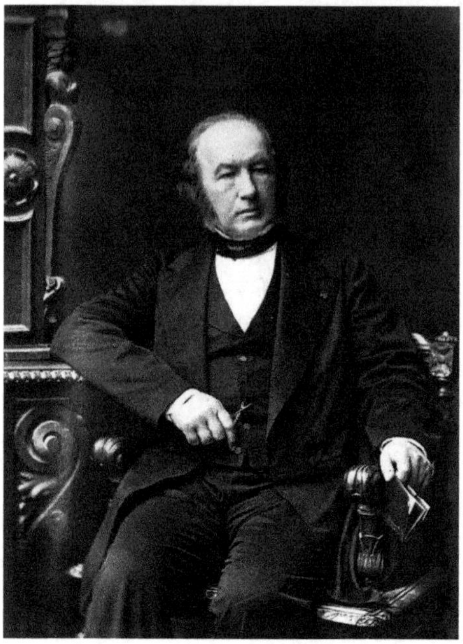

Claude Bernard, regarded as the "prince of vivisectors", argued that experiments on animals are "entirely conclusive for the toxicology and hygiene of man".

As the experimentation on animals increased, especially the practice of vivisection, so did criticism and controversy. In 1655, the advocate of Galenic physiology Edmund O'Meara said that "the miserable torture of vivisection places the body in an unnatural state." O'Meara and others argued that animal physiology could be affected by pain during vivisection, rendering results unreliable. There were also objections on an ethical basis, contending that the benefit to humans did not justify the harm to animals. Early objections to animal testing also came from another angle—many people believed that animals were inferior to humans and so different that results from animals could not be applied to humans.

On the other side of the debate, those in favor of animal testing held that experiments on animals were necessary to advance medical and biological knowledge. Claude Bernard—who is sometimes known as the prince of vivisectors and the father of physiology, and whose wife, Marie Françoise Martin, founded the first anti-vivisection society in France in 1883—famously wrote in 1865 that the science of life is a superb and dazzlingly lighted hall which may be reached only by passing through a long and ghastly kitchen. Arguing that experiments on animals ... are entirely conclusive for the toxicology and hygiene of man...the effects of these substances are the same on man as on animals, save for differences in degree, Bernard established animal experimentation as part of the standard scientific method.

In 1896, the physiologist and physician Dr. Walter B. Cannon said "The antivivisectionists are the second of the two types Theodore Roosevelt described when he said, 'Common sense without conscience may lead to crime, but conscience without common sense may lead to folly, which is the handmaiden of crime.'" These divisions between pro- and anti- animal testing groups first came to public attention during the brown dog affair in the early 1900s, when hundreds of medical students clashed with anti-vivisectionists and police over a memorial to a vivisected dog.

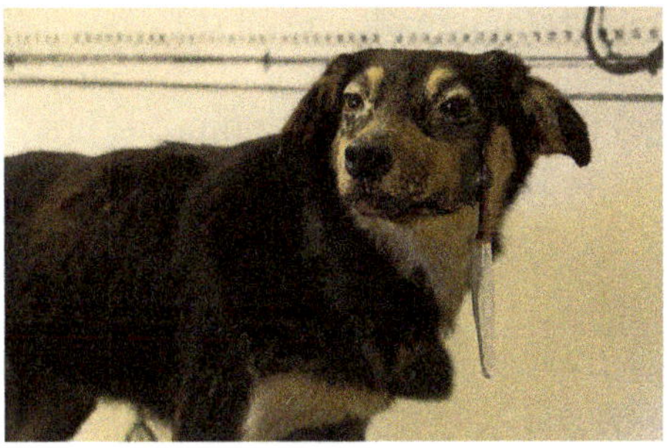

One of Pavlov's dogs with a saliva-catch container and tube surgically implanted in his muzzle, Pavlov Museum, 2005

In 1822, the first animal protection law was enacted in the British parliament, followed by the Cruelty to Animals Act (1876), the first law specifically aimed at regulating animal testing. The legislation was promoted by Charles Darwin, who wrote to Ray Lankester in March 1871: "You ask about my opinion on vivisection. I quite agree that it is justifiable for real investigations on physiology; but not for mere damnable and detestable curiosity. It is a subject which makes me sick with horror, so I will not say another word about it, else I shall not sleep to-night." In response to the lobbying by anti-vivisectionists, several organizations were set up in Britain to defend animal research: The Physiological Society was formed in 1876 to give physiologists "mutual benefit and protection", the Association for the Advancement of Medicine by Research was formed in 1882 and focused on policy-making, and the Research Defence Society (now Understanding Animal Research) was formed in 1908 to make known the facts as to experiments on animals in this country; the immense importance to the welfare of mankind of such experiments and the great saving of human life and health directly attributable to them.

Opposition to the use of animals in medical research first arose in the United States during the 1860s, when Henry Bergh founded the American Society for the Prevention of Cruelty to Animals (ASPCA), with America's first specifically anti-vivisection organization being the American AntiVivisection Society (AAVS), founded in 1883. Antivivisectionists of the era generally believed the spread of mercy was the great cause of civilization, and vivisection was cruel. However, in the USA the antivivisectionists' efforts were defeated in every legislature, overwhelmed by the superior organization and influence of the medical community. Overall, this movement had little legislative success until the passing of the Laboratory Animal Welfare Act, in 1966.

Care and use of Animals

The Three Rs

The Three Rs (3Rs) are guiding principles for more ethical use of animals in testing. These were first described by W.M.S. Russell and R.L. Burch in 1959. The 3Rs are:

- **Replacement** which refers to the preferred use of non-animal methods over animal methods whenever it is possible to achieve the same scientific aims. These methods include computer modeling.
- **Reduction** which refers to methods that enable researchers to obtain comparable levels of information from fewer animals, or to obtain more information from the same number of animals.
- **Refinement** which refers to methods that alleviate or minimize potential pain, suffering or distress, and enhance animal welfare for the animals used. These methods include non-invasive techniques.

The 3Rs have a broader scope than simply encouraging alternatives to animal testing, but aim to improve animal welfare and scientific quality where the use of animals can not be avoided. These 3Rs are now implemented in many testing establishments worldwide and have been adopted by various pieces of legislation and regulations.

Despite the widespread acceptance of the 3Rs, many countries—including Canada, Australia, Israel, the United Kingdom, and Germany—have reported rising experimental use of animals in recent years with increased use of mice and, in some cases, fish while reporting declines in the use of cats, dogs, primates, rabbits, guinea pigs, and hamsters. Along with other countries, China has also escalated its use of GM animals, resulting in an increase in overall animal use.

Regulations

The regulations that apply to animals in laboratories vary across species. In the U.S., under the provisions of the Animal Welfare Act and the *Guide for the Care and Use of Laboratory Animals* (the *Guide*), published by the National Academy of Sciences, any procedure can be performed on an animal if it can be successfully argued that it is scientifically justified. In general, researchers are required to consult with the institution's veterinarian and its Institutional Animal Care and Use Committee (IACUC), which every research facility is obliged to maintain. The IACUC must ensure that alternatives, including non-animal alternatives, have been considered, that the experiments are not unnecessarily duplicative, and that pain relief is given unless it would interfere with the study. The IACUCs regulate all vertebrates in testing at institutions receiving federal funds in the USA. Although the provisions of the Animal Welfare Act do not include purpose-bred rodents and birds, these species are equally regulated under Public Health Service policies that govern the IACUCs. Animal Welfare Act (AWA) regulations are enforced by the

USDA, whereas Public Health Service regulations are enforced by OLAW and in many cases by AAALAC.

According to the 2014 U.S. Department of Agriculture Office of the Inspector General (OIG) report —which looked at the oversight of animal use during a three-year period— "some Institutional Animal Care and Use Committees ...did not adequately approve, monitor, or report on experimental procedures on animals." The OIG found that "as a result, animals are not always receiving basic humane care and treatment and, in some cases, pain and distress are not minimized during and after experimental procedures." According to the report, within a three-year period, nearly half of all American laboratories with regulated species were cited for AWA violations relating to improper IACUC oversight. The USDA OIG made similar findings in a 2005 report. Others have criticized the composition of IACUCs, asserting that the committees are predominantly made up of animal researchers and university representatives who may be biased against animal welfare concerns.

Larry Carbone, a laboratory animal veterinarian, writes that, in his experience, IACUCs take their work very seriously regardless of the species involved, though the use of non-human primates always raises what he calls a "red flag of special concern." A study published in *Science* magazine in July 2001 confirmed the low reliability of IACUC reviews of animal experiments. Funded by the National Science Foundation, the three-year study found that animal-use committees that do not know the specifics of the university and personnel do not make the same approval decisions as those made by animal-use committees that do know the university and personnel. Specifically, blinded committees more often ask for more information rather than approving studies.

Scientists in India are protesting a recent guideline issued by the University Grants Commission to ban the use of live animals in universities and laboratories.

Numbers

Accurate global figures for animal testing are difficult to obtain; it has been estimated that 100 million vertebrates are experimented on around the world every year, 10–11 million of them in the EU. The Nuffield Council on Bioethics reports that global annual estimates range from 50 to 100 million animals. None of the figures include invertebrates such as shrimp and fruit flies.

According to the US Department of Agriculture (USDA), the total number of animals used in the US during 2014 was 834,453, down from almost 1.2 million in 2005, however, this number does not include rats and mice, which make up around 90% of research animals. By comparing with EU data, where all vertebrate species are counted, Speaking of Research estimated that around 12 million vertebrates were used in research in the US in 2014. A 2015 article published in the *Journal of Medical Ethics*, argued that the use of animals in the US has dramatically increased in recent years. Researchers found this increase is largely the result of an increased reliance on genetically modified mice in animal studies.

In 1995, researchers at Tufts University Center for Animals and Public Policy estimated that 14–21 million animals were used in American laboratories in 1992, a reduction from a high of 50 million used in 1970. In 1986, the U.S. Congress Office of Technology Assessment reported that estimates of the animals used in the U.S. range from 10 million to upwards of 100 million each year, and that their own best estimate was at least 17 million to 22 million.

In GB, Home Office figures show that 3.87 million procedures were carried out in 2014. 3,246 procedures used non-human primates, down over 50% since 1988. A "procedure" refers here to an experiment that might last minutes, several months, or years. Most animals are used in only one procedure: animals are frequently euthanized after the experiment; however death is the endpoint of some procedures. The procedures conducted on animals in GB in 2014 were categorised as -

- 9% (180 thousand) were assessed as sub-threshold
- 7% (133 thousand) were assessed as non-recovery
- 51% (980 thousand) were assessed as mild
- 25% (483 thousand) were assessed as moderate
- 8% (150 thousand) were assessed as severe

A 'severe' procedure would be, for instance, any test where death is the end-point or fatalities are expected, whereas a 'mild' procedure would be something like a blood test or an MRI scan.

Invertebrates

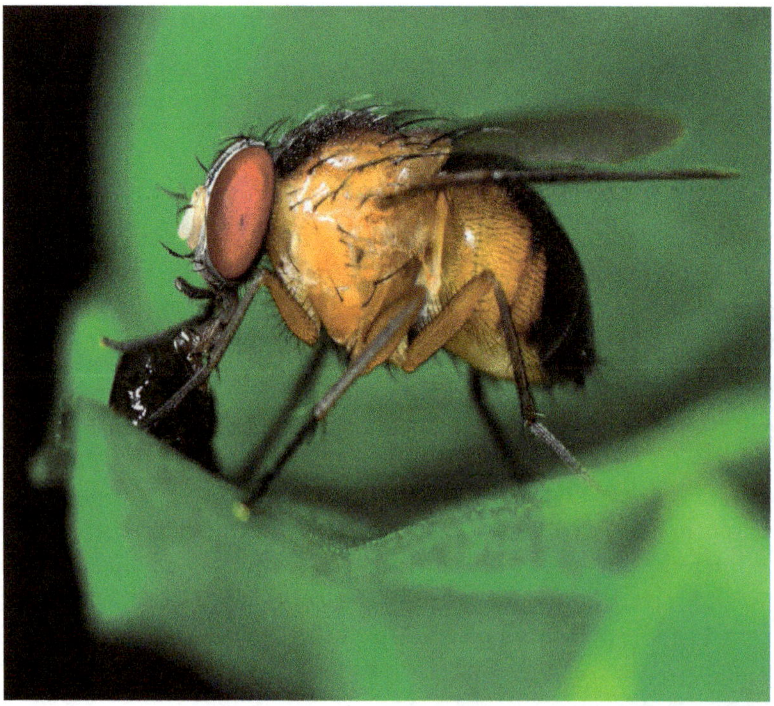

Fruit flies are an invertebrate commonly used in animal testing.

Although many more invertebrates than vertebrates are used in animal testing, these studies are largely unregulated by law. The most frequently used invertebrate species are *Drosophila melanogaster*, a fruit fly, and *Caenorhabditis elegans*, a nematode worm. In the case of *C. elegans*, the worm's body is completely transparent and the precise lineage of all the organism's cells is known, while studies in the fly *D. melanogaster* can use an amazing array of genetic tools. These invertebrates offer some advantages over vertebrates in animal testing, including their short life cycle and the ease with which large numbers may be housed and studied. However, the lack of an adaptive immune system and their simple organs prevent worms from being used in several aspects of medical research such as vaccine development. Similarly, the fruit fly immune system differs greatly from that of humans, and diseases in insects can be different from diseases in vertebrates; however, fruit flies and waxworms can be useful in studies to identify novel virulence factors or pharmacologically active compounds.

Several invertebrate systems are considered acceptable alternatives to vertebrates in early-stage discovery screens. Because of similarities between the innate immune system of insects and mammals, insects can replace mammals in some types of studies. *Drosophila melanogaster* and the *Galleria mellonella* waxworm have been particularly important for analysis of virulence traits of mammalian pathogens. Waxworms and other insects have also proven valuable for the identification of pharmaceutical compounds with favorable bioavailability. The decision to adopt such models generally involves accepting a lower degree of biological similarity with mammals for significant gains in experimental throughput.

Vertebrates

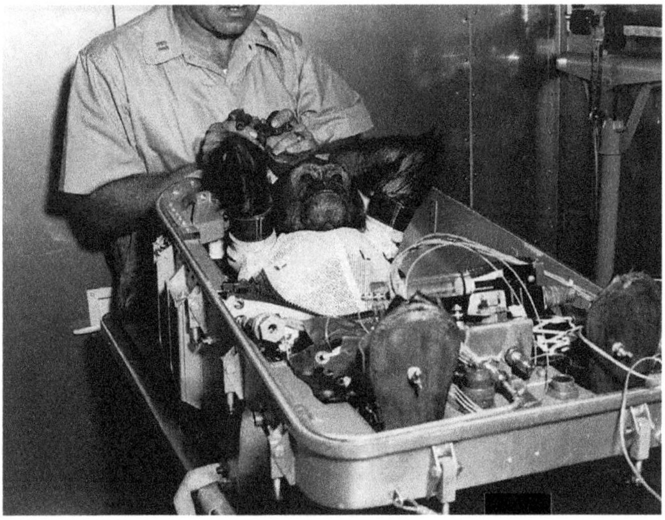

Enos the space chimp before insertion into the Mercury-Atlas 5 capsule in 1961

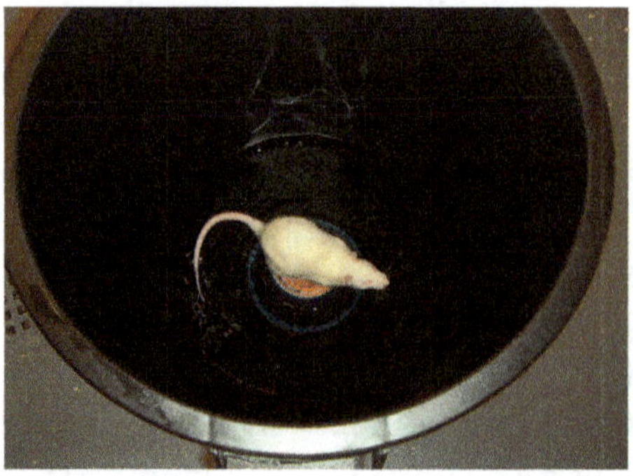

This rat is being deprived of restful sleep using a single platform ("flower pot") technique. The water is within 1 cm of the small flower pot bottom platform where the rat sits. At the onset of sleep, the rat would either fall into the water only to clamber back to the pot to avoid drowning, or its nose would become submerged into the water shocking it back to an awakened state.

In the U.S., the numbers of rats and mice used is estimated to be between 20 and 100 million a year.Other rodents commonly used are guinea pigs, hamsters, and gerbils. Mice are the most commonly used vertebrate species because of their size, low cost, ease of handling, and fast reproduction rate. Mice are widely considered to be the best model of inherited human disease and share 99% of their genes with humans. With the advent of genetic engineering technology, genetically modified mice can be generated to order and can provide models for a range of human diseases. Rats are also widely used for physiology, toxicology and cancer research, but genetic manipulation is much harder in rats than in mice, which limits the use of these rodents in basic science. Nearly 200,000 fish and 20,000 amphibians were used in the UK in 2004. The main species used is the zebrafish, *Danio rerio*, which are translucent during their embryonic stage, and the African clawed frog, *Xenopus laevis*. Over 20,000 rabbits were used for animal testing in the UK in 2004. Albino rabbits are used in eye irritancy tests (Draize test) because rabbits have less tear flow than other animals, and the lack of eye pigment in albinos make the effects easier to visualize. Rabbits are also frequently used for the production of polyclonal antibodies.

Cats

Cats are most commonly used in neurological research. 24,221 cats were used in the U.S. in 2013, around half of whom were used in experiments which have the potential to cause "pain and/or distress" though only 0.3% of cat experiments involved potential pain which was not relieved by anesthetics/analgesics.

Dogs

Dogs are widely used in biomedical research, testing, and education—particularly beagles, because they are gentle and easy to handle, and to allow for comparisons with historical data from beagles (a Reduction technique). They are used as models for human and veterinary diseases in cardiology, endocrinology, and bone and joint studies, research that tends to be highly invasive, according to the Humane Society of the United States. The most common use of dogs is in the safety assessment of new medicines for human or veterinary use as a second species following testing in rodents, in accordance with the regulations set out in the International Conference on Harmonisation of Technical Requirements for Registration of Pharmaceuticals for Human Use. The U.S. Department of Agriculture's Animal Welfare Report shows that 67,772 dogs were used in USDA-registered facilities in 2013.

Non-Human Primates

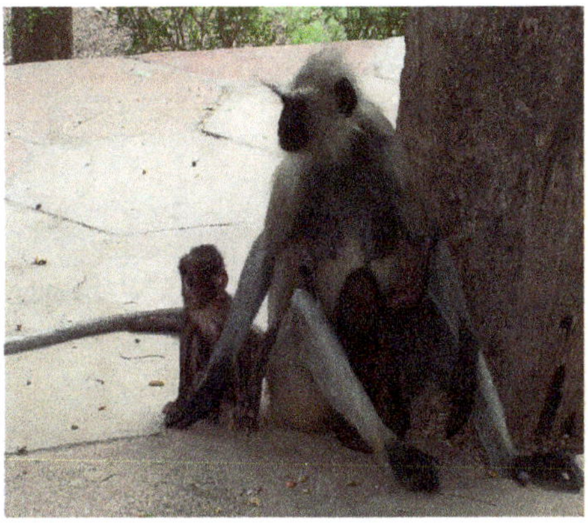

Non-human primates (NHPs) are used in toxicology tests, studies of AIDS and hepatitis, studies of neurology, behavior and cognition, reproduction, genetics, and xenotransplantation. They are caught in the wild or purpose-bred. In the United States and China, most primates are domestically purpose-bred, whereas in Europe the majority are imported purpose-bred. The European Commission reported that in 2011, 6,012 monkeys were experimented on in European laboratories. According to the U.S. Department of Agriculture, there were 105,665 monkeys in U.S. laboratories in 2014. 23,465 monkeys were imported into the U.S. in 2014 including 929 who were caught in the wild. Most of the NHPs used in experiments are macaques; but marmosets, spider monkeys, and squirrel monkeys are also used, and baboons and chimpanzees are used in the US. As of 2015, there are approximately 730 chimpanzees in U.S. laboratories.

In one survey, it was found that 89% of singly-housed primates exhibited self-injurious or abnormal stereotypyical behaviors including pacing, rocking, hair pulling, and biting among others.

The first transgenic primate was produced in 2001, with the development of a method that could introduce new genes into a rhesus macaque.This transgenic technology is now being applied in the search for a treatment for the genetic disorder Huntington's disease. Notable studies on non-human primates have been part of the polio vaccine development, and development of Deep Brain Stimulation, and their current heaviest non-toxicological use occurs in the monkey AIDS model, SIV. In 2008 a proposal to ban all primates experiments in the EU has sparked a vigorous debate.

Sources

Animals used by laboratories are largely supplied by specialist dealers. Sources differ for vertebrate and invertebrate animals. Most laboratories breed and raise flies and worms themselves, using strains and mutants supplied from a few main stock centers. For vertebrates, sources include breeders and dealers like Covance and Charles River Laboratories who supply purpose-bred and wild-caught animals; businesses that trade in wild animals such as Nafovanny; and dealers who supply animals sourced from pounds, auctions, and newspaper ads. Animal shelters also supply the laboratories directly. Large centers also exist to distribute strains of genetically modified animals; the International Knockout Mouse Consortium, for example, aims to provide knockout mice for every gene in the mouse genome.

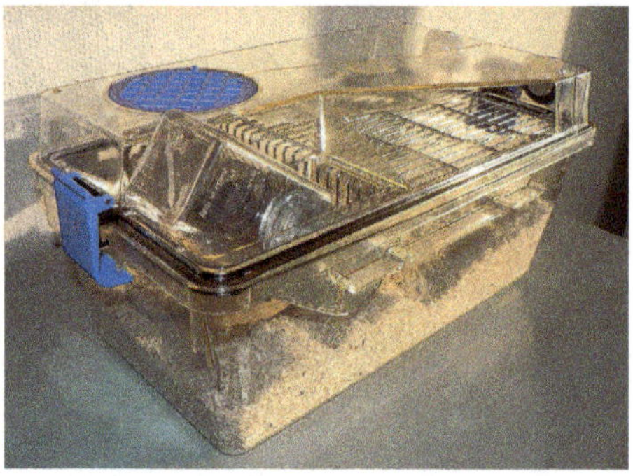

A laboratory mouse cage. Mice are either bred commercially, or raised in the laboratory.

In the U.S., Class A breeders are licensed by the U.S. Department of Agriculture (USDA) to sell animals for research purposes, while Class B dealers are licensed to buy animals from "random sources" such as auctions, pound seizure, and newspaper ads. Some Class B dealers have been accused of kidnapping pets and illegally trapping strays, a practice known as *bunching*. It was in part out of public concern over the sale of pets to research facilities that the 1966 Laboratory Animal Welfare Act was ushered in—the Senate Committee on Commerce reported in 1966 that stolen pets had been retrieved from Veterans Administration facilities, the Mayo Institute, the University of Pennsylvania, Stanford University, and Harvard and Yale Medical Schools. The USDA recovered at least a dozen stolen pets during a raid on a Class B dealer in Arkansas in 2003.

Four states in the U.S.—Minnesota, Utah, Oklahoma, and Iowa—require their shelters to provide animals to research facilities. Fourteen states explicitly prohibit the practice, while the remainder either allow it or have no relevant legislation.

In the European Union, animal sources are governed by *Council Directive 86/609/EEC*, which requires lab animals to be specially bred, unless the animal has been lawfully imported and is not a wild animal or a stray. The latter requirement may also be exempted by special arrangement. In 2010 the Directive was revised with EU Directive 2010/63/EU. In the UK, most animals used in experiments are bred for the purpose under the 1988 Animal Protection Act, but wild-caught primates may be used if exceptional and specific justification can be established. The United States also allows the use of wild-caught primates; between 1995 and 1999, 1,580 wild baboons were imported into the U.S. Over half the primates imported between 1995 and 2000 were handled by Charles River Laboratories, or by Covance, which is the single largest importer of primates into the U.S.

Pain and Suffering

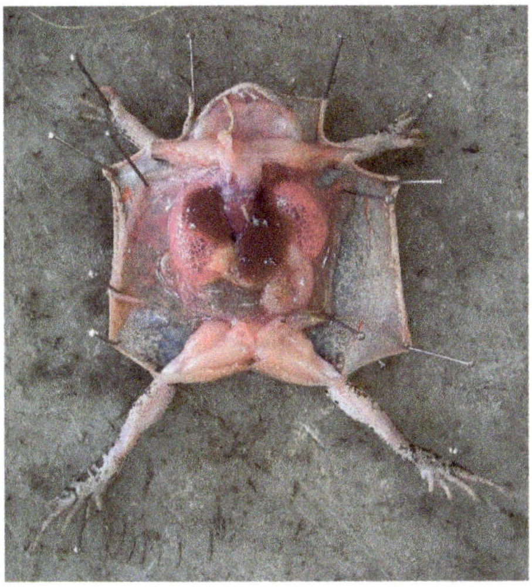

Prior to dissection for educational purposes, chloroform was administered to this common sand frog to induce anesthesia and death.

The extent to which animal testing causes pain and suffering, and the capacity of animals to experience and comprehend them, is the subject of much debate.

According to the USDA, in 2005 about 668,000 animals (57%) (not including rats, mice, birds, or invertebrates) were used in procedures that did not include more than momentary pain or distress. About 425,000 (36%) were used in procedures in which pain or distress was relieved by anesthesia, while 85,000 (7%) were used in studies that would cause pain or distress that would not be relieved.

In the UK, research projects are classified as mild, moderate, and substantial in terms of the suffering the researchers conducting the study say they may cause; a fourth category of unclassified means the animal was anesthetized and killed without recovering consciousness, according to the researchers. In December 2001, 1,296 (39%) of project licenses in force were classified as mild, 1,811 (55%) as moderate, 63 (2%) as substantial, and 139 (4%) as unclassified. There have, however, been suggestions of systemic underestimation of procedure severity.

The idea that animals might not feel pain as human beings feel it traces back to the 17th-century French philosopher, René Descartes, who argued that animals do not experience pain and suffering because they lack consciousness. Bernard Rollin of Colorado State University, the principal author of two U.S. federal laws regulating pain relief for animals, writes that researchers remained unsure into the 1980s as to whether animals experience pain, and that veterinarians trained in the U.S. before 1989 were simply taught to ignore animal pain. In his interactions with scientists and other veterinarians, he was regularly asked to prove that animals are conscious, and to provide scientifically acceptable grounds for claiming that they feel pain. Carbone writes that the view that animals feel pain differently is now a minority view. Academic reviews of the topic are more equivocal, noting that although the argument that animals have at least simple conscious thoughts and feelings has strong support, some critics continue to question how reliably animal mental states can be determined. The ability of invertebrates to experience pain and suffering is less clear, however, legislation in several countries (e.g. U.K., New Zealand, Norway) protects some invertebrate species if they are being used in animal testing.

In the U.S., the defining text on animal welfare regulation in animal testing is the *Guide for the Care and Use of Laboratory Animals*. This defines the parameters that govern animal testing in the U.S. It states "The ability to experience and respond to pain is widespread in the animal kingdom...Pain is a stressor and, if not relieved, can lead to unacceptable levels of stress and distress in animals." The Guide states that the ability to recognize the symptoms of pain in different species is vital in efficiently applying pain relief and that it is essential for the people caring for and using animals to be entirely familiar with these symptoms. On the subject of analgesics used to relieve pain, the Guide states "The selection of the most appropriate analgesic or anesthetic should reflect professional judgment as to which best meets clinical and humane requirements without compromising the scientific aspects of the research protocol". Accordingly, all issues of animal pain and distress, and their potential treatment with analgesia and anesthesia, are required regulatory issues in receiving animal protocol approval.

Euthanasia

Regulations require that scientists use as few animals as possible, especially for terminal experiments. However, while policy makers consider suffering to be the central issue and see animal euthanasia as a way to reduce suffering, others, such as the RSPCA, argue that the lives of laboratory animals have intrinsic value. Regulations focus on whether particular methods cause pain and suffering, not whether their death is undesirable in itself. The animals are euthanized at the end of studies for sample collection or post-mortem examination; during studies if their pain or suffering falls into certain categories regarded as unacceptable, such as depression, infection that is unresponsive to treatment, or the failure of large animals to eat for five days; or when they are unsuitable for breeding or unwanted for some other reason.

Methods of euthanizing laboratory animals are chosen to induce rapid unconsciousness and death without pain or distress. The methods that are preferred are those published by councils of veterinarians. The animal can be made to inhale a gas, such as carbon monoxide and carbon dioxide, by being placed in a chamber, or by use of a face mask, with or without prior sedation or anesthesia. Sedatives or anesthetics such as barbiturates can be given intravenously, or inhalant anesthetics may be used. Amphibians and fish may be immersed in water containing an anesthetic such as tricaine. Physical methods are also used, with or without sedation or anesthesia depending on the method. Recommended methods include decapitation (beheading) for small rodents or rabbits. Cervical dislocation (breaking the neck or spine) may be used for birds, mice, and immature rats and rabbits. Maceration (grinding into small pieces) is used on 1 day old chicks. High-intensity microwave irradiation of the brain can preserve brain tissue and induce death in less than 1 second, but this is currently only used on rodents. Captive bolts may be used, typically on dogs, ruminants, horses, pigs and rabbits. It causes death by a concussion to the brain. Gunshot may be used, but only in cases where a penetrating captive bolt may not be used. Some physical methods are only acceptable after the animal is unconscious. Electrocution may be used for cattle, sheep, swine, foxes, and mink after the animals are unconscious, often by a prior electrical stun. Pithing (inserting a tool into the base of the brain) is usable on animals already unconscious. Slow or rapid freezing, or inducing air embolism are acceptable only with prior anesthesia to induce unconsciousness.

Research Classification

Pure Research

Basic or pure research investigates how organisms behave, develop, and function. Those opposed to animal testing object that pure research may have little or no practical purpose, but researchers argue that it forms the necessary basis for the development of applied research, rendering the distinction between pure and applied research—research that has a specific practical aim—unclear. Pure research uses larger numbers and a greater variety of animals than applied research. Fruit flies, nematode worms, mice and rats together account for the vast majority, though small numbers of other species are used, ranging from sea slugs through to armadillos. Examples of the types of animals and experiments used in basic research include:

- Studies on *embryogenesis* and *developmental biology*. Mutants are created by adding transposons into their genomes, or specific genes are deleted by gene targeting. By studying the changes in development these changes produce, scientists aim to understand both how organisms normally develop, and what can go wrong in this process. These studies are particularly powerful since the basic controls of development, such as the homeobox genes, have similar functions in organisms as diverse as fruit flies and man.
- Experiments into *behavior*, to understand how organisms detect and interact with each other and their environment, in which fruit flies, worms, mice, and rats are all widely used. Studies of brain function, such as memory and social behavior, often use rats and birds. For some species, behavioral research is combined with enrichment strategies for animals in captivity because it allows them to engage in a wider range of activities.
- Breeding experiments to study *evolution* and *genetics*. Laboratory mice, flies, fish, and worms are inbred through many generations to create strains with defined characteristics.These provide animals of a known genetic background, an important tool for genetic analyses. Larger mammals are rarely bred specifically for such studies due to their slow rate of reproduction, though some scientists

take advantage of inbred domesticated animals, such as dog or cattle breeds, for comparative purposes. Scientists studying how animals evolve use many animal species to see how variations in where and how an organism lives (their niche) produce adaptations in their physiology and morphology. As an example, sticklebacks are now being used to study how many and which types of mutations are selected to produce adaptations in animals' morphology during the evolution of new species.

Applied Research

Applied research aims to solve specific and practical problems. Compared to pure research, which is largely academic in origin, applied research is usually carried out in the pharmaceutical industry, or by universities in commercial partnerships. These may involve the use of animal models of diseases or conditions, which are often discovered or generated by pure research programmes. In turn, such applied studies may be an early stage in the drug discovery process. Examples include:

- Genetic modification of animals to study disease. Transgenic animals have specific genes inserted, modified or removed, to mimic specific conditions such as single gene disorders, such as Huntington's disease. Other models mimic complex, multifactorial diseases with genetic components, such as diabetes, or even transgenic mice that carry the same mutations that occur during the development of cancer. These models allow investigations on how and why the disease develops, as well as providing ways to develop and test new treatments. The vast majority of these transgenic models of human disease are lines of mice, the mammalian species in which genetic modification is most efficient. Smaller numbers of other animals are also used, including rats, pigs, sheep, fish, birds, and amphibians.
- Studies on models of naturally occurring disease and condition. Certain domestic and wild animals have a natural propensity or predisposition for certain conditions that are also found in humans. Cats are used as a model to develop immunodeficiency virus vaccines and to study leukemia because their natural predisposition to FIV and Feline leukemia virus.Certain breeds of dog suffer from narcolepsy making them the major model used to study the human condition. Armadillos and humans are among only a few animal species that naturally suffer from leprosy; as the bacteria responsible for this disease cannot yet be grown in culture, armadillos are the primary source of bacilli used in leprosy vaccines.
- Studies on induced animal models of human diseases. Here, an animal is treated so that it develops pathology and symptoms that resemble a human disease. Examples include restricting blood flow to the brain to induce stroke, or giving neurotoxins that cause damage similar to that seen in Parkinson's disease. Such studies can be difficult to interpret, and it is argued that they are not always comparable to human diseases. For example, although such models are now widely used to study Parkinson's disease, the British anti-vivisection interest group BUAV argues that these models only superficially resemble the disease

symptoms, without the same time course or cellular pathology. In contrast, scientists assessing the usefulness of animal models of Parkinson's disease, as well as the medical research charity *The Parkinson's Appeal*, state that these models were invaluable and that they led to improved surgical treatments such as pallidotomy, new drug treatments such as levodopa, and later deep brain stimulation.

- Animal testing has also included the use of placebo testing. In these cases animals are treated with a substance that produces no pharmacological effect, but is administered in order to determine any biological alterations due to the experience of a substance being administered, and the results are compared with those obtained with an active compound.

Xenotransplantation

Xenotransplantation research involves transplanting tissues or organs from one species to another, as a way to overcome the shortage of human organs for use in organ transplants. Current research involves using primates as the recipients of organs from pigs that have been genetically modified to reduce the primates' immune response against the pig tissue.Although transplant rejection remains a problem, recent clinical trials that involved implanting pig insulin-secreting cells into diabetics did reduce these people's need for insulin.

Documents released to the news media by the animal rights organization Uncaged Campaigns showed that, between 1994 and 2000, wild baboons imported to the UK from Africa by Imutran Ltd, a subsidiary of Novartis Pharma AG, in conjunction with Cambridge University and Huntingdon Life Sciences, to be used in experiments that involved grafting pig tissues, suffered serious and sometimes fatal injuries. A scandal occurred when it was revealed that the company had communicated with the British government in an attempt to avoid regulation.

Toxicology Testing

Toxicology testing, also known as safety testing, is conducted by pharmaceutical companies testing drugs, or by contract animal testing facilities, such as Huntingdon Life Sciences, on behalf of a wide variety of customers. According to 2005 EU figures, around one million animals are used every year in Europe in toxicology tests; which are about 10% of all procedures. According to *Nature*, 5,000 animals are used for each chemical being tested, with 12,000 needed to test pesticides. The tests are conducted without anesthesia, because interactions between drugs can affect how animals detoxify chemicals, and may interfere with the results.

Toxicology tests are used to examine finished products such as pesticides, medications, food additives, packing materials, and air freshener, or their chemical ingredients. Most tests involve testing ingredients rather than finished products, but according to BUAV, manufacturers believe these tests overestimate the toxic effects of substances; they therefore repeat the tests using their finished products to obtain a less toxic label.

The substances are applied to the skin or dripped into the eyes; injected intravenously, intramuscularly, or subcutaneously; inhaled either by placing a mask over the animals and restraining them, or by placing them in an inhalation chamber; or administered orally, through a tube into the stomach, or simply in the animal's food. Doses may be given once, repeated regularly for many months, or for the lifespan of the animal.

There are several different types of acute toxicity tests. The LD_{50} ("Lethal Dose 50%") test is used to evaluate the toxicity of a substance by determining the dose required to kill 50% of the test animal population. This test was removed from OECD international guidelines in 2002, replaced by methods such as the fixed dose procedure, which use fewer animals and cause less suffering. Abbott writes that, as of 2005, the LD50 acute toxicity test ... still accounts for one-third of all animal toxicity tests worldwide.

Irritancy can be measured using the Draize test, where a test substance is applied to an animal's eyes or skin, usually an albino rabbit. For Draize eye testing, the test involves observing the effects of the substance at intervals and grading any damage or irritation, but the test should be halted and the animal killed if it shows continuing signs of severe pain or distress. The Humane Society of the United States writes that the procedure can cause redness, ulceration, hemorrhaging, cloudiness, or even blindness. This test has also been criticized by scientists for being cruel and inaccurate, subjective, over-sensitive, and failing to reflect human exposures in the real world. Although no accepted *in vitro* alternatives exist, a modified form of the Draize test called the *low volume eye test* may reduce suffering and provide more realistic results and this was adopted as the new standard in September 2009. However, the Draize test will still be used for substances that are not severe irritants.

The most stringent tests are reserved for drugs and foodstuffs. For these, a number of tests are performed, lasting less than a month (acute), one to three months (subchronic), and more than three months (chronic) to test general toxicity (damage to organs), eye and skin irritancy, mutagenicity, carcinogenicity, teratogenicity, and reproductive problems. The cost of the full complement of tests is several million dollars per substance and it may take three or four years to complete.

These toxicity tests provide, in the words of a 2006 United States National Academy of Sciences report, "critical information for assessing hazard and risk potential". Animal tests may overestimate risk, with false positive results being a particular problem, but false positives appear not to be prohibitively common. Variability in results arises from using the effects of high doses of chemicals in small numbers of laboratory animals to try to predict the effects of low doses in large numbers of humans. Although relationships do exist, opinion is divided on how to use data on one species to predict the exact level of risk in another.

Scientists face growing pressure to move away from using traditional animal toxicity tests to determine whether manufactured chemicals are safe. Among variety of approaches to toxicity evaluation the ones which have attracted increasing interests are in vitro cell-based sensing methods applying fluorescence.

Cosmetics Testing

The "Leaping Bunny" logo: Products in Europe that are not tested on animals carry this symbol.

Cosmetics testing on animals is particularly controversial. Such tests, which are still conducted in the U.S., involve general toxicity, eye and skin irritancy, phototoxicity (toxicity triggered by ultraviolet light) and mutagenicity.

Cosmetics testing on animals is banned in India, the European Union, Israel and Norway while legislation in the U.S. and Brazil is currently considering similar bans. In 2002, after 13 years of discussion, the European Union agreed to phase in a near-total ban on the sale of animal-tested cosmetics by 2009, and to ban all cosmetics-related animal testing. France, which is home to the world's largest cosmetics company, L'Oreal, has protested the proposed ban by lodging a case at the European Court of Justice in Luxembourg, asking that the ban be quashed. The ban is also opposed by the European Federation for Cosmetics Ingredients, which represents 70 companies in Switzerland, Belgium, France, Germany, and Italy. In October 2014, India passed stricter laws that also ban the importation of any cosmetic products that are tested on animals.

Drug Testing

Before the early 20th century, laws regulating drugs were lax. Currently, all new pharmaceuticals undergo rigorous animal testing before being licensed for human use. Tests on pharmaceutical products involve:

- *metabolic tests*, investigating pharmacokinetics—how drugs are absorbed, metabolized and excreted by the body when introduced orally, intravenously, intraperitoneally, intramuscularly, or transdermally.
- *toxicology tests*, which gauge acute, sub-acute, and chronic toxicity. Acute toxicity is studied by using a rising dose until signs of toxicity become apparent. Current European legislation demands that "acute toxicity tests must be carried out in two or more mammalian species" covering "at least two different routes of administration". Sub-acute toxicity is where the drug is given to the animals for four to six weeks in doses below the level at which it causes rapid poisoning, in order to discover if any toxic drug metabolites build up over time. Testing for chronic toxicity can last up to two years and, in the European Union, is required to involve two species of mammals, one of which must be non-rodent.

- *efficacy studies*, which test whether experimental drugs work by inducing the appropriate illness in animals. The drug is then administered in a double-blind controlled trial, which allows researchers to determine the effect of the drug and the dose-response curve.
- Specific tests on *reproductive function*, *embryonic toxicity*, or *carcinogenic potential* can all be required by law, depending on the result of other studies and the type of drug being tested.

Education

It is estimated that 20 million animals are used annually for educational purposes in the United States including, classroom observational exercises, dissections and live-animal surgeries. Frogs, fetal pigs, perch, cats, earthworms, grasshoppers, crayfish and starfish are commonly used in classroom dissections. Alternatives to the use of animals in classroom dissections are widely used, with many U.S. States and school districts mandating students be offered the choice to not dissect. Citing the wide availability of alternatives and the decimation of local frog species, India banned dissections in 2014.

The Sonoran Arthropod Institute hosts an annual Invertebrates in Education and Conservation Conference to discuss the use of invertebrates in education. There also are efforts in many countries to find alternatives to using animals in education. The NORINA database, maintained by Norecopa, lists products that may be used as alternatives or supplements to animal use in education, and in the training of personnel who work with animals. These include alternatives to dissection in schools. InterNICHE has a similar database and a loans system.

In November 2013, the US-based company Backyard Brains released for sale to the public what they call the Roboroach, an electronic backpack that can be attached to cockroaches. The operator is required to amputate a cockroach's antennae, use sandpaper to wear down the shell, insert a wire into the thorax, and then glue the electrodes and circuit board onto the insect's back. A mobile phone app can then be used to control it via Bluetooth. It has been suggested that the use of such a device may be a teaching aid that can promote interest in science. The makers of the Roboroach have been funded by the National Institute of Mental Health and state that the device is intended to encourage children to become interested in neuroscience.

Defense

Animals are used by the military to develop weapons, vaccines, battlefield surgical techniques, and defensive clothing. For example, in 2008 the United States Defense Advanced Research Projects Agency used live pigs to study the effects of improvised explosive device explosions on internal organs, especially the brain.

In the US military, goats are commonly used to train combat medics. (Goats have become the main animal species used for this purpose after the Pentagon phased out using dogs for medical training in the 1980s.) While modern mannequins used in medical training are quite efficient in simulating the behavior of a human body, some trainees feel that “the goat exercise provides a sense of urgency that only real life trauma can provide. Nevertheless, in 2014, the U.S. Coast Guard announced that it would reduce the number of animals it uses in its training exercises by half after PETA released video showing Guard members cutting off the limbs of unconscious goats with tree trimmers and inflicting other injuries with a shotgun, pistol, ax and a scalpel. That same year, citing the availability of human simulators and other alternatives, the Department of Defense announced it would begin reducing the amount of animals it uses in various training programs. In 2013, several Navy medical centers stopped using ferrets in intubation exercises after complaints from PETA.

Besides the US, six out of 28 NATO countries, including Poland and Denmark, use live animals for combat medic training.

Ethics

Viewpoints

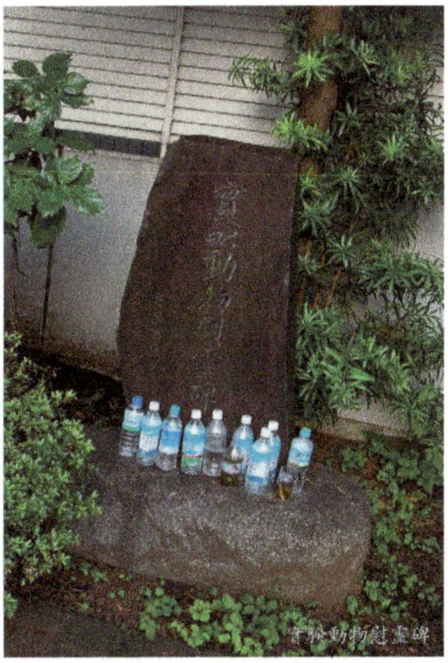

Monument for animals used in testing at Keio University

The moral and ethical questions raised by performing experiments on animals are subject to debate, and viewpoints have shifted significantly over the 20th century. There remain disagreements about which procedures are useful for which purposes, as well as disagreements over which ethical principles apply to which species.

A 2015 Gallup poll found that 67% of Americans were “very concerned” or “somewhat concerned” about animals used in research. A Pew poll taken the same year found 50% of American adults opposed the use of animals in research.

Still, a wide range of viewpoints exist. The view that animals have moral rights (animal rights) is a philosophical position proposed by Tom Regan, among others, who argues that animals are beings with beliefs and desires, and as such are the "subjects of a life" with moral value and therefore moral rights.Regan still sees ethical differences between killing human and non-human animals, and argues that to save the former it is permissible to kill the latter. Likewise, a "moral dilemma" view suggests that avoiding potential benefit to humans is unacceptable on similar grounds, and holds the issue to be a dilemma in balancing such harm to humans to the harm done to animals in research. In contrast, an abolitionist view in animal rights holds that there is no moral justification for any harmful research on animals that is not to the benefit of the individual animal. Bernard Rollin argues that benefits to human beings cannot outweigh animal suffering, and that human beings have no moral right to use an animal in ways that do not benefit that individual. Another prominent position is that of philosopher Peter Singer, who argues that there are no grounds to include a being's species in considerations of whether their suffering is important in utilitarian moral considerations. Malcolm Macleod and collaborators argue that most controlled animal studies do not employ randomization, allocation concealment, and blinding outcome assessment, and that failure to employ these features exaggerates the apparent benefit of drugs tested in animals, leading to a failure to translate much animal research for human benefit.

Governments such as the Netherlands and New Zealand have responded to the public's concerns by outlawing invasive experiments on certain classes of non-human primates, particularly the great apes. In 2015, captive chimpanzees in the U.S. were added to the Endangered Species Act adding new road blocks to those wishing to experiment on them. Similarly, citing ethical considerations and the availability of alternative research methods, the U.S. NIH announced in 2013 that it would dramatically reduce and eventually phase out experiments on chimpanzees.

The British government has required that the cost to animals in an experiment be weighed against the gain in knowledge. Some medical schools and agencies in China, Japan, and South Korea have built cenotaphs for killed animals. In Japan there are also annual memorial services (*Ireisai* 慰霊祭) for animals sacrificed at medical school.

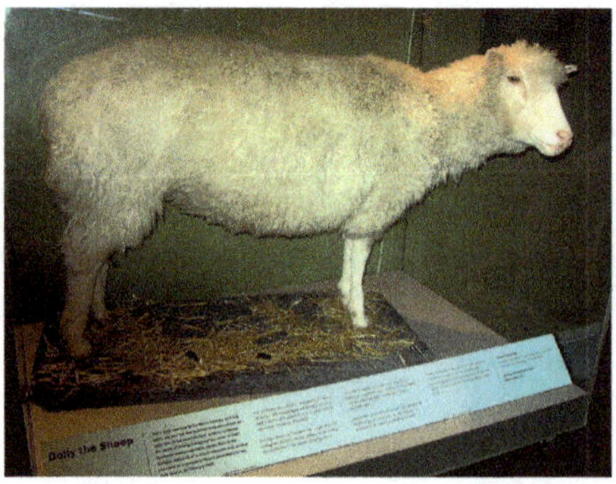

Dolly the sheep: the first clone produced from the somatic cells of an adult mammal

Various specific cases of animal testing have drawn attention, including both instances of beneficial scientific research, and instances of alleged ethical violations by those performing the tests. The fundamental properties of muscle physiology were determined with work done using frog muscles (including the force generating mechanism of all muscle, the length-tension relationship, and the force-velocity curve), and frogs are still the preferred model organism due to the long survival of muscles *in vitro* and the possibility of isolating intact single-fiber preparations (not possible in other organisms). Modern physical therapy and the understanding and treatment of muscular disorders is based on this work and subsequent work in mice (often engineered to express disease states such as muscular dystrophy). In February 1997 a team at the Roslin Institute in Scotland announced the birth of Dolly the sheep, the first mammal to be cloned from an adult somatic cell.

Concerns have been raised over the mistreatment of primates undergoing testing. In 1985 the case of Britches, a macaque monkey at the University of California, Riverside, gained public attention. He had his eyelids sewn shut and a sonar sensor on his head as part of an experiment to test sensory substitution devices for blind people. The laboratory was raided by Animal Liberation Front in 1985, removing Britches and 466 other animals. The National Institutes of Health conducted an eight-month investigation and concluded, however, that no corrective action was necessary. During the 2000s other cases have made headlines, including experiments at the University of Cambridge and Columbia University in 2002. In 2004 and 2005, undercover footage of staff of Covance's, a contract research organization that provides animal testing services, Virginia lab was shot by People for the Ethical Treatment of Animals (PETA). Following release of the footage, the U.S. Department of Agriculture fined Covance $8,720 for 16 citations, three of which involved lab monkeys; the other citations involved administrative issues and equipment. In 1997 PETA filmed staff from Huntingdon Life Sciences, showing dogs being mistreated. The employees responsible were dismissed, with two given community service orders and ordered to pay £250 costs, the first lab technicians to have been prosecuted for animal cruelty in the UK.

Threats to Researchers

In 2006, a primate researcher at the University of California, Los Angeles (UCLA) shut down the experiments in his lab after threats from animal rights activists. The researcher had received a grant to use 30 macaque monkeys for vision experiments; each monkey was anesthetized for a single physiological experiment lasting up to 120 hours, and then euthanized. The researcher's name, phone number, and address were posted on the website of the Primate Freedom Project. Demonstrations were held in front of his home. A Molotov cocktail was placed on the porch of what was believed to be the home of another UCLA primate researcher; instead, it was accidentally left on the porch of an elderly woman unrelated to the university. The Animal Liberation Front claimed responsibility for the attack. As a result of the campaign, the researcher sent an email to the Primate Freedom Project stating "you win," and "please don't bother my family anymore." In another incident at UCLA in June 2007, the Animal Liberation Brigade placed a bomb under the car of a UCLA children's ophthalmologist who experiments on cats and rhesus monkeys; the bomb had a faulty fuse and did not detonate. UCLA is now refusing Freedom of Information Act requests for animal medical records.

These attacks—as well as similar incidents that caused the Southern Poverty Law Center to declare in 2002 that the animal rights movement had "clearly taken a turn toward the more extreme"—prompted the US government to pass the Animal Enterprise Terrorism Act and the UK government to add the offense of "Intimidation of persons connected with animal research organisation" to the Serious Organised Crime and Police Act 2005. Such legislation and the arrest and imprisonment of extremists may have decreased the incidence of attacks.

Alternatives to Animal Testing

Many scientists and governments state that animal testing should cause as little suffering to animals as possible, and that animal tests should only be performed where necessary. The "Three Rs" are guiding principles for the use of animals in research in most countries. Whilst replacement of animals, i.e. alternatives to animal testing, is one of the principles, their scope is much broader. Although such principles have been welcomed as a step forwards by some animal welfare groups, they have also been criticized as both outdated by current research, and of little practical effect in improving animal welfare.

The scientists and engineers at Harvard's Wyss Institute have created "organs-on-a-chip", including the "lung-on-a-chip" and "gut-on-a-chip". These tiny devices contain human cells in a 3-dimensional system that mimics human organs. The chips can be used instead of animals in *in vitro* disease research, drug testing, and toxicity testing. Researchers have also begun using 3-D bioprinters to create human cells for *in vitro* testing.

Another non-animal research method is *in silico* or computer simulation and mathematical modeling which seeks to investigate and ultimately predict toxicity and drug affects in humans without using animals. This is done by investigating test compounds on a molecular level using recent advances in technological capabilities with the ultimate goal of creating treatments unique to each patient.

EpiOcular a form of in vitro is on the uprising of alternatives.

Microdosing is another alternative to the use of animals in experimentation. Microdosing is a process whereby volunteers are administered a small dose of a test compound allowing researchers to investigate its pharmacological affects without harming the volunteers. Microdosing can replace the use of animals in pre-clinical drug screening and can reduce the number of animals used in safety and toxicity testing.

Additional alternative methods include positron emission tomography (PET), which allows scanning of the human brain *in vivo*, and comparative epidemiological studies of disease risk factors among human populations.

Simulators and computer programs have also replaced the use of animals in dissection, teaching and training exercises.

Official bodies such as the European Centre for the Validation of Alternative Test Methods of the European Commission, the Interagency Coordinating Committee for the Validation of Alternative Methods in the US, ZEBET in Germany, and the Japanese Center for the Validation of Alternative Methods (among others) also promote and disseminate the 3Rs. These bodies are mainly driven by responding to regulatory requirements, such as supporting the cosmetics testing ban in the EU by validating alternative methods.

The European Partnership for Alternative Approaches to Animal Testing serves as a liaison between the European Commission and industries. The European Consensus Platform for Alternatives coordinates efforts amongst EU member states.

Academic centers also investigate alternatives, including the Center for Alternatives to Animal Testing at the Johns Hopkins University and the NC3Rs in the UK.

Farm Animals

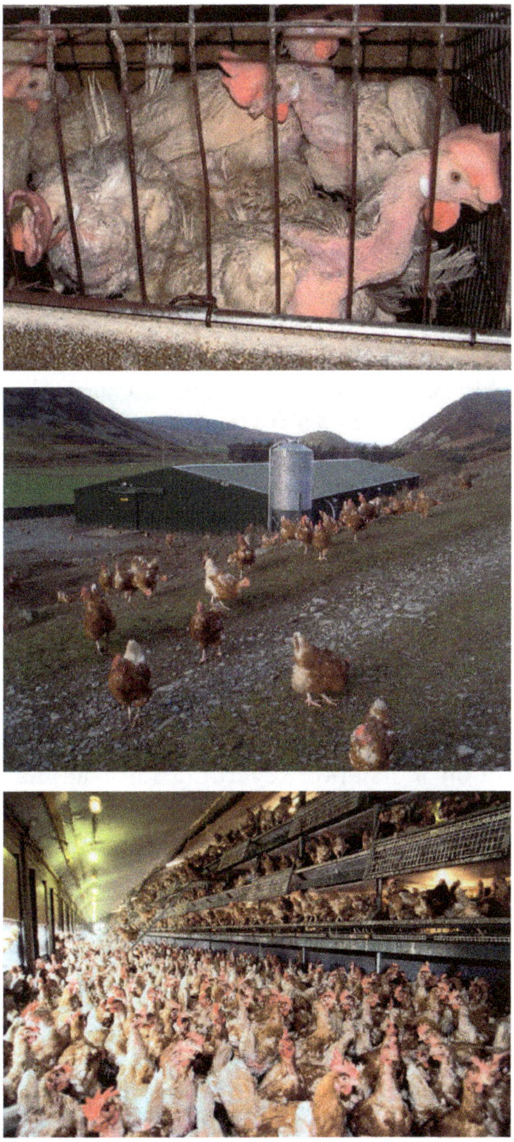

The welfare of egg laying hens in battery cages (top) can be compared with the welfare of free range hens (middle and bottom) which are given access to the outdoors. However, animal welfare groups argue that the vast majority of free-range hens are still intensively confined (bottom) and are rarely able to go outdoors.

A major concern for the welfare of farm animals is factory farming in which large numbers of animals are reared in confinement at high stocking densities. Issues include the limited opportunities for natural behaviors, for example, in battery cages, veal and gestation crates, instead producing abnormal behaviors such as tail-biting, cannibalism, and feather pecking, and routine invasive procedures such as beak trimming, castration, and ear notching. More extensive methods of farming, e.g. free range, can also raise welfare concerns such as the mulesing of sheep, predation of stock by wild animals, and biosecurity.

Farm animals are artificially selected for production parameters which sometimes impinge on the animals' welfare. For example, broiler chickens are bred to be very large to produce the greatest quantity of meat per animal. Broilers bred for fast growth have a high incidence of leg deformities because the large breast muscles cause distortions of the developing legs and pelvis, and the birds cannot support their increased body weight. As a consequence, they frequently become lame or suffer from broken legs. The increased body weight also puts a strain on their hearts and lungs, and ascites often develops. In the UK alone, up to 20 million broilers each year die from the stress of catching and transport before reaching the slaughterhouse.

Another concern about the welfare of farm animals is the method of slaughter, especially ritual slaughter. While the killing of animals need not necessarily involve suffering, the general public considers that killing an animal reduces its welfare. This leads to further concerns about premature slaughtering such as chick culling by the laying hen industry, in which males are slaughtered immediately after hatching because they are superfluous; this policy occurs in other farm animal industries such as the production of goat and cattle milk, raising the same concerns.

European Union laws

The European Commission's activities in this area start with the recognition that animals are sentient beings. The general aim is to ensure that animals do not endure avoidable pain or suffering, and obliges the owner/keeper of animals to respect minimum welfare requirements.European Union legislation regarding farm animal welfare is regularly re-drafted according to science-based evidence and cultural views.For example, in 2009, legislation was passed which aimed to reduce animal suffering during slaughter and on January 1, 2012, the European Union Council Directive 1999/74/EC came into act, which means that conventional battery cages for laying hens are now banned across the Union.

United Kingdom Laws

The Animal Welfare Act 2006 makes owners and keepers responsible for ensuring that the welfare needs of their animals are met. These include the need: for a suitable environment (place to live), for a suitable diet, to exhibit normal behavior patterns, to be housed with, or apart from, other animals (if applicable), and to be protected from pain, injury, suffering and disease. Anyone who is cruel to an animal, or does not provide for its welfare needs, may be banned from owning animals, fined up to £20,000 and/or sent to prison.

In the UK, the welfare of research animals being used for "regulated procedures" was historically protected by the Animals (Scientific Procedures) Act 1986 (ASPA) which is administrated by the Home Office. The Act defines "regulated procedures" as animal experiments that could potentially cause "pain, suffering, distress or lasting harm" to "protected animals". Initially, "protected animals" encompassed all living vertebrates other than humans, but, in 1993, an amendment added a single invertebrate species, the common octopus.

Primates, cats, dogs, and horses have additional protection over other vertebrates under the Act. Revised legislation came into force in January 2013. This has been expanded to protect "...all living vertebrates, other than man, and any living cephalopod. Fish and amphibia are protected once they can feed independently and cephalopods at the point when they hatch. Embryonic and foetal forms of mammals, birds and reptiles are protected during the last third of their gestation or incubation period." The definition of regulated procedures was also expanded: "A procedure is regulated if it is carried out on a protected animal and may cause that animal a level of pain, suffering, distress or lasting harm equivalent to, or higher than, that caused by inserting a hypodermic needle according to good veterinary practice." It also includes modifying the genes of a protected animal if this causes the animal pain, suffering, distress, or lasting harm. The ASPA also considers other issues such as animal sources, housing conditions, identification methods, and the humane killing of animals.

This legislation is widely regarded as the strictest in the world. Those applying for a license must explain why such research cannot be done through non-animal methods. The project must also pass an ethical review panel which aims to decide if the potential benefits outweigh any suffering for the animals involved.

United States Laws

In the United States, a federal law called the Humane Slaughter Act was designed to decrease suffering of livestock during slaughter.

The Georgia Animal Protection Act of 1986 was a state law enacted in response to the inhumane treatment of companion animals by a pet store chain in Atlanta. The Act provided for the licensing and regulation of pet shops, stables, kennels, and animal shelters, and established, for the first time, minimum standards of care. Additional provisions, called the Humane Euthanasia Act, were added in 1990, and then further expanded and strengthened with the Animal Protection Act of 2000.

In 2002, voters passed (by a margin of 55% for and 45% against) Amendment 10 to the Florida Constitution banning the confinement of pregnant pigs in gestation crates. In 2006, Arizona voters passed Proposition 204 with 62% support; the legislation prohibits the confinement of calves in veal crates and breeding sows in gestation crates. In 2007, the Governor of Oregon signed legislation prohibiting the confinement of pigs in gestation crates and in 2008, the Governor of Colorado signed legislation that phased out both gestation crates and veal crates. Also during 2008, California passed Proposition 2, known as the "Prevention of Farm Animal Cruelty Act", which orders new space requirements for farm animals starting in 2015.

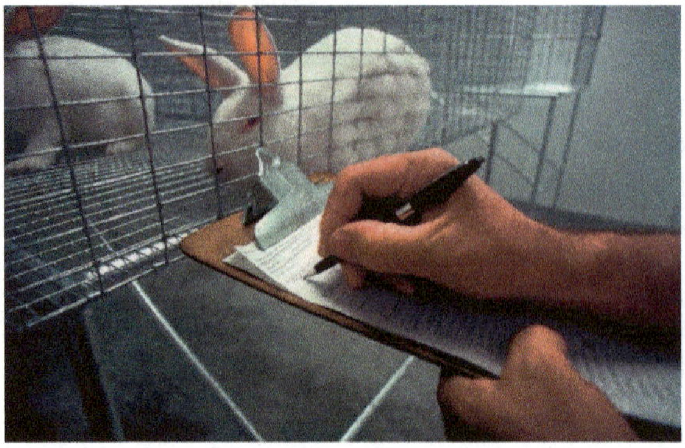

The use of animals in laboratories remains controversial. Animal welfare advocates push for enforced standards to ensure the health and safety of those animals used for tests.

In the US, every institution that uses vertebrate animals for federally funded laboratory research must have an Institutional Animal Care and Use Committee (IACUC). Each local IACUC reviews research protocols and conducts evaluations of the institution's animal care and use which includes the results of inspections of facilities that are required by law. The IACUC committee must assess the steps taken to "enhance animal well-being" before research can take place. This includes research on farm animals.

According to the National Institutes of Health Office of Laboratory Animal Welfare, researchers must try to minimize distress in animals whenever possible: "Animals used in research and testing may experience pain from induced diseases, procedures, and toxicity. The Public Health Service (PHS) Policy and Animal Welfare Regulations (AWRs) state that procedures that cause more than momentary or slight pain or distress should be performed with appropriate sedation, analgesia, or anesthesia.

However, research and testing studies sometimes involve pain that cannot be relieved with such agents because they would interfere with the scientific objectives of the study. Accordingly, federal regulations require that IACUCs determine that discomfort to animals will be limited to that which is unavoidable for the conduct of scientifically valuable research, and that unrelieved pain and distress will only continue for the duration necessary to accomplish the scientific objectives. The PHS Policy and AWRs further state that animals that would otherwise suffer severe or chronic pain and distress that cannot be relieved should be painlessly killed at the end of the procedure, or if appropriate, during the procedure."

The National Research Council's Guide for the Care and Use of Laboratory Animals also serves as a guide to improve welfare for animals used in research in the US. The Federation of Animal Science Societies' Guide for the Care and Use of Agricultural Animals in Research and Teaching is a resource addressing welfare concerns in farm animal research. Laboratory animals in the US are also protected under the Animal Welfare Act. The United States Department of Agriculture Animal and Plant Health Inspection Service (APHIS) enforces the Animal Welfare Act. APHIS inspects animal research facilities regularly and reports are published online.

According to the U.S. Department of Agriculture (USDA), the total number of animals used in the U.S. in 2005 was almost 1.2 million, but this does not include rats, mice, and birds which are not covered by welfare legislation but make up approximately 90% of research animals.

Criticisms

Animals as Automatons

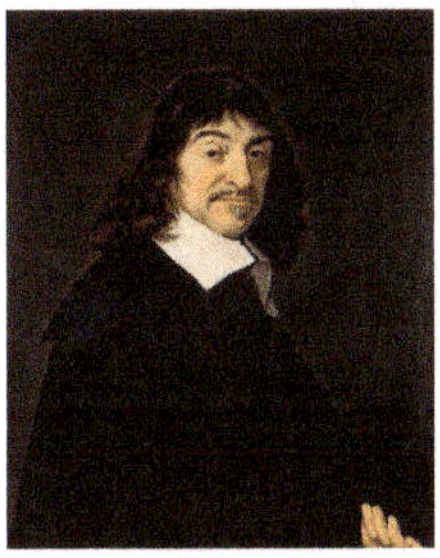

René Descartes asserted that animals are not conscious and behave as automatons.

At one time, many people denied that non-human animals could feel anything and believed that they were incapable of conscious thought, thus the concept of animal welfare was meaningless. For example, many Cartesians were of this opinion. René Descartes wrote in the early 1600s that animals act "without consciousness", much like a machine. In addition, there are accounts of Descartes visiting slaughter houses to observe how animals died. Believing that the animals were devoid of sentience, Descartes thought the death throes of animals was akin to "taking apart a spring-driven clock." In the *Discourse*, published in 1637, Descartes wrote that the ability to reason and use language involves being able to respond in complex ways to all the "contingencies of life", something that animals "clearly cannot do." He argued from this that any sounds animals make do not constitute language, but are simply "automatic responses to external stimuli."

Animal Rights

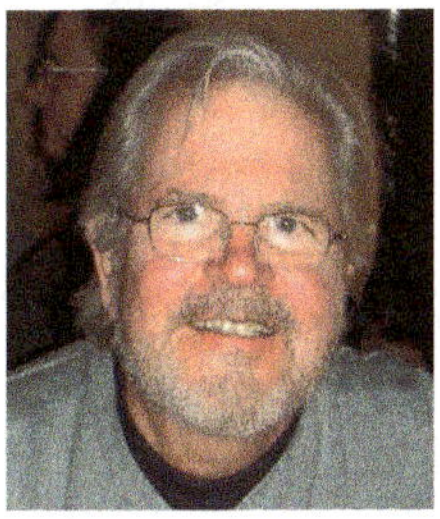

American philosopher Tom Regan has criticized the animal welfare movement for not going far enough to protect animals' interests.

Animal right advocates, such as Gary L. Francione and Tom Regan, argue that the animal welfare position (advocating for the betterment of the condition of animals, but without abolishing animal use) is inconsistent in logic and ethically unacceptable. However, there are some animal right groups, such as PETA, which support animal welfare measures in the short term to alleviate animal suffering until all animal use is ended.

According to PETA's Ingrid Newkirk in an interview with *Wikinews*, there are two issues in animal welfare and animal rights. "If I only could have one thing, it would be to end suffering", said Newkirk. "If you could take things from animals and kill animals all day long without causing them suffering, then I would take it... Everybody should be able to agree that animals should not suffer if you kill them or steal from them by taking the fur off their backs or take their eggs, whatever. But you shouldn't put them through torture to do that."

Abolitionism holds that focusing on animal welfare not only fails to challenge animal suffering, but may actually prolong it by making the exercise of property rights over animals appear less unattractive. The abolitionists' objective is to secure a moral and legal paradigm shift, whereby animals are no longer regarded as property.

ANIMAL WELFARE ORGANIZATIONS

Global

World Animal Protection was founded in 1981 to protection animals around the globe.

World Organisation for Animal Health (OIE): The intergovernmental organisation responsible for improving animal health worldwide. The OIE has been established "for the purpose of projects of international public utility relating to the control of animal diseases, including those affecting humans and the promotion of animal welfare and animal production food safety."

World Animal Protection: Protects animals across the globe. World Animal Protection's objectives include helping people understand the critical importance of good animal welfare, encouraging nations to commit to animal-friendly practices, and building the scientific case for the better treatment of animals. They are global in a sense that they have consultative status at the Council of Europe and collaborate with national governments, the United Nations, the Food and Agriculture Organization and the World Organization for Animal Health.

Non-Governmental Organizations

Canadian Council on Animal Care: The national organization responsible for overseeing the care and use of animals involved in Canadian Science.

Canadian Federation of Humane Societies (CFHS): The only national organization representing humane societies and SPCAs in Canada. They provide leadership on animal welfare issues and spread the message across Canada.

The Canadian Veterinary Medical Association: Brings in veterinary involvement to animal welfare. Their objective is to share this concern of animals with all members of the profession, with the general public, with government at all levels, and with other organizations such as the CFHS, which have similar concerns.

Compassion in World Farming: Founded over 40 years ago in 1967 by a British farmer who became horrified by the development of modern, intensive factory farming. "Today we campaign peacefully to end all cruel factory farming practices. We believe that the biggest cause of cruelty on the planet deserves a focused, specialised approach – so we only work on farm animal welfare."

The Movement for Compassionate Living: Exists to- "Promote simple vegan living and self-reliance as a remedy against the exploitation of humans, animals and the Earth. Promote the use of trees and vegan-organic farming to meet the needs of society for food and natural resources. Promote a land-based society where as much of our food and resources as possible are produced locally."

National Animal Interest Alliance: An animal welfare organization in the United States founded in 1991 promotes the welfare of animals, strengthens the human-animal bond, and safeguards the rights of responsible animal owners, enthusiasts and professionals through research, public information and sound public policy. They host an online library of information about various animal-related subjects serving as a resource for groups and individuals dedicated to responsible animal care and well-being.

National Farm Animal Care Council: Their objectives are to facilitate collaboration among members with respect to farm animal care issues in Canada, to facilitate information sharing and communication, and to monitor trends and initiatives in both the domestic and international market place.

National Office of Animal Health: A British organisation that represents its members drawn from the animal medicines industry.

Ontario Society for the Prevention of Cruelty to Animals: A registered charity comprising over 50 communities.

Royal Society for the Prevention of Cruelty to Animals: A well-known animal welfare charity in England and Wales, founded in 1824.

Universities Federation for Animal Welfare: A UK registered charity, established in 1926, that works to develop and promote improvements in the welfare of all animals through scientific and educational activity worldwide.

CRUELTY TO ANIMALS

Cruelty to animals, also called **animal abuse** or **animal neglect**, is the intentional infliction by humans of suffering or harm upon any non-human animal, regardless of whether the act is against the law. More narrowly, it can be the causing of harm or suffering for specific gain, such as killing animals for food or for their fur; opinions differ about the extent of cruelty associated with a given method of slaughter. Cruelty to animals sometimes encompasses inflicting harm or suffering for personal amusement, as in zoosadism.

Laws concerning animal cruelty are designed to prevent needless cruelty. Divergent approaches to such laws occur in different jurisdictions throughout the world. For example, some laws govern methods of killing animals for food, clothing, or other products, and other laws concern the keeping of animals for entertainment, education, research, or pets. Cruelty to animals is not the same thing as disrespect towards animals.

In broad terms, there are three conceptual approaches to the issue of cruelty to animals. The animal welfare position holds that there is nothing inherently wrong with using animals for human purposes, such as food, clothing, entertainment, and research, but that it should be done in a way that minimizes unnecessary pain and suffering, sometimes referred to as "humane" treatment.

Utilitarian advocates argue from the position of costs and benefits and vary in their conclusions as to the allowable treatment of animals. Some utilitarians argue for a weaker approach which is closer to the animal welfare position, whereas others argue for a position that is similar to animal rights. Animal rights theorists criticize these positions, arguing that the words "unnecessary" and "humane" are subject to widely differing interpretations, and that animals have basic rights. They say that the only way to ensure protection for animals is to end their status as property and to ensure that they are never used as commodities.

Definition and Viewpoints

Before modern biology revealed similarities between humans and animals, some thinkers considered humans completely distinct from animals; the controversy over animal welfare was virtually non-existent. Certain thinkers, however, still viewed cruelty against animals as an injustice. Renaissance polymath Leonardo da Vinci's regard for animal welfare, for example, is well-documented. He was particularly troubled by the sight of birds in captivity, and (according to biographer Giorgio Vasari) once purchased caged birds in order to set them free. Da Vinci also expressed anger within his notebooks with the fact that humans use their strength and power to raise animals for slaughter.

René Descartes contrarily believed that non-humans are automata, complex machines with no soul, mind, or reason. In Cartesian dualism, consciousness was unique to human among all other animals and linked to physical matter by divine grace. However, close analysis shows that many human features such as complex sign usage, tool use, and self-consciousness can be found in some animals.

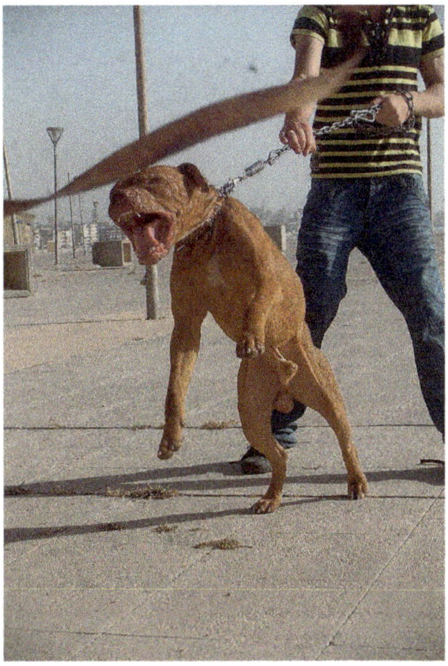

Man beating a chained pitbull terrier with a strap. The strap is visible in the foreground.

Charles Darwin, by presenting the theory of evolution, revolutionized the way that humans viewed their relationship with other species. Darwin believed that not only did human beings have a direct kinship with other animals, but the latter had social, mental and moral lives too. Later, in *The Descent of Man* (1871), he wrote: "There is no fundamental difference between man and the higher mammals in their mental faculties."

Some philosophers and intellectuals, such as Peter Singer and Tom Regan, have argued that animals' ability to feel pain as humans does make their well-being worthy of equal consideration. There are many precursors of this train of thought. Jeremy Bentham, the founder of utilitarianism, famously wrote in his *An Introduction to the Principles of*

"The question is not, can they reason nor can they talk? but, can they suffer?"

These arguments have prompted some to suggest that animals' well-being should enter a social welfare function directly, not just indirectly via its effect only on human well-being.

In one survey of United States homeowners, 68% of respondents said they actually consider the price of meat a more important issue. Worldwide meat overconsumption is another factor that contributes to the miserable situation of farm animals.

Forms

Neglect

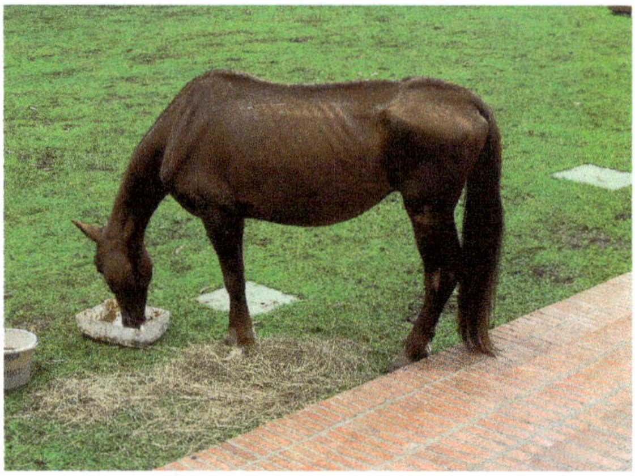

A starved and bruised horse eating at a veterinary clinic after rescue.

Animal cruelty can be broken down into two main categories: active and passive. Passive cruelty is typified by cases of neglect, in which the cruelty is a lack of action rather than the action itself. Examples of neglect are starvation, dehydration, parasite infestations, allowing a collar to grow into an animal's skin, inadequate shelter in extreme weather conditions, and failure to seek veterinary care when necessary. In many cases of neglect in which an investigator believes that the cruelty occurred out of ignorance, the investigator may attempt to educate the pet owner, then revisit the situation. In more severe cases, exigent circumstances may require that the animal be removed for veterinary care.

Industrial Animal Farming

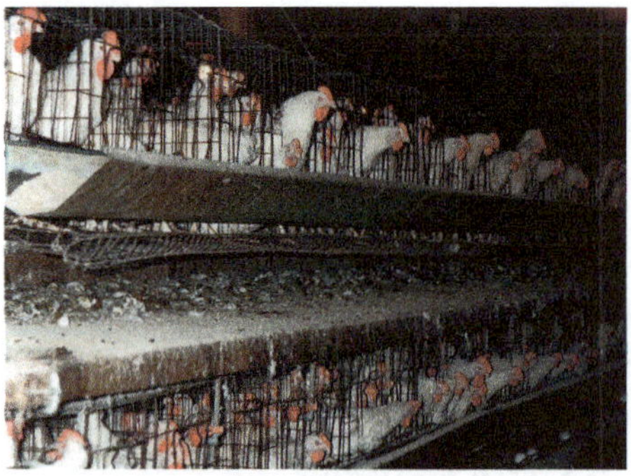

Egg laying hens in a crowded cage.

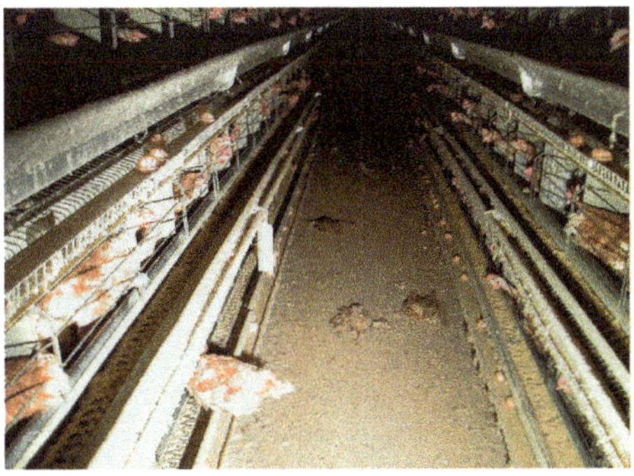

A chicken egg production facility.

Farm animals are generally produced in large, industrial facilities that house thousands of animals at high densities; these are sometimes called factory farms. The industrial nature of these facilities means that many routine procedures or animal husbandry practices impinge on the welfare of the animals and could arguably be considered as "cruelty". It has been suggested the number of animals hunted, kept as companions, used in laboratories, reared for the fur industry, raced, and used in zoos and circuses, is insignificant compared to farm animals, and therefore the "animal welfare issue" is numerically reducible to the "farm animal welfare issue". Similarly, it has been suggested by campaign groups that chickens, cows, pigs, and other farm animals are among the most numerous animals subjected to cruelty. For example, because male chickens do not lay eggs, newly hatched males are culled using macerators or grinders.

The American Veterinary Medical Association accepts maceration subject to certain conditions, but recommends alternative methods of culling as more humane. Egg-laying hens are then transferred to "battery cages where they are kept in high densities. Matheny and Leahy attribute osteoporosis in hens to this caging method. Broiler chicken suffer similar situations, in which they are fed steroids to grow at a super-fast speed, so fast that their bones, heart and lungs often cannot keep up. Broiler chickens under six weeks old suffer painful crippling due to fast growth rates, whilst one in a hundred of these very young birds dies of heart failure.

To reduce aggression in overcrowded conditions, shortly after birth piglets are castrated, their tails are amputated, and their teeth clipped. Calves are sometimes raised in veal crates, which are small stalls that basically immobilize calves during their growth, reducing costs and preventing muscle development, making the resulting meat a pale color, preferred by consumers.

Animal cruelty such as soring, which is illegal, sometimes occurs on farms and ranches, as does lawful but cruel treatment such as livestock branding. Since Ag-gag laws prohibit video or photographic documentation of farm activities, these practices have been documented by secret photography taken by whistleblowers or undercover operatives from such organizations as Mercy for Animals and the Humane Society of the United States posing as employees. Agricultural organizations such as the American Farm Bureau Federation have successfully advocated for laws that tightly restrict secret photography or concealing information from farm employers.

The following are lists of invasive procedures which cause pain, routinely performed on farm animals, and housing conditions that routinely cause animal welfare concerns. It is arguable whether these practices are **cruelty to animals**.

Welfare concerns of farm animals		
Species	**Invasive procedures**	**Housing**
Cattle	• Branding • Castration • Dehorning • Ear tagging • Nose ringing • Restraint • Tail docking • Tongue resection (calves)	• High stocking density (feedlots) • Restricted movement (feedlots) • Veal crates
Pigs	• Castration • Ear docking • Ear tagging • Ear notching • Nose ringing • Tail docking • Tattooing • Teeth cutting • Tusk trimming	• Gestation crates • High stocking density • Restricted movement
Egg laying hens	• Beak-trimming • Blinders • Dubbing	• High stocking density • Restricted movement
Broiler chickens	• Beak-trimming	• High stocking density • Restricted movement

Domestic turkey	• Beak-trimming • Desnooding • Detoeing • Devocalization • Spur removal • Toe clipping	• High stocking density • Restricted movement
Goats and sheep	• Ear tagging • Ear notching • Dehorning • Marking • Mulesing • Tail docking • Teeth grinding	• High stocking density (fine wool industry, live export) • Restricted movement (fine wool industry, live export)

'Blinders' or 'spectacles' are included as some versions require a pin to pierce the nasal septum.

- 'Dubbing' is the procedure of removing the comb, wattles and sometimes earlobes of poultry. Removing the wattles is sometimes called "dewattling".
- 'Desnooding' is the removal of the snood, a fleshy appendage on the forehead of turkeys.
- 'Marking' is the simultaneous mulesing, castration and tail docking of lambs.
- 'Mulesing' is the removal of strips of wool-bearing skin from around the breech (buttocks) of a sheep to prevent flystrike (myiasis)

Psychological Disorders and the Link to Human Violence

There are studies providing evidence of a link between animal cruelty and violence towards humans.

Conviction statistics are thought by some to show people convicted for animal cruelty to be more likely to be violent to humans, leading experts to believe that decreasing animal abuse will, in turn, decrease domestic violence. Meanwhile, others explain apparent correlation by criminal courts more often convicting the former for the latter crime as a self-fulfilling prophecy, without any actual link between the two types of actions. Others argue that psychiatry and other authorities outside of courts keep records of who have been cruel to animals and can make biased guesses about whether or not they did violence to humans thereafter and also that they conversely record people who have been violent to humans and can be more biased towards later assuming them to have been cruel to animals, explaining apparent links by institutional bias without link between the actions themselves.

Intentional acts of cruelty can lead to multiple years behind bars. These acts (of intentional animal cruelty or non-accidental injury) may be indicators of serious psychological problems. According to the American Humane Association, 13% of intentional animal abuse cases involve domestic violence. As many as 71% of pet-owning women seeking shelter at safe houses have reported that their partner had threatened and/or actually hurt or killed one or more of their pets; 32% of these women reported that one or more of their children had also hurt or killed pets. Battered women report that they are prevented from leaving their abusers because they fear what will happen to the animals in their absence. Animal abuse is sometimes used as a form of intimidation in domestic disputes.

One of the known warning signs of certain psychopathologies, including antisocial personality disorder, also known as psychopathic personality disorder, is a history of torturing pets and small animals, a behavior known as zoosadism. According to *The New York Times*, "the FBI has found that a history of cruelty to animals is one of the traits that regularly appears in its computer records of serial rapists and murderers, and the standard diagnostic and treatment manual for psychiatric and emotional disorders lists cruelty to animals a diagnostic criterion for conduct disorders. A survey of psychiatric patients who had repeatedly tortured dogs and cats found all of them had high levels of aggression toward people as well, including one patient who had murdered a young boy. Robert K. Ressler, an agent with the Federal Bureau of Investigation's behavioral sciences unit, studied serial killers and noted,Murderers like this (Jeffrey Dahmer) very often start out by killing and torturing animals as kids.

Cruelty to animals is one of the three components of the Macdonald triad, indicators of violent antisocial behavior in children and adolescents. According to the studies used to form this model, cruelty to animals is a common (but not universal) behavior in children and adolescents who grow up to become serial killers and other violent criminals.

It has also been found that children who are cruel to animals have often witnessed or been victims of abuse themselves. In two separate studies cited by the Humane Society of the United States, roughly one-third of families suffering from domestic abuse indicated that at least one child had hurt or killed a pet.

Cultural Rituals

Many times, when Asiatic elephants are captured in Thailand, handlers use a technique known as the training crush, in which handlers use sleep-deprivation, hunger, and thirst to ‹break' the elephants' spirit and make them submissive to their owners; moreover, handlers drive nails into the elephants' ears and feet. The practice of cruelty to animals for divination purposes is found in ancient cultures, and some modern religions such as Santeria continue to do animal sacrifices for healing and other rituals. Taghairm was performed by ancient Scots to summon devils.

TV and Film Making

Animal cruelty has long been an issue with the art form of filmmaking, with even some big-budget Hollywood films receiving criticism for allegedly harmful—and sometimes lethal—treatment of animals during production.

The American Humane Association (AHA) has been associated with monitoring American filmmaking since after the release of the 1939 film *Jesse James*, in which a horse was pushed off a plank and drowned in a body of water after having fallen 40 feet into it. Initially, monitoring of animal cruelty was a partnership between the AHA and officials in the Hays Office through the Motion Picture Production Code. Provisions in the code discouraged "apparent cruelty to children and animals", and because the Hays Office had the power to enforce this clause, the American Humane Association (AHA) often had access to sets to assess adherence to it. However, because the American Humane Association's Hollywood office depended on the Hays Office for the right to monitor sets, the closure of the Hays Office in 1966 corresponded with an increase in animal cruelty on movie sets.

By 1977, a three-year contract was in place between the Screen Actors Guild (SAG) and the American Federation of Television and Radio Artists which specified that the American Humane Association should be "consulted in the use of animals 'when appropriate'", but the contract did not provide a structure for what "appropriate" meant, and had no enforcement powers. This contract expired in 1980.

One of the most infamous examples of animal cruelty in film was Michael Cimino's legendary flop *Heaven's Gate* (1980), in which numerous animals were brutalized and even killed during production. Cimino allegedly killed chickens and bled horses from the neck to gather samples of their blood to smear on actors for *Heaven's Gate*, and also allegedly had a horse blown up with dynamite while shooting a battle sequence, the shot of which made it into the film. This film played a large part in renewed scrutiny of animal cruelty in films, and led to renewed official on-set jurisdiction to monitor the treatment of animals by the AHA in 1980.

After the release of the film *Reds* (1981), the star and director of the picture, Warren Beatty apologized for his Spanish film crew's use of tripwires on horses while filming a battle scene, when Beatty wasn't present. Tripwires were used against horses when *Rambo III* (1988) and *The 13th Warrior* (1999) were being filmed. An ox was sliced nearly in half during production of *Apocalypse Now* (1979), while a donkey was bled to death for dramatic effect for the Danish film *Manderlay* (2005), in a scene later cut from the film.

There is a case of cruelty to animals in the South Korean film *The Isle* (2000), according to its director Kim Ki-Duk. In the film, a real frog is skinned alive while fish are mutilated. Seven animals were killed for the camera in the controversial Italian film *Cannibal Holocaust* (1980). The images in the film include the slow and graphic beheading and ripping apart of a turtle, a monkey being beheaded and its brains being consumed by natives and a spider being chopped apart. *Cannibal Holocaust* was only one film in a collective of similarly themed movies (cannibal films) that featured unstaged animal cruelty. Their influences were rooted in the films of Mondo filmmakers, which sometimes contained similar content. In several countries, such as the UK, *Cannibal Holocaust* was only allowed for release with most of the animal cruelty edited out.

More recently, the video sharing site YouTube has been criticized for hosting thousands of videos of real life animal cruelty, especially the feeding of one animal to another for the purposes of entertainment and spectacle. Although some of these videos have been flagged as inappropriate by users, YouTube has generally declined to remove them, unlike videos which include copyright infringement.

The Screen Actors Guild (SAG) has contracted with the American Humane Association (AHA) for monitoring of animal use during filming or while on the set. Compliance with this arrangement is voluntary and only applies to films made in the United States. Films monitored by the American Humane Association may bear one of their end-credit messages. Many productions, including those made in the US, do not advise AHA or SAG of animal use in films, so there is no oversight.

Simulations of animal cruelty exist on television, too. On the September 23, 1999 edition of WWE Smackdown!, a plot line had professional wrestler Big Boss Man trick fellow wrestler Al Snow into appearing to eat his pet chihuahua Pepper.

Circuses

The use of animals in the circus has been controversial since animal welfare groups have documented instances of animal cruelty during the training of performing animals. Numerous instances of animal abuse in circuses have been documented such as confining enclosures, lack of regular veterinary care, abusive training methods and lack of oversight by regulating bodies. Animal trainers have argued that some criticism is not based in fact, including beliefs that shouting makes the animals believe the trainer is going to hurt them, that caging is cruel and common, and the harm caused by the use of whips, chains or training implements.

Some circuses now present animal-free acts. Bolivia has enacted what animal rights activists called the world's first ban on all animals in circuses.

Bullfighting

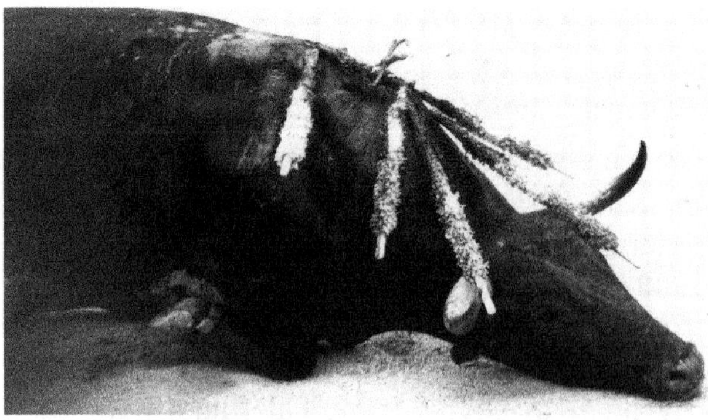

A bull dying in a bullfight.

Bullfighting is criticized by animal rights or animal welfare activists, referring to it as a cruel or barbaric blood sport in which the bull suffers severe stress and a slow, torturous death. A number of activist groups undertake anti-bullfighting actions in Spain and other countries. In Spanish, opposition to bullfighting is referred to as *antitaurismo*.

The Bulletpoint Bullfight warns that bullfighting is "not for the squeamish", advising spectators to "be prepared for blood". It details prolonged and profuse bleeding caused by horse-mounted lancers, the charging by the bull of a blindfolded, armored horse who is "sometimes doped up, and unaware of the proximity of the bull", the placing of barbed darts by banderilleros, followed by the matador's fatal sword thrust. It stresses that these procedures are a normal part of bullfighting and that death is rarely instantaneous. It further warns those attending bullfights to "be prepared to witness various failed attempts at killing the animal before it lies down."

Toro Embolado

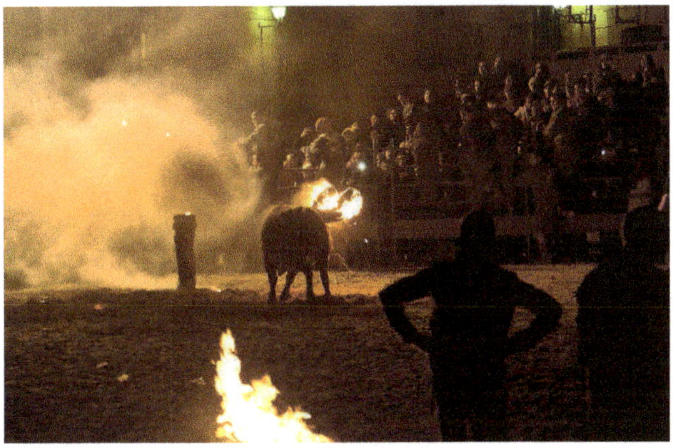

The Toro Jubilo, Madrid, 2014.

The "Toro Jubilo" or Toro embolado in Soria, Medinaceli, Spain, is a festival associated with animal cruelty. During this festival, balls of pitch are attached to a bull's horns and set on fire. The bull is then released into the streets and can do nothing but run around in pain, often smashing into walls in an attempt to douse the fire. These fiery balls can burn for hours, and they burn the bull's horns, body, and eyes – all while spectators cheer and run around the victim. The animal rights group PACMA has described the fiesta as "a clear example of animal mistreatment", and PETA calls it "a sadistic festival".

Crush Films

Animal snuff films, known as crush films can be found on the Internet. These films depict instances of animal cruelty, and/or pornographic acts with animals, usually involving the death of an animal, including insects, mice, rats, guinea pigs, hamsters, monkeys, birds, cats, and dogs. In 1999, the U.S. government banned the depiction of animal cruelty; however, the law was overturned by the 3rd U.S. Circuit Court of Appeals which ruled that the category "depiction of animal cruelty contained in the law was not an exception to First Amendment protections. In an 8–1 decision handed down in April 2010, the U.S.

Supreme Court agreed with the lower court's ruling, but on the grounds that the law was unconstitutionally broad. The case itself did not involve crush films, but rather, a video that in part depicted dogfighting.

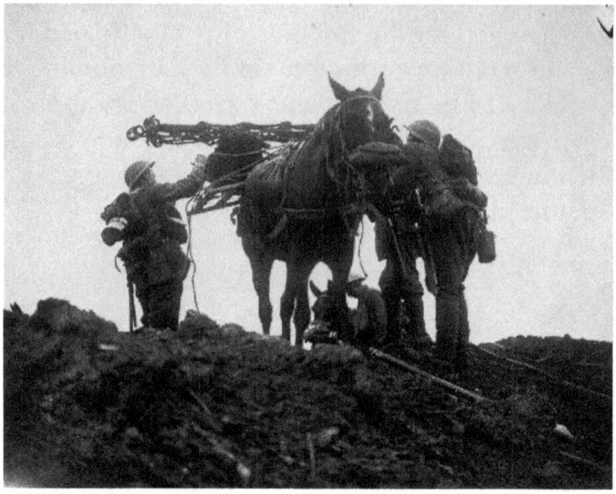

A horse with a gas mask during World War I.

Warfare

Military animals are creatures that have been employed by humankind for use in warfare. They are a specific application of working animals. Examples include horses, dogs and dolphins. Only recently has the involvement of animals in war been questioned, and practices such as using animals for fighting, as living bombs (as in the use of exploding donkeys) or for military testing purposes (such as during the Bikini atomic experiments) may now be criticised for being cruel.

Princess Anne, the Princess Royal, the patron of the British Animals in War Memorial, stated that animals adapt to what humans want them to do, but that they will not do things that they don't want to, despite training. Animal participation in human conflict was commemorated in the United Kingdom in 2004 with the erection of the Animals in War Memorial in Hyde Park, London.

In 2008 a video of a US Marine throwing a puppy over a cliff during the Iraq conflict was popularised as an internet phenomenon and attracted widespread criticism of the soldier's actions for being an act of cruelty.

Unnecessary Scientific Experiments or Demonstrations

Under all three of the conceptual approaches to animal cruelty discussed above, performing unnecessary experiments or demonstrations upon animals that cause them substantial pain or distress may be viewed as cruelty. Due to changes in ethical standards, this type of cruelty tends to be less common today than it used to be in the past. For example, schoolroom demonstrations of oxygen depletion routinely suffocated birds by placing them under a glass cover, and animals were suffocated in the Cave of Dogs to demonstrate the density and toxicity of carbon dioxide to curious travellers on the Grand Tour.

No Pet Policies and Abandonment

Many apartment complexes and rental homes institute no pet policies. No pet policies are a leading cause of animal abandonment, which is considered a crime in many jurisdictions. In many cases, abandoned pets have to be euthanized due to the strain they put on animal shelters and rescue groups. Abandoned animals often become feral or contribute to feral populations. In particular, feral dogs can pose a serious threat to pets, children, and livestock. Feral cats are known to hunt endangered birds and have interbred with wild cat populations.

In Ontario, Canada, no pet policies are outlawed under the Ontario Landlord and Tenant Act and are considered invalid even when a tenant signs a lease including a no pets clause.Similar legislation has also been considered in Manitoba.

Laws by Country

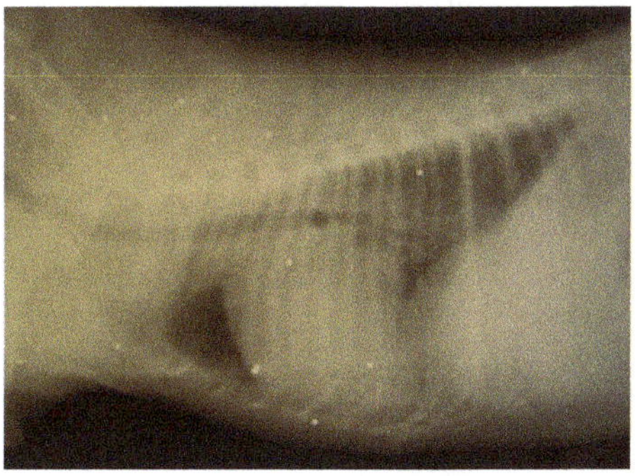

Chest X-ray of a cat that has been shot. White spots are lead shot.

Many jurisdictions around the world have enacted statutes which forbid cruelty to some animals but these vary by country and in some cases by the use or practice.

Africa

Egypt

Egyptian law states that anyone who inhumanely beats or intentionally kills any domesticated animal may be jailed or fined. The Egyptian Society for the Prevention of Cruelty to Animals was established by the British over a hundred years ago, and is currently administered by the Egyptians. The SPCA was instrumental in promoting a 1997 ban on bullfighting in Egypt.

In ancient Egyptian law, the killers of cats or dogs were executed.

South Sudan

The Criminal Code of South Sudan has laws against maltreatment of animals. The laws read:

196. Ill-treatment of Domestic Animal.

Whoever cruelly beats, tortures or otherwise willfully ill-treats any tame, domestic or wild animal, which has previously been deprived of its liberty, or arranges, promotes or organizes fights between cocks, rams, bulls or other domestic animals or encourages such acts, commits an offence, and upon conviction, shall be sentenced to imprisonment for a term not exceeding two months or with a fine.

197. Riding and Neglect of Animal.

Whoever wantonly rides, overdrives or overloads any animal or intentionally drugs or employs any animal, which by reason of age, sickness, wounds or infirmity is not in a condition to work, or neglects any animal in such a manner as to cause it unnecessary suffering, commits an offence, and upon conviction, shall be sentenced to imprisonment for a term not exceeding one month or with a fine or with both.

Americas

Argentina

In Argentina, National Law 14346 sanctions with from 15 days to one year in prison those who mistreat or inflict acts of cruelty on animals.

Brazil

Canada

In Canada, it is an offence under the Criminal Code to intentionally cause unnecessary pain, suffering or injury to an animal. Poisoning animals is specifically prohibited. It is also an offence to threaten to harm an animal belonging to someone else. Most provinces and Territories also have their own animal protection legislation.

The Animal Legal Defense Fund releases an annual report ranking the animal protection laws of every province and territory based on their relative strength and general comprehensiveness. In 2014, the top four jurisdictions were Manitoba, British Columbia, Ontario and Nova Scotia. The worst four were Saskatchewan, Northwest Territories, Quebec, and Nunavut.

Chile

Law 20380 established sanctions including fines, from 2 to 30 Mensual Tributary Units, and prison, from 541 days to 3 years, for those involved in acts of animal cruelty. Also, it promotes animal care through school education, and establishes a Bioethics Committee to define policies related to experiments with animals.

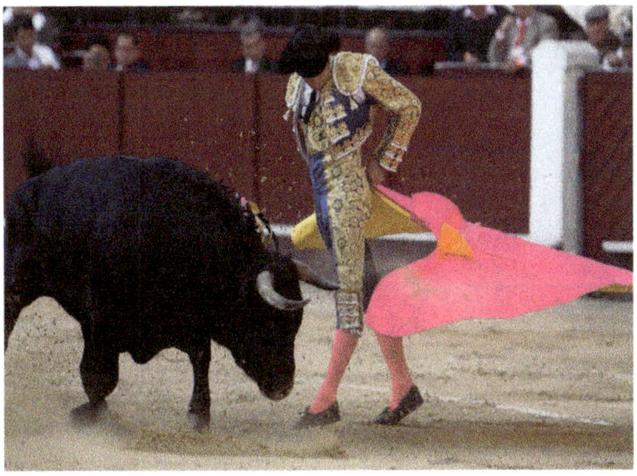

A bull fight in Bogotá, a legacy of Spanish culture. Despite being criticized by numerous organizations in Colombia, the practice of bullfighting remains legal.

Colombia

In Colombia, there is little control over cruel behaviors against animals, and the government has proposed that bullfighting be declared a "Cultural Heritage; other cruel activities like cockfighting are given the same legal treatment.

Costa Rica

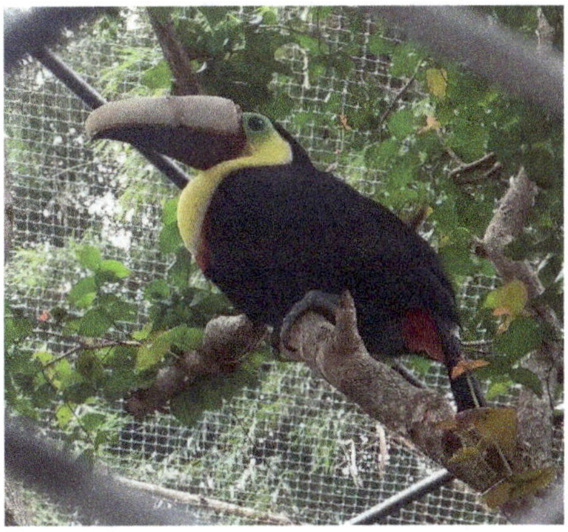

Toucan Grecia with 3D printed prosthetic beak after losing half its beak from a beating by youth.

A new bill has been presented to the Costa Rican legisletive assembly to better define animal cruelty and establish harsher punishments for the abuse of animals. Exceptions for events deemed "traditional", such as horse parades, rodeos and Tico-style bullfights are not provided in the bill's draft which may see motions filed against its passing. The bill had stalled its motion through legislators until notorious toucan Grecia was found having lost half its top beak. The news and images of the injured toucan produced enough contributions to create a 3D printing prosthesis for the bird and rallies in the country's capital for action in relation to the animal cruelty bill.

Mexico

The current policy of Mexico, in civil law, condemns physical harm to animals as property damage to the owners of the abused animal, considering the animals as owned property.

In criminal law, the situation is different. In December 2012, the Legislative Assembly of the Federal District reformed the existing Penal Code of Mexico City, establishing abuse and cruelty to animals as criminal offenses, provided the animals are not deemed to be plagues or pests. Abandoned animals are not considered to be plagues. A subsequent reform was entered into force on January 31, 2013, by a decree published in the Official Gazette of the Federal District. The law provides penalties of 6 months to 2 years imprisonment, and a fine of 50 to 100 days at minimum wage, to persons who cause obvious injury to an animal, and the penalty is increased by one half if those injuries endanger its life. The penalty rises to 2 to 4 years of prison, and a fine of 200 to 400 days at minimum wage, if the person intentionally causes the death of an animal.

This law is considered to extend throughout the rest of the 31 constituent states of the country. In addition, The Law of Animal Protection of the Federal District is wide-ranging, based on banning unnecessary suffering. Similar laws now exist in most states.

United States

The primary federal law relating to animal care and conditions in the US is the Animal Welfare Act of 1966, amended in 1970, 1976, 1985, 1990, 2002 and 2007. It is the only Federal law in the United States that regulates the treatment of animals in research, exhibition, transport, and by dealers. Other laws, policies, and guidelines may include additional species coverage or specifications for animal care and use, but all refer to the Animal Welfare Act as the minimum acceptable standard.

The AWA has been criticized by animal rights groups for excluding birds, rats and mice bred for research, and animals raised for food or fiber as well as all cold-blooded animals.

The Animal Legal Defense Fund releases an annual report ranking the animal protection laws of every state based on their relative strength and general comprehensiveness. In 2013's report, the top five states for their strong anti-cruelty laws were Illinois, Maine, Michigan, Oregon, and California.The five states with the weakest animal cruelty laws in 2013 were Kentucky, Iowa, South Dakota, New Mexico, and Wyoming.

In Massachusetts and New York, agents of humane societies and associations may be appointed as special officers to enforce statutes outlawing animal cruelty.

In 2004, a Florida legislator proposed a ban on "cruelty to bovines," stating: "A person who, for the purpose of practice, entertainment, or sport, intentionally fells, trips, or otherwise causes a cow to fall or lose its balance by means of roping, lassoing, dragging, or otherwise touching the tail of the cow commits a misdemeanor of the first degree." The proposal did not become law.

In the United States, ear cropping, tail docking, rodeo sports, and other acts are legal and sometimes condoned. Penalties for cruelty can be minimal, if pursued. Currently, 46 of the 50 states have enacted felony penalties for certain forms of animal abuse. However, in most jurisdictions, animal cruelty is most commonly charged as a misdemeanor offense. In one recent California case, a felony conviction for animal cruelty could theoretically net a 25-year to life sentence due to their three-strikes law, which increases sentences based on prior felony convictions.

In 2003, West Hollywood, California passed an ordinance banning declawing of house cats. In 2007, Norfolk, Virginia passed legislation only allowing the procedure for medical reasons. However, most jurisdictions allow the procedure.

In April 2013, Texas Federal Court Judge Sim Lake ruled that the Animal Crush Video Prohibition Act of 2010, which criminalized the recording, sale, and transport of videos depicting animal cruelty as obscenity, is in violation of the First Amendment. Judge Lake noted that obscenity tests require an explicitly sexual depiction, which the criminalized videos lack. This follows the precedent set by United States v. Stevens, which additionally held that restrictions on the possession of animal cruelty videos were unconstitutional.

State Welfare Laws

Several states have enacted or considered laws in support of humane farming.

- On November 5, 2002, Florida voters passed Amendment 10 by a margin of 55% for, amending the Florida Constitution to ban the confinement of pregnant pigs in gestation crates.
- On January 14, 2004, the bill AB-732 died in the California Assembly's Agriculture Committee. The bill would have banned gestation and veal crates, eventually being amended to include only veal crates. On May 9, 2007, the bill AB-594 was withdrawn from the California State Assembly. The bill had been effectively killed in the Assembly Agriculture Committee, by replacing the contents of the bill with language concerning tobacco cessation coverage under Medi-Cal. AB-594 was very similar to the current language of Proposition 2.
- On November 7, 2006, Arizona voters passed Proposition 204 with 62% support. The measure prohibits the confinement of calves in veal crates and breeding sows in gestation crates.
- On June 28, 2007, Oregon Governor Ted Kulongoski signed a measure into law prohibiting the confinement of pigs in gestation crates (SB 694, 74th Leg. Assembly, Regular Session).

- In January 2008, Nebraska State Senate bill LB 1148, to ban the use of gestation crates for pig farmers, was withdrawn within 5 days amidst controversy.
- On May 14, 2008, Colorado Governor Bill Ritter signed into law a bill, SB 201, that phases out gestation crates and veal crates.

Venezuela

Venezuela published a "Law for Protection of Domestic Fauna free and in captivity" in 2010, defining responsibilities and sanctions about animal care and ownership. Animal cruelty acts are fined, but are not a cause for imprisonment. The law also forbids the possession, breeding and reproduction of pit bull dogs, among similar breeds that are alleged to be aggressive and dangerous. It elicited reactions from dog owners, who said that aggressiveness in dogs is determined more by treatment by the owner than by the breed itself.

China

As of 2006 there were no laws in China governing acts of cruelty to animals. There are no government supported charitable organizations like the RSPCA, which monitors the cases on animal cruelty. All kinds of animal abuses, such as to fish, tigers, and bears, are to be reported for law enforcement and animal welfare.

Despite the absence of a unified law against animal mistreatment, the World Animal Protection notes that some legislation protecting the welfare of animals exists in certain contexts, especially ones used in research and in zoos.

In September 2009, legislation was drafted to address deliberate cruelty to animals in China. If passed, the legislation would offer some protection to pets, captive wildlife and animals used in laboratories, as well as regulating how farm animals are raised, transported and slaughtered.

In certain jurisdictions such as Fuzhou, dog control officers may kill any unaccompanied dogs on sight. The People's Republic of China is currently in the process of making changes to its stray-dog population laws in the capital city, Beijing. Mr. Zheng Gang who is the director of the Internal and Judicial Committee which comes under the Beijing Municipal People's Congress (BMPC), supports the new draft of the Beijing Municipal Regulation on Dogs from the local government. This new law is due to replace the current Beijing Municipal Regulation on Dog Ownership, introduced in 1889. The current regulation talks of "strictly" limiting dog ownership and controlling the number of dogs in the city. The new draft focuses instead on "strict management and combining restrictions with management."

Hong Kong

As of 2010, Hong Kong has supplemented or replaced the laws against cruelty with a positive approach using laws that specify how animals should be treated. The government department primarily responsible for animal welfare in Hong Kong is the Agriculture,

Fisheries and Conservation Department (AFCD).

Laws enforced by the AFCD include these:

- the Prevention of Cruelty to Animals Ordinance (also enforced by the police)
- the Public Health (Animals and Birds) Ordinance (including regulations for licences imposed on livestock keepers and animal traders and a Code of Standards for Licensed Animal Traders)
- the Dogs and Cats Ordinance
- the Pounds Ordinance
- the Rabies Ordinance
- the Wild Animals Protection Ordinance

In addition, the Food and Environmental Hygiene Department (FEHD) does the following:

- enforces the Public Health and Municipal Services Ordinance, which includes regulations for slaughterhouses and wet markets
- publishes a Code of Practice for the Welfare of Food Animals (which describes their transport)
- publishes Operational Guidelines for the Welfare of Food Animals at Slaughterhouses

The Department of Health does the following:

- enforces the Animals (Control of Experiments) Ordinance.
- publishes a Code of Practice for the Care and Use of Animals for Experimental Purposes

As of 2006, Hong Kong has a law titled "Prevention of Cruelty to Animals Ordinance", with a maximum 3 year imprisonment and fines of HKD$200,000.

India

The Prevention of Cruelty to Animals Act,1960 was amended in the year 1982. According to the newly amended *Indian animal welfare act, 2011* cruelty to animals is an offence and is punishable with a fine which shall not be less than ten thousand Rupees, which may extend to twenty five thousand Rupees or with imprisonment up to two years or both in the case of a first offence. In the case of second or subsequent offence, with a fine which shall not be less than fifty thousand Rupees, but may extend to one lakh Rupees and with imprisonment with a term which shall not be less than one year but may extend to three years. This amendment is currently awaiting ratification from the Government of India. The 1962 Act in the meanwhile is the one that is practiced as of now. The maximum penalty under the 1962 Act is Rs. 50 (under $1). Many organizations, including ones such as the local SPCA, PFA and Fosterdopt are actively involved in assisting the general population in reporting cruelty cases to the police and helping bring the perpetrator to justice. Due to this, much of change has been observed through the subcontinent.

Israel

Japan

In Japan, the 1973 Welfare and Management of Animals Act (amended in 1999 and 2005) stipulates that "no person shall kill, injure, or inflict cruelty to animals without due course", and in particular, criminalises cruelty to all mammals, birds, and reptiles possessed by persons; as well as cattle, horses, goats, sheep, pigs, dogs, cats, pigeons, domestic rabbits, chickens, and domestic ducks regardless of whether they are in captivity.

- Killing or injuring without due reason: up to one year's imprisonment with labour or a fine of up to one million yen
- Cruelty such as causing debilitation by discontinuing feeding or watering without due reason: a fine of up to five hundred thousand yen
- Abandonment: a fine of up to five hundred thousand yen

Separate national and local ordinances exist with regards to ensuring health and safety of animals handled by pet shops and other businesses.

Animal experiments are regulated by the 2000 Law for the Humane Treatment and Management of Animals, which was amended in 2006. This law requires those using animals to follow the principles outlined in the 3Rs and use as few animals as possible, and cause minimal distress and suffering. Regulation is at a local level based on national guidelines, but there are no governmental inspections of institutions and no reporting requirement for the numbers of animals used.

Malaysia

Saudi Arabia

Veterinarian Lana Dunn and several Saudi nationals report that there are no laws to protect animals from cruelty since the term is not well-defined within the Saudi legal system. They point to a lack of a governing body to supervise conditions for animals, particularly in pet stores and in the exotic animal trade with East Africa.

South Korea

South Korea's animal welfare laws are weak by international standards.

Taiwan

The Taiwanese Animal Protection Act was passed in 1998, imposing fines up to NT$250,000 for cruelty. Criminal penalties for animal cruelty were enacted in 2007, including a maximum of 1 year imprisonment.

Thailand

Thailand introduced its first animal welfare law in 2014. The *Cruelty Prevention and Welfare of Animal Act, B.E. 2557 (2014)* came into being on 27 December 2014.

Europe

European Union

The European Union Council Directive 1999/74/EC is a directive passed by the European Union on the minimum standards for keeping egg laying hens which effectively bans conventional battery cages. The directive, passed in 1999, banned conventional battery cages in the EU from January 1, 2012 after a 13-year phase-out.

It is also illegal in many parts of Europe to declaw a cat.

France

In France, cruelty to animals is punishable by imprisonment of two years and a financial penalty (30,000 €).

Germany

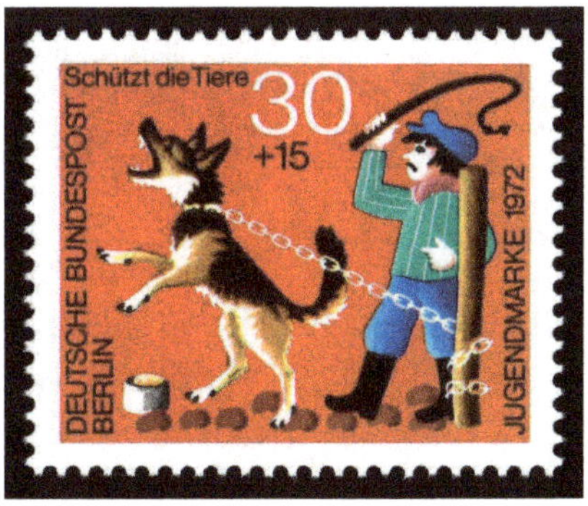

A German stamp depicting a man beating a chained dog. In the upper left corner it reads: protect the animals.

In Germany, killing animals or causing significant pain (or prolonged or repeated pain) to them is punishable by imprisonment of up to three years or a financial penalty. If the animal is of foreign origin, the act may also be punishable as criminal damage.

Italy

Acts of cruelty against animals can be punished with imprisonment, for a minimum of three months up to a maximum of three years, and with a fine ranging from a minimum of 3,000 Euros to a maximum of 160,000 Euros, as for the law n°189/2004.

Ireland

The *Animal Health and Welfare Act 2013* came into force in 2014, improving animal protection.

Portugal

Since 1 October 2014, violence against animals has been a crime in Portugal. Legislation published in the *Diário da Républica* on August 29 criminalizes the mistreatment of animals, and indicates that "those who, without reasonable cause, inflict pain, suffering, or any other hardship to a companion animal abuse" are to be subject to imprisonment of up to one year. If such acts result in the "death of the animal", the "deprivation of an important organ or member", or "serious and permanent impairment of its capacity of locomotion", those responsible will be punished by imprisonment up to two years.

As for pets, the new law provides that whoever, having the duty to store, monitor or pet watch, abandons them, thereby putting in danger their food and the provision of care owed faces up to six months imprisonment.

Sweden

In Sweden cruelty to animals is punishable by financial penalty and the owner will lose the right to own the animals, and the animals will be removed from the owner.

Switzerland

The Swiss animal protection laws are among the strictest in the world, comprehensively regulating the treatment of animals including the size of rabbit cages, and the amount of exercise that must be provided to dogs.

In the canton of Zurich an animal lawyer, Antoine Goetschel, is employed by the canton government to represent the interests of animals in animal cruelty cases.

Turkey

Under Turkey's Animal Protection Law No. 5199, cruelty to animals is considered a misdemeanor, punishable by a fine only, with no jail time or a black mark on one's criminal record. HAYTAP, the Animal Rights Federation in Turkey, believes that the present law does not contain a strong enough punishment for animal abusers.

United Kingdom

In the United Kingdom, cruelty to animals is a criminal offence for which one may be jailed for up to 6 months.

On August 18, 1911, the House of Commons introduced the Protection of Animals Act 1911 (c.27) following lobbying by the Royal Society for the Prevention of Cruelty to Animals (RSPCA). The maximum punishment was 6 months of hard labour with a fine of 25 pounds.

In the London Police Act 1839, fighting or baiting Lions, Bears, Badgers, Cocks, Dogs, or other Animals was prohibited in London, with a penalty of up to one month imprisonment, with possible hard labour, or up to five pounds. The law laid numerous restrictions on how, when, and where animals could be driven, wagons unloaded, etc.. It also prohibited owners from letting mad dogs run loose and gave police the right to destroy any dog suspected of being rabid or any dog bitten by a suspected rabid dog. The same law prohibited the use of dogs for drawing carts.

Up until then, dogs were used for delivering milk, bread, fish, meat, fruit, vegetables, animal food (the cat's-meat man), and other items for sale and for collecting refuse (the rag-and-bone man). As Nigel Rothfels notes, the prohibition against dogs pulling carts in or near London caused most of the dogs to be killed by their owners as they went from being contributors to the family income to unaffordable expenses. Cart dogs were replaced by people with handcarts. About 150,000 dogs were killed or abandoned. Erica Fudge quotes Hilda Kean:

At the heart of nineteenth-century animal welfare campaigns is the middle-class desire not to be able to see cruelty.

—Hilda Kean, Animal Rights, 1998

The Protection of Animals Act 1911 extended the ban on draft dogs to the rest of the kingdom. As many as 600,000 dogs were killed or abandoned.

The Protection of Animals Act 1911 has since been largely superseded by the Animal Welfare Act 2006, which also superseded and consolidated more than 20 other pieces of legislation, including the Protection of Animals Act 1934 and the Abandonment of Animals Act 1960. The Act introduced the new welfare offence, which means that animal owners have a positive duty of care, and outlaws neglecting to provide for their animals' basic needs, such as access to adequate nutrition and veterinary care.

Under the Criminal Damage Act 1971, domestic animals can be classed as property that is capable of being damaged or destroyed. A charge of criminal damage may be appropriate for the injury or death of an animal owned by someone other than the defendant, although prosecution under the Animal Welfare Act 2006 may also be appropriate.

Oceania

Australia

In Australia, all states and territories have enacted legislation governing animal welfare. The legislations are:

- Animal Welfare Act 1992 (ACT)
- Prevention of Cruelty to Animals Act 1979 (NSW)
- Animal Welfare Act (NT)
- Animal Care and Protection Act 2001 (Qld)
- Animal Welfare Act 1985 (SA)
- Animal Welfare Act 1993 (Tas)

- Prevention of Cruelty to Animals Act 1986 (Vic)
- Animal Welfare Act 2002 (WA)

Welfare laws have been criticized as not adequately protecting animals. Whilst police maintain an overall jurisdiction in prosecution of criminal matters, in many states officers of the RSPCA and other animal welfare charities are accorded authority to investigate and prosecute animal cruelty offenses.

REFERENCES

1. Grandin, Temple (2013). "Animals are not things: A view on animal welfare based on neurological complexity" (PDF). Trans-Scripts 3: An Interdisciplinary Online Journal in Humanities And Social Sciences at UC Irvine. UC Irvine. Retrieved 20 December 2013.
2. Hewson, C.J. (2003). "What is animal welfare? Common definitions and their practical consequences". The Canadian Veterinary Journal. 44 (6): 496–499. PMC 340178 . PMID 12839246.
3. Broom, D.M. (1991). "Animal welfare: concepts and measurement". Journal of Animal Science. 69 (10): 4167–75. PMID 1778832.
4. "Draft of the Universal Declaration on Animal Welfare"(PDF). media.animalmatter.org. Archived from the original(PDF) on 2012-02-27.
5. "The Cambridge Declaration on Consciousness" (PDF). Retrieved 26 May 2015.
6. "Scientists Finally Conclude Nonhuman Animals Are Conscious Beings". Retrieved 26 May 2015.
7. "Do animals have consciousness?". Retrieved 26 May 2015.
8. Garner, R. (2005). Animal Ethics. Polity Press.
9. Regan, T. (1983). The Case for Animal Rights. University of California Press.
10. Francione, G.L. (1996). Rain Without Thunder: The Ideology of the Animal Rights Movement. ISBN 978-1-56639-461-1.
11. Francione, G. (1995). Animals, Property, and the Law. Temple University Press.
12. "What is Animal Welfare and why is it important? - The difference between Animal Rights & Animal Welfare.". National Animal Interest Alliance. Retrieved 2014-06-27.
13. Webster, J (2008). Animal Welfare: Limping Towards Eden. John Wiley and Sons. p. 6.
14. Duncan, I.J.H. (1996). "Animal welfare defined in terms of feelings". Acta Agriculturae Scandinavica, Section A. 27: 29–35.
15. Dawkins, M.S. (1980). Animal Suffering: The Science Of Animal Welfare. Chapman & Hall, London.
16. Duncan, I.J.H. (2005). "Science-based assessment of animal welfare: farm animals". Rev. Sci. Tech. Off. Int. Epiz. 24 (2): 483–492.
17. Dawkins, M.S. (1990). "From an animal's point of view: Motivation, fitness

and animal welfare". Behavioral and Brain Sciences. 13: 1–61. doi:10.1017/s0140525x00077104.

18. Ng, Yew-Kwang (1995). "Towards welfare biology: Evolutionary economics of animal consciousness and suffering". Journal of Biology and Philosophy. 10 (3): 255–285. doi:10.1007/BF00852469.
19. Animal. medical-dictionary.thefreedictionary.com. Retrieved 28 November 2010.
20. "What is animal welfare?". American Veterinary Medical Association. Retrieved April 2, 2013.
21. "OIE A new definition for the Terrestrial Animal Health Code: 'animal welfare'" (PDF). Terrestrial Animal Health Code. OIE. Retrieved 20 December 2013.
22. Broom, D.M. (1996). "Animal welfare defined in terms of attempts to cope with the environment". Acta Agriculturae Scandinavica, Section A. 27: 22–28.
23. John Webster. Animal Welfare: Limping Towards Eden. 2008. Page 5
24. Linda J. Keeling, Jeff Rushen and Ian Duncan. Understanding animal welfare. Animal Welfare. 2011 Page 13. edited by Michael C. Appleby, Barry O. Hughes, Joy A. Mench. Books.google.com.au. Retrieved 2014-01-03.
25. Bekoff, Marc (2009-09-24). "Animal Emotions, Animal Sentience, Animal Welfare, and Animal Rights. Marc Bekoff". Psychologytoday.com. Retrieved 2014-01-03.
26. Fearnley-Whittingstall, Hugh (2009). "My meat manifesto". Retrieved October 21, 2013.
27. Garner, Robert. Animal Ethics. Polity Press, 2005, pp. 15-16.
28. Garner, Robert. (2005). Animal Ethics. Polity Press. p. 72
29. Nozick, Robert (1974). Anarchy, State, and Utopia.
30. Garner 2005, p. 15;
31. Singer, P. (1975). Animal Liberation. Random House.
32. Taylor, A. (2003). Animals and Ethics. Broadview Press. p. 88.
33. De Villiers, J-H. (2013). "Rights theory, welfarism, and the "new welfarist" amalgamation: A critical perspective". Retrieved October 20, 2013.
34. "How do we do research with animals?". Understanding Animal Research. 2013. Retrieved October 21, 2013.
35. Phillips 2009. pp 60-63.
36. Euroballot (2007). "Attitudes of EU citizens towards animal welfare" (PDF). European Commission. Retrieved October 21, 2013.
37. Phillips 2009. p 60.
38. "Animal Rights History". Retrieved November 8, 2011.
39. "AWIC". Retrieved November 8, 2011.
40. Phillips 2009. p 56.
41. "Five Freedoms". Farm Animal Welfare Council. 2009. Archived from the

original on October 5, 2013. Retrieved October 21, 2013.

42. Universal Declaration on Animal Welfare ArchivedMarch 28, 2014, at the Wayback Machine. Compassion in World Farming
43. Back a Universal Declaration on Animal Welfare World Animal Protection
44. Sherwin, C.M.; Richards, G.J.; Nicol, C.J. (2010). "Comparison of the welfare of layer hens in 4 housing systems in the UK". British Poultry Science. 51: 488–499. doi:10.1080/00071668.2010.502518.
45. Fraser, D. (2008). Understanding Animal Welfare: The Science in its Cultural Context. John Wiley and Sons. p. 8.
46. Laws, N.; Ganswindt, A.; Heistermann, M.; Harris, M.; Harris, S.; Sherwin, C. (2007). "A case study: Fecal corticosteroid and behavior as indicators of welfare during relocation of an Asian elephant". Journal of Applied Animal Welfare Science. 10: 349–358. doi:10.1080/10888700701555600.
47. "RSPCA says egg industry is 'misleading the public' on free range". Retrieved 26 May 2015.
48. "What The Rise Of Cage-Free Eggs Means For Chickens". Retrieved 26 May 2015.
49. "Farm Fresh? Natural? Eggs Not Always What They're Cracked Up To Be". Retrieved 26 May 2015.
50. "Compassion in World Farming – Meat chickens – Welfare issues". Compassion In World Farming. Retrieved October 22, 2013.
51. Phillips 2009. p 10.
52. "EUROPA - Animal Health & Welfare - Animal Welfare - References". Retrieved 14 June 2015.
53. "Animal Welfare". ESDAW. Retrieved 14 Junc 2015.
54. Glue. "EU & Animal Welfare - What We Do - Eurogroup For Animals". Retrieved 14 June 2015.
55. "European Commission" (PDF). Official Journal of the European Union. 2009-11-18. Retrieved 2011-06-30.
56. "Animal welfare act 2006". The National Archive. 2006. Retrieved October 22, 2013.
57. Department for Environment, Food and Rural Affairs (2013). "Animal welfare". Retrieved October 22, 2013.
58. "The Animals (Scientific Procedures) Act(Amendment) Order 1993". August 23, 1993. Retrieved February 22, 2013.
59. "Draft guidance on the operation of the Animals 1 (Scientific Procedures) Act 1986 (as amended)" (PDF). Home Office (UK). 2013. Retrieved July 18, 2013.
60. "Regulations". Retrieved 2012-11-20.
61. "United States Code". Office of the Law Revision Counsel. 2011-01-07. Archived from the original on 8 July 2011. Retrieved 2011-06-30.

62. "Animal Protection - Ga Dept of Agriculture". Agr.georgia.gov. Retrieved 2012-10-16.
63. "Georgia Humane Euthansia Act, O.C.G.A. §4-11-5.1". Animal Law Coalition. Retrieved 2012-10-16.
64. "Georgia Animal Protection Act". Animallaw.info. Retrieved 2012-10-16.
65. "PorkNet Newsletter". MetaFarms.com, Inc. 2002-11-07. Archived from the original on 2006-03-14. Retrieved 2008-07-03.
66. "Back door activists gain momentum". Learfield Communications, Inc. 2007-07-05. Retrieved 2008-07-03.
67. "Farm Sanctuary Applauds Colorado for Passing Legislation Phasing out Veal and Gestation Crates". Reuters. 2008-05-14. Retrieved 2008-07-03.
68. "Farm Animal Welfare Measure Becomes Law". Federation of Animal Science Societies (FASS). 2008-05-14. Archived from the original on 15 June 2008. Retrieved 2008-07-03.
69. "Research Regulations". Retrieved 2012-10-22.
70. cftp://ftp.grants.nih.gov/IACUC/GuideBook.pdf
71. "Research Animals | Animal Welfare Information Center". Awic.nal.usda.gov. 1985-11-20. Archived from the originalon 2012-10-17. Retrieved 2012-10-16.
72. "AGGuideCovers2010.indd" (PDF). Archived from the original (PDF) on 2012-12-12. Retrieved 2012-10-16.
73. http://acissearch.aphis.usda.gov/LPASearch/faces/CustomerSearch.jspx
74. "2005 Report on Enforcement of the Animal Welfare Act"(PDF). U.S. Department of Agriculture.
75. The humane care and treatment of laboratory animals. National Association of Biomedical Research
76. Trull, F. L. (1999). "More Regulation of Rodents". Science. 284 (5419): 1463. Bibcode:1999Sci...284.1463T. doi:10.1126/science.284.5419.1463.
77. Midgley, M. (May 24, 1999). "Descartes Prisoners". The New Statesman. Archived from the original on December 2, 2008.
78. Honderich, T., ed. (1995). The Oxford Companion to Philosophy. Oxford University Press. pp. 188–192, Cottingham, J., Descartes, René. Discourse on the Method (1637).
79. Interview with Ingrid Newkirk, David Shankbone, Wikinews, November 20, 2007.
80. "World Organisation for Animal Health (OIE)". World Organisation for Animal Health. 2013. Retrieved October 22, 2013.
81. "World Animal Protection history". World Animal Protection. Retrieved June 18, 2014.
82. "Provincial and territorial legislation concerning farm animal welfare". Government of Canada. 2013. Archived from the original on March 7, 2013. Retrieved October 22, 2013.

83. “Compassion in World Farming - The farm animal welfare charity”. Ciwf.org.uk. 2011-12-16. Retrieved 2014-01-03.
84. “The Movement for Compassionate Living | Home Page”. Mclveganway.org.uk. Retrieved 2014-01-03.
85. “Animal Welfare Principals”. National Animal Interest Alliance. Retrieved 2014-06-02.
86. “Ontario SPCA”. Ontario Society for the Prevention of Cruelty to Animals. Retrieved March 20, 2013.

CHAPTER 6

Veterinary Ethics

Chapter Contents

Veterinary ethics is the application of ethical theories, principles, and rules by professionals and paraprofessionals in resolving ethical dilemmas in the practice of veterinary care. In order to resolve ethical dilemmas, a minimum understanding of and exposure to moral theories is essential. Aesculapian authority and professionalism confer on veterinarians the right to treat animals and the expectation from the public that veterinarians will act in the interest of the animal, client, and the public. Branches of veterinary ethics are described with a greater focus on normative ethics, or theories are discussed.

INTRODUCTION

Veterinary Ethics is a system of moral principles that apply values and judgements to the practice of veterinary medicine. As a scholarly discipline, veterinary ethics encompasses its practical application in clinical settings as well as work on its history, philosophy, theology, and sociology. Veterinary ethics combines veterinary professional ethics and the subject of animal ethics. It can be interpreted as a critical reflection on the provision of veterinary services in support of the profession's responsibilities to animal kind and mankind.

Animal welfare has been a subject that is studied in great depth, it largely looks at the ways in which an animal may suffer in particular circumstances or how their lives may be enriched. Animal ethics is another well documented subject where philosophers, since Aristotle, have commented on its importance. Often referred to as "the animal problem' the questions that seem to be asked in this field are at their foundation trying to determine what the morally relevant difference is between animals and humans, and if there is no difference how do we justify treating animals a certain way and if there is a difference then what is it about this difference that allows us to treat animals in a certain way.

Veterinary ethics is a modern subject that does not have a defined start point. As it combines the study of animal welfare and animal ethics as its root and uses information from this as data for its deliberations it could be said to have a long history, however as an academic discipline it is only recently that works have been published on the topic.

The two academics seen to have written on veterinary ethics for the longest are Bernard Rollin (Colorado State University) and Jerrold Tannenbaum (University of California, Davis).They can be seen as the founders of the subject in veterinary ethics. Currently, most veterinary schools teach veterinary ethics and it is often combined in teaching with animal welfare or with law.

RELATIONS WITH MEDICAL ETHICS

The subject is very similar to that of human medical ethics in that the study of the relationship between the doctor and the patient relates closely to that of the veterinary surgeon and animal owner. However, the subject differs greatly in the consideration of the uses of animals, while a doctor's duty may to preserve life at nearly all cost, the veterinary surgeon needs to adapt their attitude to health and longetivity of life to the purpose of the animal (E.g., farm animals).

Much of what is understood in the field of professionalism and professional responsibilities in confidentiality, preserving autonomy, beneficence, truth-telling, whistleblowing, informed consent and communication is largely lifted from the research done in the medical profession. The difference between the human patients and the animal patients does not interfere with the professionalism discussion between doctors and human patients and vets with their clients.

Another major difference between veterinary ethics and human medical ethics is the interplay with law. Human medical ethics has driven changes in the law and, to a lesser degree, vice versa. Largely involving cases of human rights a wide ranging variety of high-profile legal challenges in many countries have involved the use of ethics to encourage changes in law (for example, assisted suicide, abortion, duty of care, rights to refuse treatment). Veterinary ethics does not have such a strong interplay. It is rare to have an animal based legal challenge reaching high into the legal system. Cases involving challenges to professionalism and duty of care are largely dealt with via the veterinary governing bodies.

The veterinary profession remains largely self-regulating across the world (*e.g.*, by the RCVS and AVMA). This has caused some controversy as to why the veterinary profession remains one of the few remaining self-regulating professions. Bernard Rollin wrote on this the difficulty in keeping public confidence while remaining self-regulating, trust and impartiality are critical but most importantly is the need for a profession to self-sacrificial by putting the clients needs above that of the profession or professional's need.

"Every profession—be it medicine, law, or agriculture—is given freedom by the social ethic to pursue its aims. In return, society basically says to professions it does not understand well enough to regulate, "You regulate yourselves the way we would regulate you if we understood what you do, which we don't. But we will know if you don't self-regulate properly and then we will hammer you with draconian rules and regulate you, despite our lack of understanding."

Principles of Veterinary Medical Ethics

The American Veterinary Medical Association (AVMA) regularly reviews and updates policies and procedures including a document considered the principles of ethics. The AVMA Judicial Council acts as the group in charge of insuring the principles are current. Much like the human medical code, veterinarians are expected to "adhere to a progressive code of ethical conduct known as the Principles of Veterinary Medical Ethics (PVME)". In February 2015 the AVMA adopted the newest version of the "Principles of Veterinary Medical Ethics" which has been approved by the AVMA House of Delegates. The contents of the principles were "modeled after the American Medical Association's Code of Ethics". Overall there are eight main principles. They are as follows:

- A veterinarian shall be dedicated to providing competent veterinary medical care, with compassion and respect for animal welfare and human health
- A veterinarian shall provide veterinary medical clinical care under the terms of a veterinarian-client-patient relationship (VCPR).
- A veterinarian shall uphold the standards of professionalism, be honest in all professional interactions, and report veterinarians who are deficient in character or competence to the appropriate entities.
- A veterinarian shall respect the law and also recognize a responsibility to seek changes to laws and regulations which are contrary to the best interests of the patient and public health.
- A veterinarian shall respect the rights of clients, colleagues, and other health professionals, and shall safeguard medical information within the confines of the law.
- A veterinarian shall continue to study, apply and advance scientific knowledge, maintain a commitment to veterinary medical education, make relevant information available to clients, colleagues, the public, and obtain consultation or referral when indicated.
- A veterinarian shall, in the provision of appropriate patient care, except in emergencies, be free to choose whom to serve, with whom to associate, and the environment in which to provide veterinary medical care.

- A veterinarian shall recognize a responsibility to participate in activities contributing to the improvement of the community and the betterment of public health.
- List obtained from "Principles of Veterinary Medical Ethics" revised.

The full details of the updates to the Principles of Veterinary Medical Ethics can be found on the American Veterinary Medical Association web site located in the knowledge base article titled "Principles of Veterinary Medical Ethics of the AVMA".

KEY TOPICS

The Key topics within veterinary ethics are:

- Euthanasia
- Informed consent
- Complementary and Alternative Medicine
- Cosmetic interventions
- Non-therapeutic mutilations
- Negligence
- Professionalism
- Religious influences
- Research ethics
- Confidentiality
- Selective breeding
- Professional Regulation

Key Texts

- An Introduction to Veterinary Medical Ethics: Theory and Cases by Bernard E. Rollin
- Veterinary Ethics: An Introduction by Giles Legood
- Veterinary Ethics: Animal Welfare, Client Relations, Competition & Collegiality: Animal Welfare, Client Relations, Competition and Collegiality by Jerrold Tannenbaum JD
- Law and Ethics of the Veterinary Profession by James F. Wilson and Joanne L. Garbe
- Law and ethics of the veterinary profession by James F Wilson
- Principles of Veterinary Medical Ethics of the AVMA as adopted by the AVMA Judicial Council

Conferences

- The Universities Federation for Animal Welfare (UFAW) offer yearly conferences on animal welfare which may be of interest to veterinary ethicists.
- The Institute of Medical Ethics also offer conferences, often several times a year, on the issues of ethics that affect doctors. However, as many of these are transferable to veterinary ethics it may also provide an interesting.
- The Animal Welfare Science, Ethics and Law Veterinary Association (AWSELVA) have regularly meetings on the all the subjects in its title.
- The First International Conference of Veterinary and Animal Ethics has just been announced, with bursaries available for students attendees.
- American Veterinary Medical Association Leadership Conference and House of Delegates
- American Veterinary Medical Association Annual Convention
- Pet Health Awareness Events

REFERENCES

1. "Mr Martin Whiting".
2. "The Moral Status of Animals".
3. "Home - Philosophy". Philosophy.
4. "Faculty - UC Davis School of Veterinary Medicine".
5. An Introduction to Veterinary Medical Ethics: Theory and Cases by Bernard E. Rollin
6. "Archived copy" (PDF). Archived from the original (PDF) on July 15, 2011. Retrieved February 13, 2011.
7. "Principles of Veterinary Medical Ethics of the AVMA".
8. ""Principles of Veterinary Medical Ethics" revised".
9. ""Principles of Veterinary Medical Ethics" revised".
10. "Principles of Veterinary Medical Ethics of the AVMA".
11. "Homepage - UFAW".
12. "IME".
13. "Home".
14. "Archived copy". Retrieved February 13, 2011.
15. "2016 AVMA Veterinary Leadership Conference & House of Delegates Winter Session".
16. "AVMA Annual Convention".
17. "Pet Health Awareness Events 2016".

CHAPTER 7

Veterinary Surgery

Chapter Contents

A veterinary surgeon is a veterinarian who specializes in surgery. Most vets in the United States can do basic surgery, but as veterinary medicine becomes more involved and more specialized, many vet practices are now turning to specially trained veterinary surgeons for major surgeries on animals.

INTRODUCTION

Veterinary surgery is surgery performed on animals by veterinarians, whereby the procedures fall into three broad categories: orthopaedics (bones, joints, muscles), soft tissue surgery (skin, body cavities, cardiovascular system, GI/urogenital/respiratory tracts), and neurosurgery. Advanced surgical procedures such as joint replacement (total hip, knee and elbow replacement), fracture repair, stabilization of cranial cruciate ligament deficiency, oncologic (cancer) surgery, herniated disc treatment, complicated gastrointestinal or urogenital procedures, kidney transplant, skin grafts, complicated wound management, minimally invasive procedures (arthroscopy, laparoscopy, thoracoscopy), etc. are performed by Veterinary Surgeons (as registered in their jurisdiction). Most general practice veterinarians perform routine surgery neuters (spay and castration), minor mass excisions, etc., some also perform additional procedures.

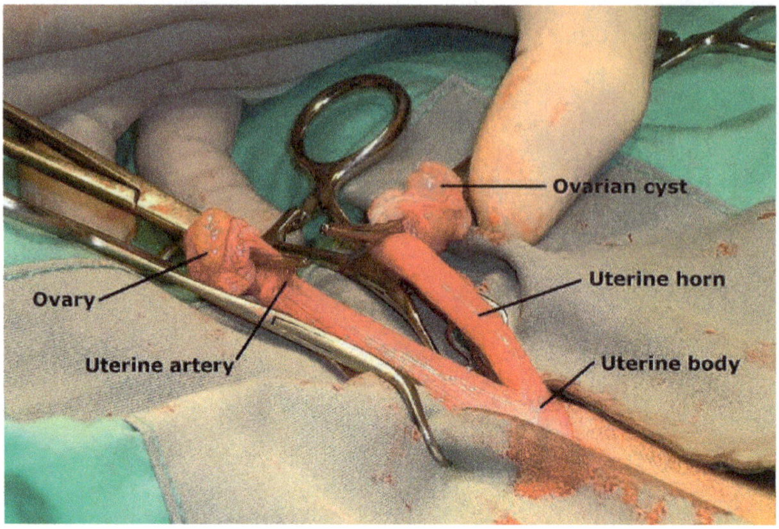

A cat spay

The goal of veterinary surgery may be quite different in pets and in farm animals. In the former, situation is a bit like in human beings, and more and more complex operations are performed, with sophisticated anaesthesia techniques. In the latter, the cost of the operation must not exceed the economic benefit in surgically treating the illness.

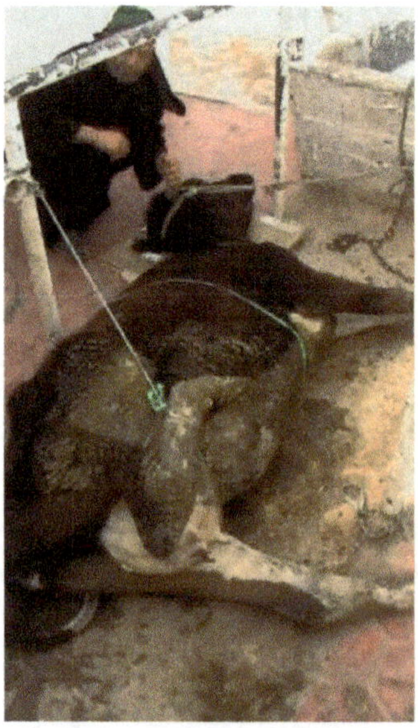

Preparing a cow for udder surgery in field conditions: the physical restraint with a set of ropes is necessary next to xylazine tranquilisation

Specialization in Surgery

In the United States, Canada and Europe, veterinary surgery is one of 20 veterinary specialties recognized by the American Veterinary Medical Association respectively the European Board of Veterinary Specialisation. Those wishing to become board certified must undergo a one-year clinical internship program followed by three years of intensive training in a residency program under direct supervision of Board Certified Veterinary Surgeons, including performance of a large number of surgical procedures in such categories as abdominal surgery, surgical treatment of angular limb deformities, arthroscopic surgery, surgery of the foot, fracture fixation, ophthalmic surgery, urogenital surgery, and upper respiratory surgery, etc. Once the minimum requirements of training are met residents are required to pass a rigorous certification examination before being admitted as members (Diplomates) of the American College of Veterinary Surgeons or European College of Veterinary Surgeons

Veterinary Anesthesia

Anesthesia in animals has many similarities to human anesthesia, but some differences as well. Local anesthesia is primarily used for wound closure and removal of small tumors. Lidocaine, mepivacaine, and bupivacaine are the most commonly used local anesthetics used in veterinary medicine. Sedation without general anesthesia is used for more involved procedures. Sedatives commonly used include acepromazine, hydromorphine, midazolam, diazepam, xylazine, and medetomidine. α2 agonists like xylazine and medetomidine are especially useful because they can be reversed, xylazine by yohimbine and medetomidine by atipamezole. Xylazine is approved for use in dogs, cats, horses, deer, and elk in the United States, while medetomidine is only approved for dogs. Most surgeries in ruminants can be performed with regional anesthesia.

General anesthesia is commonly used in animals for major surgery. Animals are often premedicated intravenously or intramuscularly with a sedative, analgesic, and anticholinergic agent (dogs frequently receive buprenorphine, acepromazine, and glycopyrrolate). The next step is induction, usually with an intravenous drug. Dogs and cats commonly receive thiopental (no longer allowed in the UK), ketamine with diazepam, tiletamine with zolazepam (usually just in cats), and/or propofol. Alfaxalone is a steroid anaesthetic used in many practices in the UK to induce anaesthesia in cats and sometimes dogs. It is similar in physiological effect but different in composition to the now withdrawn Saffan. Horses commonly receive thiopental and guaifenesin. Following induction, the animal is intubated with an endotracheal tube and maintained on a gas anesthetic. The most common gas anesthetics in use in veterinary medicine are isoflurane, enflurane, and halothane, although desflurane and sevoflurane are becoming more popular due to rapid induction and recovery.

Common Veterinary Surgeries

Elective Procedures

Elective procedures are those performed on a non-emergency basis, and which do not involve immediately life-threatening conditions. These are in contrast to emergency procedures.

Sterilization Surgery

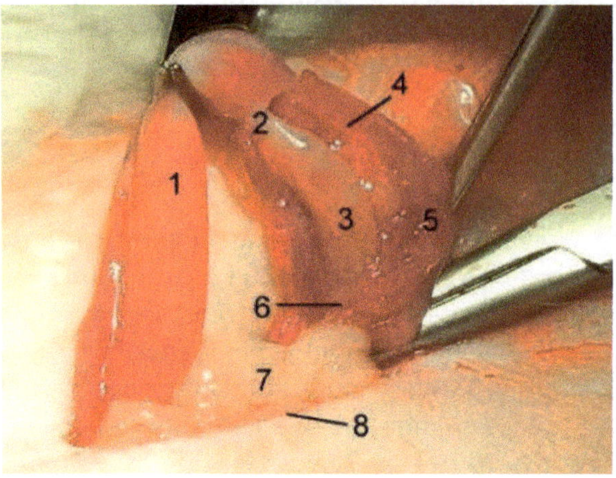

A cat spay

One of the most common elective surgical procedures in animals are those that render animals incapable of reproducing. Neutering in animals describes spaying or castration (also please see castration). To spay (medical term: ovariectomy or ovario-hysterectomy) is to completely remove the ovaries and often the uterus of a female animal. In a dog, this is accomplished through a ventral midline incision into the abdomen. In a cat, this is accomplished either by a ventral midline abdominal incision, or by a flank incision (more common in the UK). With an ovariectomy ligatures are placed on the blood vessels above and below the ovary and the organ is removed. With an ovariohysterectomy, the ligaments of the uterus and ovaries are broken down and the blood vessels are ligated and both organs are removed. The body wall, subcutis, and skin are sutured. To castrate (medical term: orchiectomy) is to remove the testicles of a male animal. Different techniques are used depending on the type of animal, including ligation of the spermatic cord with suture material, placing a rubber band around the cord to restrict blood flow to the testes, or crushing the cord with a specialized instrument like the Burdizzo.

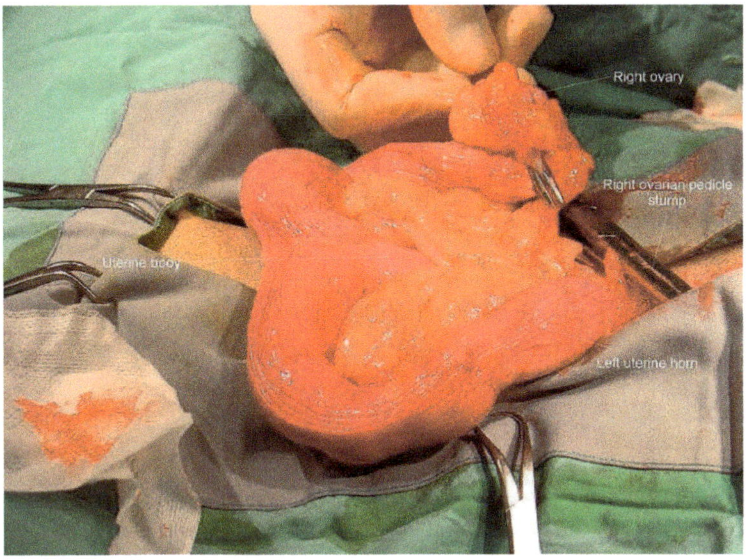

Pyometra surgery

Neutering is usually performed to prevent breeding, prevent unwanted behavior, or decrease risk of future medical problems. Neutering is also performed as an emergency procedure to treat certain reproductive diseases, like pyometra and testicular torsion, and it is used to treat ovarian, uterine, and testicular cancer. It is also recommended in cases of cryptorchidism to prevent torsion and malignant transformation of the testicles. Please see spaying and neutering for more information on the advantages and disadvantages of this procedure.

Laser surgery offers a number of benefits, including reduced risk of infection, less post-operative pain and swelling, reduced bleeding and improved visibility of the surgical field. Better hemostasis and visibility can in some cases minimize the need for anesthesia and/or reduce overall surgical time.

Controversial Elective Animal Procedures

Other common elective surgical procedures in the United States are declawing in cats (onychectomy), ear-cropping in dogs, tail docking in dogs, horses, and dairy cattle, and Livestock dehorning in cattle, sheep, and goats. These procedures have been controversial and recently debated among breeders, veterinary organizations, and animal welfare scientists. The controversy is different for each procedure, but issues arise based on reasons to perform the procedure, differing opinions on techniques and methods, perceived long-term benefits in individual animals, and the development of alternatives. Declawing, for example, consists of removal of the distal phalanges using either a scalpel, scissors or laser. It is typically performed to prevent property damage in house cats, but may also be performed in purebred dogs to meet certain show requirements. Some procedures are illegal in some countries (in the UK, declawing is illegal and tail docking is only allowed in working dogs) and face ethical challenges in others.

Dental Surgery

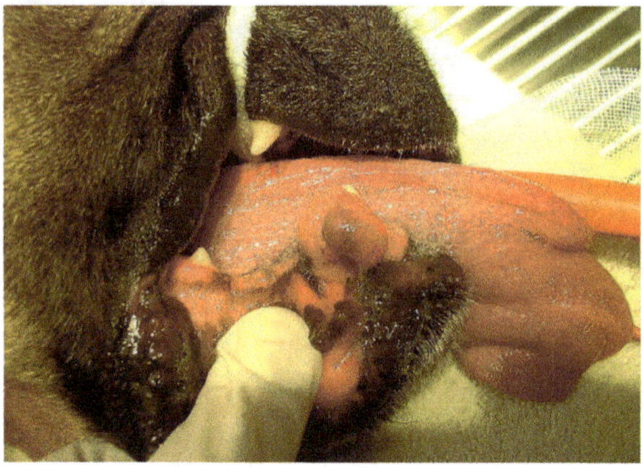

Anesthetised dog with an epulis

Common dental surgical procedures:

- Horses - Floating (grinding down) of uneven teeth edges and removal of wolf teeth.
- Dogs - Dental prophylaxis is commonly performed to remove tartar and treat periodontal disease. This procedure is usually performed under anesthesia. Other common procedures include extraction of abscessed or broken teeth, extraction of deciduous teeth, root canals, and removal of gingival hyperplasia and epulides.
- Cats - Dental prophylaxis as described above for the dog and treatment and extraction of teeth with feline odontoclastic resorptive lesions (FORLs).

Surgical Oncology

In older dogs and cats tumors are a common occurrence, and may involve any or multiple body systems: skin, musculoskeletal, gastrointestinal tract, urogentital tract, reproductive tract, cardiovascular system, spinal cord and peripheral nerves, the spleen and the lining of body cavities. Common skin tumors include lipomas, mast cell tumors, melanomas, squamous cell carcinomas, basal cell carcinomas, fibrosarcomas, and histiocytomas. Skin tumors are removed through either simple excisions or through excisions needing reconstructive plastic surgery. Common oral tumors include melanomas, fibrosarcomas, squamous cell carcinomas, which are removed with as much surrounding tissue as possible, including parts of the mandible and maxilla. Other types of cancer requiring surgery include osteosarcoma, stomach and intestinal tumors, splenic masses, and urinary bladder tumors.

Ophthalmic Surgery

Common ophthalmic surgeries in animals include:

- Enucleation of the eye to treat glaucoma or eye proptosis.
- Cataract surgery
- Entropion surgery
- Ectropion surgery
- Eyelid tumor removal
- Cherry eye surgery
- Exenteration (complete removal) of the orbit, especially for squamous cell carcinoma in the cat and cow.

Orthopedic Surgery

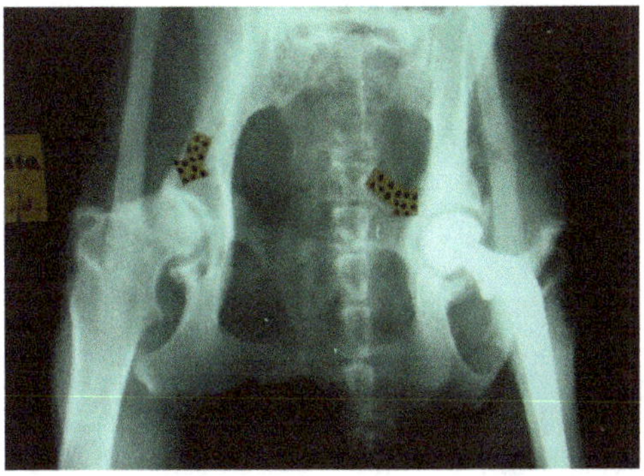

X-ray of a dog with an artificial hip to repair hip dysplasia

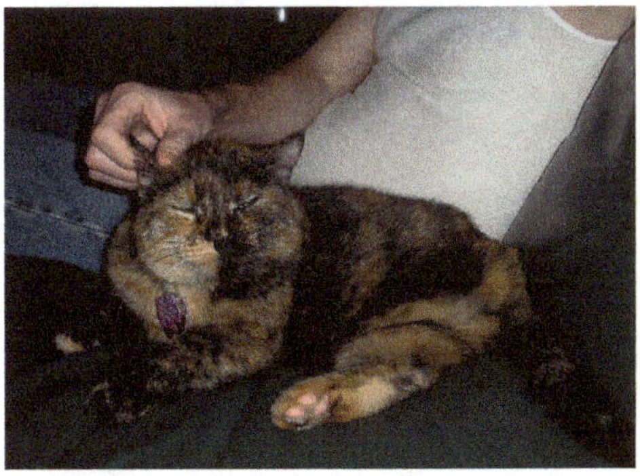

A healthy tortoise-mix cat healed and adapted quickly to her new mobility after a hind leg was amputated.

Common orthopedic surgeries in animals include:

- Ruptured anterior cruciate ligament repair
- For hip dysplasia:
- Femoral head ostectomy

- Triple pelvic osteotomy
- Hip replacement
- Leg amputation
- Bone fracture repair
- Arthroscopy
- MPL - medial patellar luxation
- APL - anterior patellar luxation

Other Common Procedures

Caesarean Section

Caesarean sections are commonly performed in dogs, cats, horses, sheep, and cattle. Usually it is done as an emergency surgery due to difficulties in the birthing process. Certain dog breeds such as Bulldogs often need to have this surgery because of the size of the puppy's head relative to the width of the bitch's birth canal.

Bloat Surgery

In dogs bloat or gastric dilatation volvulus (GDV) is a common condition where the stomach fills with gas and commonly twists. If the stomach is torsed it requires immediate surgical intervention to prevent necrosis of the stomach wall. After radiographs to confirm the GDV and blood tests to determine the lactate and general health of the dog, surgical intervention is required. The stomach is put back into its normal position, deflated and tacked (gastropexy) to the body wall. Sometimes a splenectomy or partial gastrectomy is also required.

Cystotomy

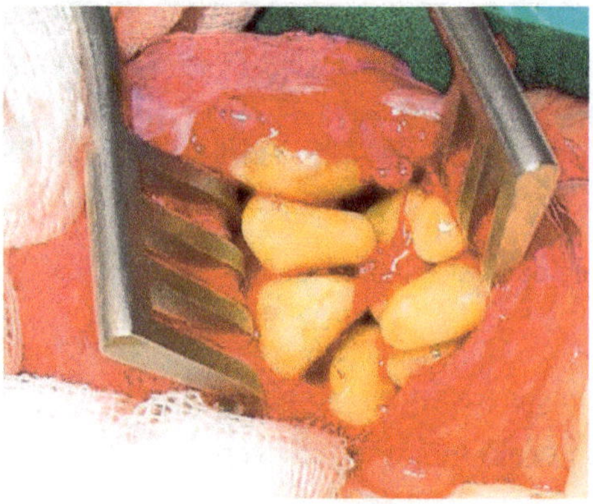

Cystotomy to remove bladder stones

A cystotomy is a surgical opening of the urinary bladder. It is commonly performed in dogs and cats to remove bladder stones or tumors.

Wound Repair

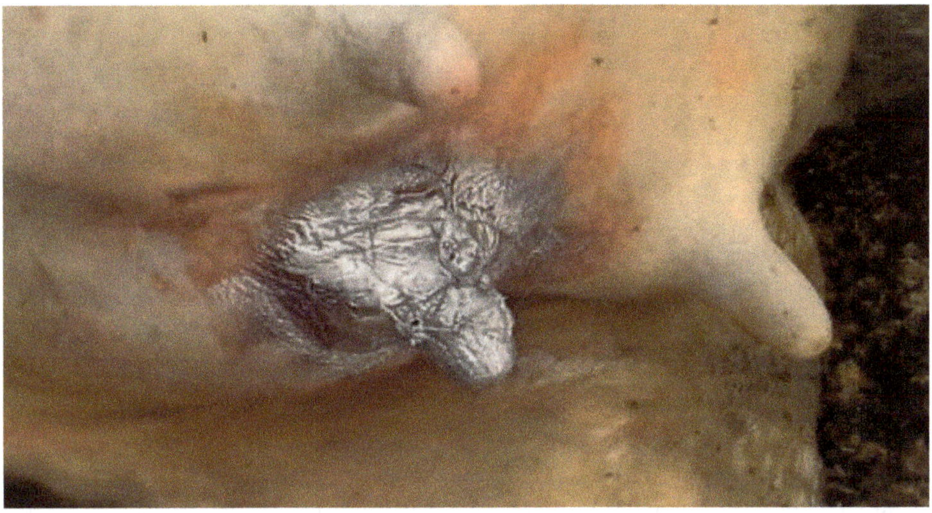

Sutured wound on the teats of a cow

Bite wounds from other animals (and rarely humans) are a common occurrence. Wounds from objects that the animal may step on or run into are also common. Usually these wounds are simple lacerations that can be easily cleaned and sutured, sometimes using a local anesthetic. Bite wounds, however, involve compressive and tensile forces in addition to shearing forces, and can cause separation of the skin from the underlying tissue and avulsion of underlying muscles. Deep puncture wounds are especially prone to infection. Deeper wounds are assessed under anesthesia and explored, lavaged, and debrided. Primary wound closure is used if all remaining tissue is healthy and free of contamination. Small puncture wounds may be left open, bandaged, and allowed to heal without surgery. A third alternative is delayed primary closure, which involves bandaging and reevaluation and surgery in three to five days.

Wounds occurring in the udder and teats of cows are more difficult to repair, due to the difficult access and sensitivity of the organ, and because deep anaesthesia may not be applied to bovines. But some practitioners have acquired a great experience in dealing them.

Foreign Body Removal

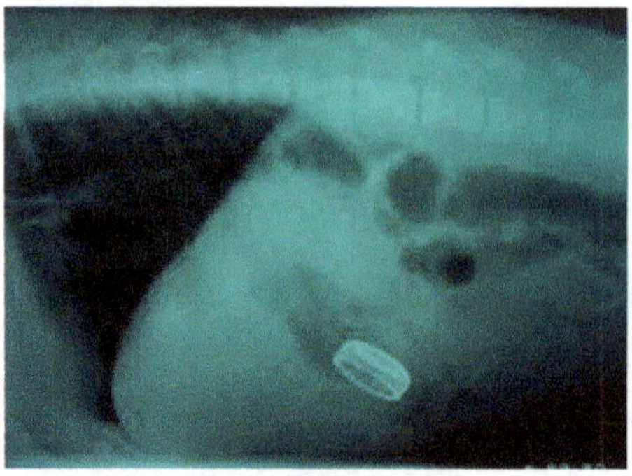

Bottle top swallowed by a dog that had to be removed surgically

A variety of non-edible objects are commonly swallowed by dogs, cats, and cattle. These foreign bodies can cause obstruction of the gastrointestinal tract causing severe vomiting and resulting electrolyte imbalances. The stomach (gastrotomy) or intestine (enterotomy) can be surgically opened to remove the foreign body. Necrotic intestine can be removed (enterectomy) and repaired with intestinal anastomosis. Foreign bodies can also be removed by endoscopy, which although requires general anesthesia does not require surgery and significantly decreases recovery time. However, endoscopic foreign body retrieval is anatomically limited to objects lodged in the esophagus, the stomach or the colon. The condition in cattle is known as hardware disease.

VETERINARY ANESTHESIA

Veterinary anesthesia is anesthesia performed on non-human animals by a veterinarian. Anesthesia is used for a wider range of circumstances in animals than in people, due to animals' inability to cooperate with certain diagnostic or therapeutic procedures. Veterinary anesthesia includes anesthesia of the major species: dogs, cats, horses, cattle, sheep, goats, and pigs, as well as all other animals requiring veterinary care such as birds, pocket pets, and wildlife.

Specialization in Anesthesia

In North America, the American College of Veterinary Anesthesia and Analgesia is one of 21 specialty organizations recognized by the American Veterinary Medical Association. The ACVAA was recognized by the AVMA in 1975, despite attempts by the AVMA to include anesthesia as a subspecialty of surgery or medicine. As of 2016, there are more than 250 Diplomates of the ACVAA. To become an ACVAA board-certified Diplomate, veterinarians must have at least one year of clinical practice experience followed by three years of anesthesia residency training under the supervision of ACVAA Diplomates, have accepted for publication a scientific peer-reviewed research article, and passed both a written and oral examination.

In Europe, the European College of Veterinary Anaesthesia and Analgesia (ECVAA) is one of 23 specialty organizations recognized by the European Board of Veterinary Specialisation. As of February 2014, there are 147 ECVA Diplomates.

Anesthesia Technicians

Evidence exists that suggests that anesthesia which is supervised by a qualified technician is safer than anesthesia without a technician. In most private veterinary practices, the technician administers and monitors anesthesia with supervision from the attending veterinarian. In many academic institutions, anesthesia technicians are involved in working with and teaching veterinary students as well as supervising anesthetized cases. The Academy of Veterinary Technician Anesthetists is a provisional specialty academy of the North American Veterinary Technician Association and is responsible for licensing technicians as being specialized in anesthesia. For a technician to become specialized, they must be a licensed technician in their state, accumulate 6000 hours of work in veterinary medicine (at least 75% of which must be in anesthesia), 40 hours of continuing education related to anesthesia, demonstrate proficiency in anesthesia skills, and pass a comprehensive written examination.

Application in Animals

Anesthesia is required for many surgical procedures which require the patient to be immobile, unaware, and without pain. Furthermore, anesthesia aims to minimize the surgical stress response. In addition, certain diagnostic procedures require anesthesia, notably stomach or airway endoscopy, bone marrow sampling, and occasionally ultrasound. Aggressive animals may require anesthesia in order to handle and perform a physical exam or obtain blood for testing. Exotic animals frequently require anesthesia for simple procedures (such as taking a radiograph or catheter placement) due to lack of domesticity. Animals may require anesthesia for therapeutic procedures, such as urinary catheterization to relieve obstruction, injection into a mass, or removing fluid from the eye to treat glaucoma.

In addition to anesthesia, analgesia is often managed by anesthesiologists or is included in the considerations for anesthesia.

Techniques in Small Animals

Cats and dogs are frequently anesthetized for surgical procedures. Small animals are most often placed under general anesthesia due to the types of procedures typically performed, the small size of the patient, their suitability to general anesthesia, and the greater degree of control. A balanced anesthesia protocol can be used whereby different drugs with different effects are used so that a high dose of just one drug can be avoided. For example, combining a sedative and an opioid will permit less inhalant anesthesia to be used, improving cardiovascular stability. A one-year study in a teaching hospital shows that dogs and cats typically experience a 1 in 9 chance of anesthetic complications, with a 1 in 233 risk of death. A larger-scale study states the risk of death in healthy dogs and cats as 1:1849 and 1:895 respectively. For sick dogs and cats, it was 1:75 and 1:71 respectively. For rabbits, the risk was 1:137 and 1:14 respectively for the healthy and sick groups.

Techniques in horses and Ruminants

Many procedures can be performed on the standing horse with heavy sedation alone. Some procedures may require general anesthesia due to the location of surgery (for example, castration). Other procedures in horses require general anesthesia using an inhalant anesthetic. Horses, due to their complex physiology as performance animals, suffer a number of difficulties that can complicate anesthesia. This results in horses having a higher risk of perioperative fatality - approximately 1:400.

Most procedures in ruminants can be performed standing under sedation and/or local anesthesia. This strategy is manageable due to the types of procedures being performed, the larger size of the patient, the relative difficulty of general anesthesia, and the cost of the procedure versus the product value of the animal.

Exotic Pets

Anesthesia of exotic animals (Guinea pigs, rabbits, birds) is challenging and the higher peri-anesthetic mortality in these species compared to dogs and cats, attests to this fact. These animals are challenging to anesthetize for a number of reasons: very little research has been carried out on safe and effective drug doses for specific species; exotic pets often 'hide' the fact that they are sick and by the time owners realize how sick the pet is the course of the disease is far advanced; the unique anatomy and physiology of exotic pets poses challenges for anesthetic management. For example, the anatomy of the respiratory system of birds, Guinea pigs, and reptiles makes it difficult to induce and maintain anesthesia solely with inhalation agents such as isoflurane and sevoflurane. Injectable drugs such as sedatives or tranquilizers are often used in these patients to facilitate induction and maintenance of anesthesia.

Anesthetic Agents

Most anesthetic agents used in human medicine are used in veterinary medicine. Alpha-2 receptor agonist drugs such as xylazine, romifidine, detomidine, and medetomidine, are used frequently in veterinary species (particularly large animal), but are rarely used in people. Guaifenesin is used as a muscle relaxant prior to anesthesia induction in some animals. Propofol is commonly used in small animal anesthesia, however it is rarely used in large animals due to the cost. 'Propoclear' is also commonly used in smaller branches of small animal surgery as it has a longer shelf life once opened than propofol whilst essentially having the same properties. Butorphanol is rarely used in people but is commonly used in all species. Ketamine, used in children for anesthesia, is used extensively in many species to induce anesthesia or cause heavy sedation. Expensive agents, such as etomidate and desflurane are rarely used outside of university hospitals. Different species have different responses to drugs. For example, horses may experience mania with morphine whereas dogs typically become sedated. Rabbits and guinea pigs are well sedated with midazolam, which can occasionally excite dogs and cats.

Gallery

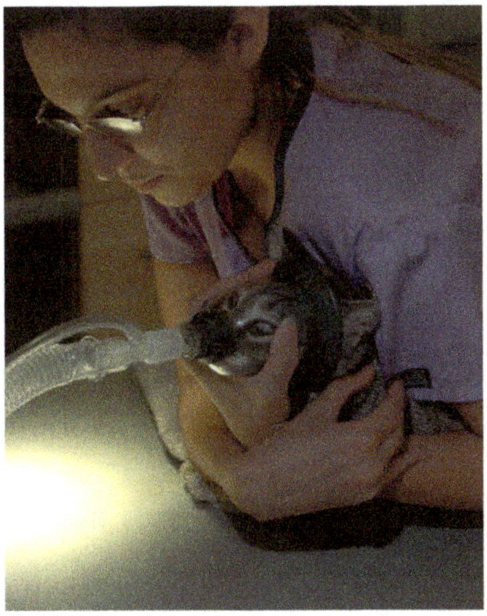

Cat masked down for spay surgery

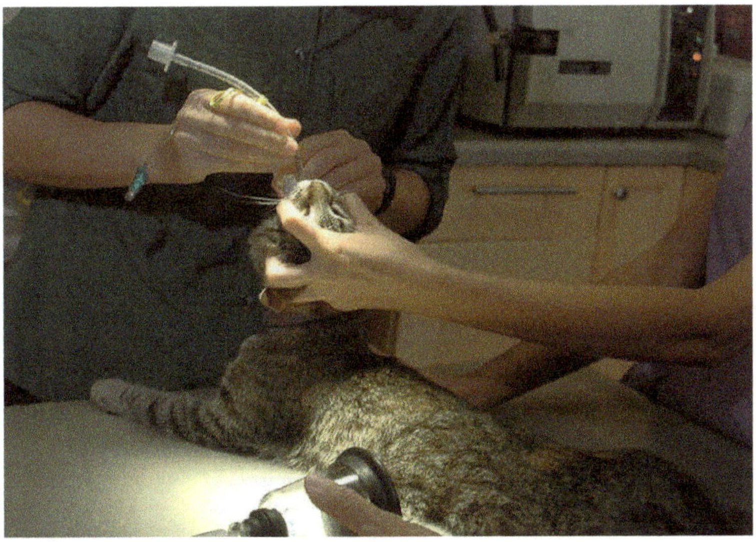

Intubated

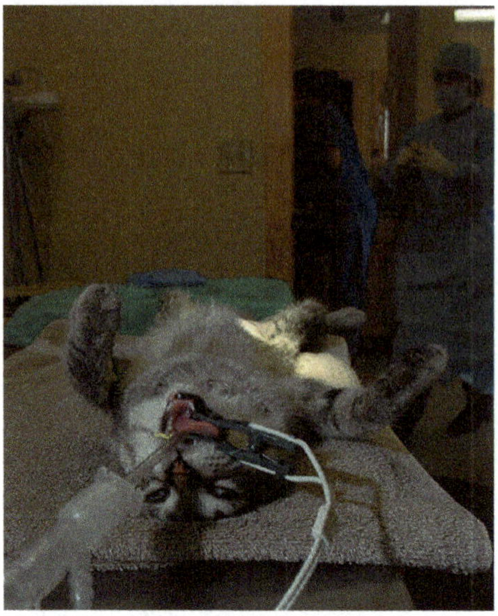

A cat intubated for spay/neuter surgery

REFERENCES

1. "Veterinary Specialty Organizations". Archived from the original on May 1, 2006. Retrieved 2006-04-06.
2. EBVS Website Archived April 14, 2015, at the Wayback Machine.
3. ACVS Residency Program[permanent dead link]
4. ECVS Website Archived March 18, 2013, at the Wayback Machine.
5. Muir, William W.; Hubbell, John A. E. (1995). Handbook of Veterinary Anesthesia (2nd ed.). Mosby. ISBN 0-8016-7656-8.
6. Paddleford, Robert R.; Harvey, Ralph C. (1999). "Alpha2 Agonists and Antagonists". The Veterinary Clinics of North America. 29: 737–744.
7. Paddleford, Robert R. (1999). Manual of Small Animal Anesthesia (2nd ed.). W.B. Saunders Company. ISBN 0-7216-4060-5.
8. Clarke, Cathy W. (1999). "Desflurane and Sevoflurane". The Veterinary Clinics of North America. 29: 793–809.
9. N. Berger, P.H. Eeg, Veterinary Laser Surgery, Blackwell, ISBN 978-0-8138-0678-5
10. "Archived copy". Archived from the original on 2016-01-28. Retrieved 2016-03-30. Veterinary laser surgery, URL accessed March 25, 2008
11. Woolridge, Anne A.; Seahorn, Thomas L. (1999). "Proper Dental Care Is Vital For Horses". Louisiana State University Equine Veternary Research Program Newsletter. Retrieved 2006-07-29.

12. "Feline Odontoclastic Resorptive Lesions". Small Animal Dental Service. Texas A&M University Veterinary Medical Teaching Hospital. Archived from the original on 2006-08-28. Retrieved 2006-07-29.
13. Holt, David E.; Griffin, Greg (2000). "Bite Wounds in Dogs and Cats". The Veterinary Clinics of North America. 30: 669–678.
14. Grunert E. & Luhman F., Chirurgische Versorgung von Euter- und Zitzenwunden, in Buiatrik, 2. Ed. Schaper Verlag, Hannover, 1972
15. "Archived copy". Archived from the original on 2016-05-28. Retrieved 2012-12-17.

CHAPTER 8

Veterinary Virology

Chapter Contents

Veterinary virology is concerned with the study of viruses causing diseases and disorders in animals. A fully infective virus is called a viron. The genomes of viruses are smaller than those found in prokaryotic and eukaryotic cells and in most viruses the nucleic acid is present in a single molecule. The genomes of viruses are of two types: single and double-stranded and viruses can contain either RNA or DNA. Due to these viruses are of three main groups based on their nucleic acid composition: DNA viruses, RNA viruses and viruses.

INTRODUCTION

Veterinary virology is the study of viruses in non-human animals. It is an important branch of veterinary medicine.

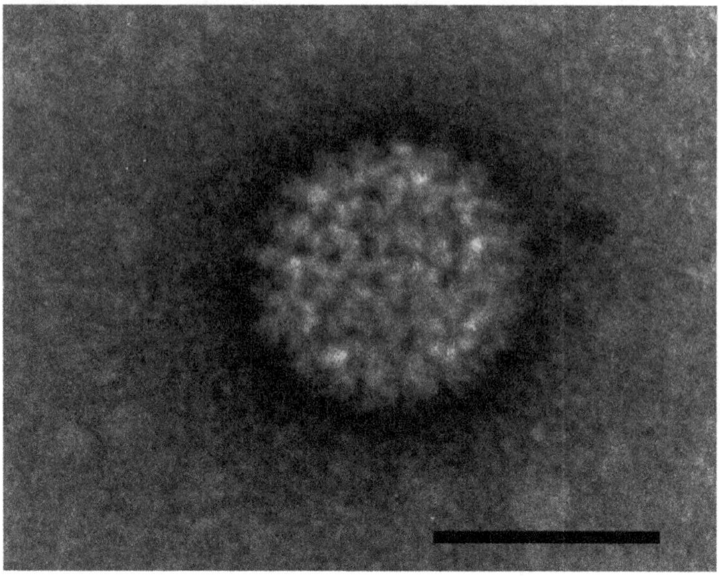

Bluetongue virus

RHABDOVIRUSES

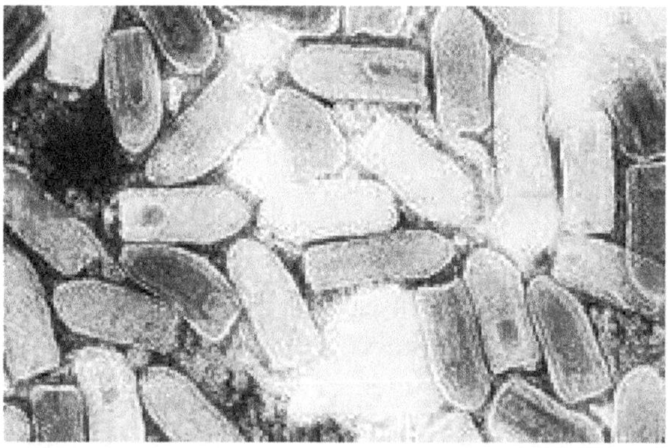

Vesicular stomatitis virus (VSV), the prototypical rhabdovirus

Rhabdoviruses are a diverse family of single stranded, negative sense RNA viruses that infect a wide range of hosts, from plants and insects, to fish and mammals. The *Rhaboviridae* family consists of six genera, two of which, cytorhabdoviruses and nucleorhabdoviruses, only infect plants. Novirhabdoviruses infect fish, and vesiculovirus, lyssavirus and ephemerovirus infect mammals, fish and invertebrates. The family includes pathogens such as rabies virus, vesicular stomatitis virus and potato yellow dwarf virus that are of public health, veterinary, and agricultural significance.

Foot-and-Mouth Disease Virus

Foot-and-mouth disease virus (FMDV) is a member of the Aphthovirus genus in the Picornaviridae family and is the cause of foot-and-mouth disease in pigs, cattle, sheep and goats. It is a non-enveloped, positive strand, RNA virus. FMDV is a highly contagious virus. It enters the body through inhalation.

Pestiviruses

Pestiviruses have a single stranded, positive-sense RNA genomes. They cause Classical swine fever (CSF) and Bovine viral diarrhea(BVD). Mucosal disease is a distinct, chronic persistent infection, whereas BVD is an acute infection.

Arteriviruses

Arteriviruses are small, enveloped, animal viruses with an icosahedral core containing a positive-sense RNA genome. The family includes equine arteritis virus (EAV), porcine reproductive and respiratory syndrome virus (PRRSV), lactate dehydrogenase elevating virus (LDV) of mice and simian haemorrhagic fever virus (SHFV).

Coronaviruses

Coronaviruses are enveloped viruses with a positive-sense RNA genome and with a nucleocapsid of helical symmetry. They infect the upper respiratory and gastrointestinal tract of mammals and birds. They are the cause of a wide range of diseases in cats, dog, pigs, rodents, cattle and humans. Transmission is by the faecal-oral route.

Toroviruses

Torovirus is a genus of viruses within the family *Coronaviridae*, subfamily *Torovirinae* that primarily infect vertebrates and include Berne virus of horses and Breda virus of cattle. They cause gastroenteritis in mammals, including humans but rarely.

INFLUENZA

Influenza is caused by RNA viruses of the family Orthomyxoviridae and affects birds and mammals.

Avian Influenza

Wild aquatic birds are the natural hosts for a large variety of influenza A viruses. Occasionally viruses are transmitted from this reservoir to other species and may then cause devastating outbreaks in domestic poultry or give rise to human influenza pandemics. *Edward J Dubovi & MacLachlan NJ (2010). Fenner's Veterinary Virology, Fourth Edition. Boston: Academic Press. p. 365. ISBN 0-12-375158-6.*

SWINE INFLUENZA

Bluetongue Virus

Bluetongue virus (BTV), a member of Orbivirus genus within the Reoviridae family causes serious disease in livestock (sheep, goat, cattle). It is non-enveloped, double-stranded RNA virus. The genome is segmented.

Circoviruses

Circoviruses are small single-stranded DNA viruses. There are to genera: gyrovirus, with one species called chicken anemia virus; and circovirus, which includes porcine circovirus types 1 and 2, psittacine beak and feather disease virus, pigeon circovirus, canary circovirus goose circovirus.

Herpesviruses

Herpesviruses are ubiquitous pathogens infecting animals and humans.

African Swine Fever Virus

African swine fever virus (ASFV) is a large double-stranded DNA virus which replicates in the cytoplasm of infected cells and is the only member of the Asfarviridae family. The virus causes a lethal haemorraghic disease in domestic pigs. Some strains can cause death of animals within as little as a week after infection. In other species, the virus causes no obvious disease. ASFV is endemic to sub-Saharan Africa and exists in the wild through a cycle of infection between ticks and wild pigs, bushpigs and warthogs.

Retroviruses

Retroviruses are established pathogens of veterinary importance. They are generally a cause of cancer or immune deficiency.

Flaviviruses

Flaviviruses constitute a family of linear, single-stranded RNA(+) viruses. Flaviviruses include the West Nile virus, dengue virus, Tick-borne Encephalitis Virus, Yellow Fever Virus, and several other viruses. Many flavivirus species can replicate in both mammalian and insect cells. Most flaviviruses are arthropod borne and multiply in both vertebrates and arthropods. The viruses in this family that are of veterinary importance include Japanese encephalitis virus, St. Louis encephalitis virus, West Nile virus, Israel turkey meningoencephalomyelitis virus, Sitiawan virus, Wesselsbron virus, yellow fever virus and the tick-borne flaviviruses e.g. louping ill virus.

Paramyxoviruses

Paramyxoviruses are a diverse family of non-segmented negative strand RNA viruses that include many highly pathogenic viruses affecting humans, animals, and birds. These include canine distemper virus (dogs), phocine distemper virus (seals), cetacean morbillivirus (dolphins and porpoises) Newcastle disease virus (birds) and rinderpest virus (cattle). Some paramyxoviruses such as the henipaviruses are zoonotic pathogens, occurring primarility in an animal hosts, but also able to infect humans.

Parvovirus

Parvoviruses are linear, non-segmented single-stranded DNA viruses, with an average genome size of 5000 nucleotides. They are classified as group II viruses in Baltimore classification of viruses. Parvoviruses are among the smallest viruses (hence the name, from Latin *parvus* meaning *small*) and are 18–28 nm in diameter.

Parvoviruses can cause disease in some animals, including starfish and humans. Because the viruses require actively dividing cells to replicate, the type of tissue infected varies with the age of the animal. The gastrointestinal tract and lymphatic system can be affected at any age, leading to vomiting, diarrhea and immunosuppression but cerebellar hypoplasia is only seen in cats that were infected in the womb or at less than two weeks of age, and disease of the myocardium is seen in puppies infected between the ages of three and eight weeks.

REFERENCES

1. Bourhy H, Gubala AJ, Weir RP, Boyle DB (2009). Mahy BWJ, van Regenmortel MHV, eds. Desk Encyclopedia Animal and Bacterial Virology. Boston: Academic Press. p. 23. ISBN 0-12-375144-6.
2. Rowlands DJ (2009). Mahy BWJ; van Regenmortel MHV, eds. Desk Encyclopedia Animal and Bacterial Virology. Boston: Academic Press. pp. 131–139. ISBN 0-12-375144-6.
3. Miarian C. Horzinek; Murphy, Frederick A.; Studdert, Michael J. (1999). Veterinary virology. Boston: Academic Press. pp. 563–568. ISBN 0-12-511340-4.
4. Brinton MA & Snijder EJ (2009). Mahy BWJ & van Regenmortel MHV, eds. Desk Encyclopedia Animal and Bacterial Virology. Boston: Academic Press. pp. 33–43. ISBN 0-12-375144-6.
5. Edward J Dubovi & MacLachlan NJ (2010). Fenner's Veterinary Virology, Fourth Edition. Boston: Academic Press. p. 395. ISBN 0-12-375158-6.
6. Glass RI, Bresee J, Jiang B, et al. (2001). "Gastroenteritis viruses: an overview". Novartis Found. Symp. Novartis Foundation Symposia. 238: 5–19; discussion 19–25. doi:10.1002/0470846534.ch2. ISBN 978-0-470-84653-7. PMID 11444035.
7. Edward J Dubovi & MacLachlan NJ (2010). Fenner's Veterinary Virology, Fourth Edition. Boston: Academic Press. p. 283. ISBN 0-12-375158-6.

8. Roy P. (2009). Mahy BWJ; van Regenmortel MHV, eds. Desk Encyclopedia Animal and Bacterial Virology. Boston: Academic Press. pp. 43–50. ISBN 0-12-375144-6.
9. Mankertz A. (2009). Mahy BWJ; van Regenmortel MHV, eds. Desk Encyclopedia Animal and Bacterial Virology. Boston: Academic Press. pp. 89–90. ISBN 0-12-375144-6.
10. Edward J Dubovi & MacLachlan NJ (2010). Fenner's Veterinary Virology, Fourth Edition. Boston: Academic Press. pp. 169–170. ISBN 0-12-375158-6.
11. Edward J Dubovi & MacLachlan NJ (2010). Fenner's Veterinary Virology, Fourth Edition. Boston: Academic Press. pp. 243–274. ISBN 0-12-375158-6.
12. Swanepoel R & Burt FJ (2009). Mahy BWJ & van Regenmortel MHV, eds. Desk Encyclopedia Animal and Bacterial Virology. Boston: Academic Press. pp. 117–124. ISBN 0-12-375144-6.
13. Edward J Dubovi & MacLachlan NJ (2010). Fenner's Veterinary Virology, Fourth Edition. Boston: Academic Press. p. 302. ISBN 0-12-375158-6.
14. Leppard, Keith; Nigel Dimmock; Easton, Andrew (2007). Introduction to Modern Virology. Blackwell Publishing Limited. p. 450. ISBN 1-4051-3645-6.
15. Fenner, Frank J.; Gibbs, E. Paul J.; Murphy, Frederick A.; Rott, Rudolph; Studdert, Michael J.; White, David O. (1993). Veterinary Virology (2nd ed.). Academic Press, Inc. ISBN 0-12-253056-X.

Index

W